LETTERS ON YOGA

PART ONE

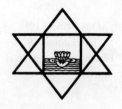

Sri Aurobindo

Letters on Yoga

PART ONE

Sri Aurobindo Ashram
Pondicherry

First Edition: 1958
Third Edition: 1970
Eighth Impression: 2004

(S. C.) Rs. 160.00
ISBN 81-7058-007-2

Lotus Press
PO Box 325
Twin Lakes, WI 53181 USA
www.lotuspress.com
lotuspress@lotuspress.com

Contents

Footnotes in this Volume on pages 50, 130, 161, 210 (2nd f n), 262, 266, 273, 288, 289, 484 are by Sri Aurobindo himself. The other footnotes are inserted by the editor.

PART ONE

PART ONE

SECTION ONE

THE SUPRAMENTAL EVOLUTION

The Supramental Evolution

THERE have been times when the seeking for spiritual attainment was, at least in certain civilisations, more intense and widespread than now or rather than it has been in the world in general during the past few centuries. For now the curve seems to be the beginning of a new turn of seeking which takes its start from what was achieved in the past and projects itself towards a greater future. But always, even in the age of the Vedas or in Egypt, the spiritual achievement or the occult knowledge was confined to a few, it was not spread in the whole mass of humanity. The mass of humanity evolves slowly, containing in itself all stages of the evolution from the material and the vital man to the mental man. A small minority has pushed beyond the barriers, opening the doors to occult and spiritual knowledge and preparing the ascent of the evolution beyond mental man into spiritual and supramental being. Sometimes this minority has exercised an enormous influence as in Vedic India, Egypt or, according to tradition, in Atlantis, and determined the civilisation of the race, giving it a strong stamp of the spiritual or the occult; sometimes they have stood apart in their secret schools or orders, not directly influencing a civilisation which was sunk in material ignorance or in chaos and darkness or in the hard external enlightenment which rejects spiritual knowledge.

The cycles of evolution tend always upward, but they are cycles and do not ascend in a straight line. The process therefore gives the impression of a series of ascents and descents, but what is essential in the gains of the evolution is kept or, even if eclipsed for a time, re-emerges in new forms suitable to the new ages. The creation has descended all the degrees of being from the Supermind to Matter and in each degree it has created a world, reign, plane or order proper to that degree. In the creating of the material world there was a plunge of this descending Consciousness into an apparent Inconscience and an emergence of it out of that Inconscience, degree by degree, until it recovers its highest spiritual and supramental summits and manifests their powers here in Matter. But even in the Inconscience there is a secret Consciousness which works, one may say, by an involved and hidden Intuition proper to itself. In each stage of Matter, in each stage of Life, this Intuition assumes a working proper to that stage and acts from behind the veil, supporting and enforcing the immediate necessities of the creative Force. There is an Intuition in Matter which holds the action of the material world from the electron to the sun and planets and their contents. There is an Intuition in Life which similarly supports and guides the play and development of Life in Matter till it is ready for the mental evolution of which man is the vehicle. In man also the creation follows the same upward process, — the Intuition within develops according to the stage he has reached in his progress. Even the precise intellect of the scientist, who is inclined to deny the separate existence or the superiority of Intuition, yet cannot really move forward unless there is behind him a mental Intuition, which enables him to take a forward step or to divine what has to be done. Intuition therefore is present at the beginning of things and in their middle as well as at their consummation.

But Intuition takes its proper form only when one goes beyond the mental into the spiritual domain, for there only it comes fully forward from behind the veil and reveals its true and complete nature. Along with the mental evolution of man there has been going forward the early process of another evolution which prepares the spiritual and supramental being. This has had two lines, one the discovery of the occult forces secret in Nature and of the hidden planes and worlds concealed from us by the world of Matter and the other the discovery of man's soul and spiritual self. If the tradition of Atlantis is correct, it is that of a progress which went to the extreme of occult knowledge, but could go no farther. In the India of Vedic times we have the record left of the other line of achievement, that of spiritual self-discovery; occult knowledge was there but kept subordinate. We may say that here in India the reign of Intuition came first, intellectual Mind developing afterwards in the later philosophy and science. But in fact the mass of men at the time, it is quite evident, lived entirely on the material plane, worshipped the Godheads of material Nature, sought from them entirely material objects. The effort of the Vedic mystics revealed to them the things behind through a power of inner sight and hearing and experience which was confined to a limited number of seers and sages and kept carefully secret from the mass of humanity — secrecy was always insisted on by the mystic. We may very well attribute this flowering of Intuition on the spiritual plane to a rapid re-emergence of essential gains brought down from a previous cycle. If we analyse the spiritual history of India we shall find that after reaching this height there was a descent which attempted to take up each lower degree of the already evolved consciousness and link it to the spiritual at the summit. The Vedic age was followed by a great outburst of intellect and philosophy which yet took spiritual truth as its basis and tried to reach it anew, not through a direct Intuition or occult process as did the Vedic seers, but by the power of the mind's reflective, speculative, logical thought; at the same time processes of yoga were developed which used the thinking mind as a means of arriving at spiritual realisation, spiritualising this mind itself at the same time. Then followed an era of the development of philosophies and yoga processes which more and more used the emotional and aesthetic being as the means of spiritual realisation and spiritualised the emotional level in man through the heart and feeling. This was accompanied by Tantric and other processes which took up the mental will, the life-will, the will of sensations and made them at once the instruments and the field of spiritualisation. In the Hathayoga and the various attempts at divinisation of the body there is also a line of endeavour which attempted to arrive at the same achievement with regard to living Matter; but this still awaits the discovery of the true characteristic method and power of Spirit in the body. We may say therefore that the universal Consciousness after its descent into Matter has conducted the evolution there along two lines, one of ascent to the discovery of the Self and Spirit, the other of descent through the already evolved levels of mind, life and body so as to bring down the spiritual consciousness into these also and to fulfil thereby some secret intention in the creation of the material universe. Our yoga is in its principle a taking up and summarising and completing of this process, an endeavour to rise to the highest possible supramental level and bring down its consciousness and power into mind, life and body.

The condition of present-day civilisation, materialistic with an externalised intellect and life-endeavour, which you find so painful, is an episode, but one which was perhaps inevitable. For if the spiritualisation of the mind, life and body is the thing to be achieved, the conscious presence of the Spirit even in the physical consciousness and material body, an age which puts Matter and the physical life in the forefront and devotes itself to the effort of the intellect to discover the truth of material existence, had perhaps to come. On one side, by materialising everything up to the intellect itself it has created the extreme difficulty of which you speak for the spiritual seeker, but, on the other hand, it has given the life in Matter an importance which the spirituality of the past was inclined to deny to it. In a way it has made the spiritualisation of it a necessity for spiritual seeking and so aided the descent movement of the evolving spiritual consciousness in the earth-nature. More than that we cannot claim for it; its conscious effect has been rather to stifle and almost extinguish the spiritual element in humanity; it is only by the divine use of the pressure of contraries and an intervention from above that there will be the spiritual outcome.

All the phases of human history may be regarded as a working out of the earth-consciousness in which each phase has its place and significance, so this materialistic intellectual phase had to come and has had, no doubt, its purpose and significance. One may also hold that one of its issues was as an experiment to see how far and whither the human consciousness would go through an intellectual and external control of Nature with physical and intellectual means only and without the intervention of any higher consciousness and knowledge — or that it may help by resistance to draw the spiritual consciousness that is growing behind all vicissitudes to attempt the control of Matter and turn it towards the Divine, as the Tantriks and Vaishnavas tried to do with the emotional and lower vital nature, not contenting themselves with the Vedantic turning of the mind towards the Supreme. But it is difficult to go farther than that or to hold that this materialism is itself a spiritual thing or that the dark, confused and violent state of contemporary Europe was an indispensable preparation for the descent of the Spirit. This darkness and violence which seems bent on destroying such light of mental idealism and desire of harmony as had succeeded in establishing itself in the mind of humanity, is obviously due to a descent of fierce and dark vital Powers which seek to possess the human world for their own, not for a spiritual purpose. It is true that such a precipitation of Asuric forces from the darker vital worlds has been predicted by some occultists as the one first result of the pressure of the Divine descent on their vital domain, but it was regarded as a circumstance of the battle, not as something helping towards the Divine Victory. The churning of Matter by the attempt of human intellect to conquer material Nature and use it for its purpose may break something of the passivity and inertia, but it is done for material ends, in a rajasic spirit, with a denial of spirituality as its mental basis. Such an attempt may end, seems to be ending indeed, in chaos and disintegration, while the new attempts at creation and reintegration seem to combine the obscure rigidity of material Nature with a resurgence of the barbaric brutality and violence of a half-animal vital Nature. How are the spiritual forces to deal with all that or make use of such a churning of the energies of the material universe? The way of the Spirit is the way of peace and light and harmony; if it has to battle, it is precisely because of the presence of such forces which seek either to extinguish or to prevent the spiritual light. In the spiritual change inertia has to be replaced by the divine peace and calm, the rajasic troubled energy by a tranquil and potent, pure and liberated dynamis, while the mind must be kept plastic for the workings of a higher Light of knowledge. How will the activity of Materialism lend itself to that change?

Materialism can hardly be spiritual in its basis, because its basic method is just the opposite of the spiritual way of doing things. The spiritual works from within outward, the way of materialism is to work from out inwards. It makes the inner a result of the outer, fundamentally a phenomenon of Matter and it works upon that view of things. It seeks to "perfect" humanity by outward means and one of its main efforts is to construct a perfect social machine which will train and oblige men to be what they ought to be. The loss of the ego in the Divine is the spiritual ideal; here it is replaced by the immolation of the individual to the military and industrial State. Where is there any spirituality in all that? Spirituality can only come by opening of the mind, vital and physical to the inmost soul, to the higher Self, to the Divine, and their sub-ordination to the spiritual forces and instrumentation as channels of the inner Light, the higher Knowledge and Power. Other things, mental, aesthetic, vital, are often misnamed 'spirituality', but they lack the essential character without which the word loses its true significance.

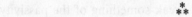

When there is a pressure on the vital world due to the preparing Descent from above, that world usually precipitates something of itself into the human. The vital world is very large and far exceeds the human in extent. But usually it dominates by influence not by descent. Of course the effort of this part of the vital world is always to maintain humanity under its sway and prevent the higher Light.

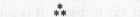

The vital descent cannot prevent the supramental — still less can the possessed nations do it by their material power, since the supramental descent is primarily a spiritual fact which will bear its necessary outward consequences. What previous vital descents have done is to falsify the Light that came down as in the history of Christianity where it took possession of the teaching and diluted it and deprived it of any widespread fulfilment. But the supermind is by definition a Light that cannot be distorted if it comes in its own right and by its own presence. It is only when it holds itself back and allows inferior Powers of consciousness to use a diminished and already deflected Truth that the knowledge can be seized by the vital Forces and made to serve their own purpose.

*
**

All that you say only amounts, on the general issue, to the fact that this is a world of slow evolution in which man has emerged out of the beast and is still not out of it, light out of darkness, and a higher consciousness out of first a dead and then a struggling and troubled unconsciousness. A spiritual consciousness is emerging and it is through this spiritual consciousness that one can meet the Divine. Religions, full of vital and mental, mixed, troubled and ignorant stuff, can only get glimpses of the Divine; positivist reason with its questioning based upon things as they are and refusing to believe in anything that may or will be cannot get any vision at all. The spiritual is a new consciousness that has to evolve and has been evolving. It is quite natural that at first and for a long time only a few should get the full light, while a greater number but still only a few compared with the mass of humanity, should get it partially. But what has been gained by the few can at a stage of the evolution be completed and more generalised and that is the attempt which we are making. But if this greater consciousness of light, peace and joy is to be gained, it cannot be by questioning and scepticism which can only fall back on what is and say: "It is impossible, what has not been in the past cannot be in the future, what is so imperfectly realised as yet cannot be better realised in the future." A faith, a will, or at least a persistent demand and aspiration are needed — a feeling that with this and this alone I can be satisfied and a push towards it that will not cease till it is done. That is why a spirit of scepticism and denial stands in the way, because they stand against the creation

of the conditions under which spiritual experience can unroll
itself.

*
**

The descent of the supermind is a long process, or at least a
process with a long preparation, and one can only say that the
work is going on sometimes with a strong pressure for completion, sometimes retarded by the things that rise from below and
have to be dealt with before further progress can be made.
The process is a spiritual evolutionary process, concentrated
into a brief period; it could be done otherwise (by what men
would regard as a miraculous intervention) only if the human
mind were more flexible and less attached to its ignorance
than it is. As we envisage it, it must manifest in a few first and
then spread, but it is not likely to overpower the earth in a
moment. It is not advisable to discuss too much what it will
do and how it will do it, because these are things the supermind
itself will fix, acting out of the Divine Truth in it, and the mind
must not try to fix for it grooves in which it will run. Naturally,
the release from subconscient ignorance and from disease, duration of life at will, and a change in the functionings of the body
must be among the ultimate elements of a supramental change;
but the details of these things must be left for the supramental
Energy to work out according to the Truth of its own nature.

The descent of the supramental is an inevitable necessity
in the logic of things and is therefore sure. It is because people
do not understand what the supermind is or realise the significance of the emergence of consciousness in a world of inconscient Matter that they are unable to realise this inevitability.
I suppose a matter-of-fact observer, if there had been one at
the time of the unrelieved reign of inanimate Matter in the
earth's beginning, would have criticised any promise of the
emergence of life in a world of dead earth and rock and mineral
as an absurdity and a chimera; so too, afterwards he would have
repeated this mistake and regarded the emergence of thought
and reason in an animal world as an absurdity and a chimera.
It is the same now with the appearance of supermind in the

stumbling mentality of this world of human consciousness and its reasoning ignorance.

It is quite possible that there have been periods of harmony on different levels, not supramental, which were afterwards disturbed — but that could only be a stage or resting place in an arc of spiritual evolution out of the Inconscience.

What is meant here is the Divine in its essential manifestation which reveals itself to us as Light and Consciousness, Power, Love and Beauty. But in its actual cosmic manifestation the Supreme, being the Infinite and not bound by any limitation, can manifest in Itself, in its consciousness of innumerable possibilities, something that seems to be the opposite of itself, something in which there can be Darkness, Inconscience, Inertia, Insensibility, Disharmony and Disintegration. It is this that we see at the basis of the material world and speak of nowadays as the Inconscient — the Inconscient Ocean of the Rigveda in which the One was hidden and arose in the form of this universe — or, as it is sometimes called, the non-being, Asat. The Ignorance which is the characteristic of our mind and life is the result of this origin in the Inconscience. Moreover, in the evolution out of inconscient existence there rise up naturally powers and beings which are interested in the maintenance of all negations of the Divine, error and unconsciousness, pain, suffering, obscurity, death, weakness, illness, disharmony, evil. Hence the perversion of the manifestation here, its inability to reveal the true essence of the Divine. Yet in this very base of this evolution all that is divine is there involved and pressing to evolve, Light, Consciousness, Power, Perfection, Beauty, Love. For in the Inconscient itself and behind the perversions of the Ignorance the Divine Consciousness lies concealed and works and must more and more appear, throwing off in the end its disguises. That is why it is said that the world is called to express the Divine.

Your statement about the supramental evolution is correct except that it does not follow that humanity as a whole will become supramental. What is more likely to happen is that the supramental principle will be established in the evolution by the descent just as the mental principle was established by the appearance of thinking Mind and Man in earthly life. There will be a race of supramental beings on the earth just as now there is a race of mental beings. Man himself will find a greater possibility of rising to the planes intermediary between his mind and supermind and making their powers effective in his life, which will mean a great change in humanity on earth, but it is not likely that the mental stage will disappear from the ascending ladder and, if so, the continued existence of a mental race will be necessary so as to form a stage between the vital and the supramental in the evolutionary movement of the Spirit.

Such a descent of higher beings as you suggest may be envisaged as a part of the process of the change. But the main part of the change will be the appearance of the supramental being and the organisation of a supramental nature here, as a mental being has appeared and a mental nature organised itself during the last stage of the evolution. I prefer nowadays not to speak of the descent of the higher beings because my experience is that it leads to a vain and often egoistic romanticism which distracts the attention from the real work, that of the realisation of the Divine and the transformation of the nature.

What we are doing, if and when we succeed, will be a beginning, not a completion. It is the foundation of a new consciousness on earth — a consciousness with infinite possibilities of manifestation. The eternal progression is in the manifestation and beyond it there is no progression.

If the redemption of the soul from the physical vesture be the object, then there is no need of supramentalisation. Spiritual Mukti and Nirvana are sufficient. If the object is to rise to supraphysical planes, then also there is no need of supramentalisation. One can enter into some heaven above by devotion to the Lord of that heaven. But that is no progression. The other worlds are typal worlds, each fixed in its own kind and type and law. Evolution takes place on the earth and therefore the earth is the proper field for progression. The beings of the other worlds do not progress from one world to another. They remain fixed to their own type.

The purely monistic Vedantist says, all is Brahman, life is a dream, an unreality, only Brahman exists. One has Nirvana or Mukti, then one lives only till the body falls — after that there is no such thing as life.

They do not believe in transformation, because mind, life and body are an ignorance, an illusion — the only reality is the featureless relationless Self or Brahman. Life is a thing of relations; in the pure Self, all life and relations disappear. What would be the use or the possibility of transforming an illusion that can never be anything else (however transformed) than an illusion? There is no such thing for them as a "Nirvanic life".

It is only some yogas that aim at a transformation of any kind except that of ignorance into knowledge. The idea varies, — sometimes a divine knowledge or power or else a divine purity or an ethical perfection or a divine love.

What has to be overcome is the opposition of the Ignorance that does not want the transformation of the nature. If that can be overcome, then old spiritual ideas will not form an obstacle.

It is not intended to supramentalise humanity at large, but to establish the principle of the supramental consciousness in the earth-evolution. If that is done, all that is needed will be evolved by the supramental Power itself. It is not therefore important that the mission should be widespread. What is important is that the thing should be done at all in however small a number; that is the only difficulty.

If the transformation of the body is complete, that means no subjection to death — it does not mean that one will be bound to keep the same body for all time. One creates a new body for oneself when one wants to change, but how it will be done cannot be said now. The present method is by physical birth — some occultists suppose that a time will come when that will not be necessary — but the question must be left for the supramental evolution to decide.

The questions about the supermind cannot be answered profitably now. Supermind cannot be described in terms that the mind will understand, because the terms will be mental and mind will understand them in a mental way and mental sense and miss their true import. It would therefore be a waste of time and energy which should be devoted to the preliminary work — psychicisation and spiritualisation of the being and nature without which no supramentalisation is possible. Let the whole dynamic nature led by the psychic make itself full of the dynamic spiritual light, peace, purity, knowledge, force; let it afterwards get experience of the intermediate spiritual planes and know, feel and act in their sense; then it will be possible to speak last of the supramental transformation.

What is a perfect technique of yoga or rather of a world-changing or Nature-changing yoga? Not one that takes a man by a little bit of him somewhere, attaches a hook, and pulls him up by a pulley into Nirvana or Paradise. The technique of a world-changing yoga has to be as multiform, sinuous, patient, all-including as the world itself. If it does not deal with all the difficulties or possibilities and carefully deal with each necessary element, has it any chance of success? And can a perfect technique which everybody can understand do that? It is not like writing a small poem in a fixed metre with a limited number of modulations. If you take the poem simile, it is the Mahabharata of a Mahabharata that has to be done. And what, compared with the limited Greek perfection, is the technique of the Mahabharata?

Next, what is the use of *vicārabuddhi* in such a case? If one has to get a new consciousness which surpasses the reasoning intellect, can one do it on lines which are to be judged and understood by the reasoning intellect, controlled at every step by it, told by the intellect what it is to do, what is the measure of its achievements, what its steps must be and what their value? If one does that, will one ever get out of the range of the reasoning intelligence into what is beyond it? And if one does, how shall others judge what one is doing by the intellectual measure? How can one judge what is beyond the ordinary consciousness when one is oneself in the ordinary consciousness? Is it not only by exceeding yourself that you can feel, experience, judge what exceeds you? What is the value of a judgment without the feeling and experience?

What the supramental will do the mind cannot foresee or lay down. The mind is ignorance seeking for the Truth, the supramental by its very definition is the Truth-Consciousness, Truth in possession of itself and fulfilling itself by its own power. In a supramental world imperfection and disharmony are bound to disappear. But what we propose just now is not to make the earth a supramental world but to bring down the supramental as a power and established consciousness in the midst of the rest — to let it work there and fulfil itself as Mind descended into Life and Matter and has worked as a Power there to fulfil itself in the midst of the rest. This will be enough to change the world and to change Nature by breaking down her present limits. But what, how, by what degrees it will do it, is a thing that ought not to be said now — when the Light is there, the Light will itself do its work — when the supramental Will stands on earth, that Will will decide. It will establish a perfection, a harmony, a Truth-creation — for the rest, well, it will be the rest — that is all.

The whole of humanity cannot be changed at once. What has to be done is to bring the Higher Consciousness down into the earth-consciousness and establish it there as a constant realised force. Just as mind and life have been established and embodied in Matter, so to establish and embody the supramental Force.

It would not be possible to change all that in a moment — we
have always said that the whole of humanity will not change the
moment there is the Descent. But what can be done is to establish the higher principle in the earth-consciousness in such a
way that it will remain and go on strengthening and spreading
itself in the earth-life. That is how a new principle in the evolution must necessarily work.

It [the world] wants and it does not want something that it
has not got. All that the supramental could give, the inner
mind of the world would like to have, but its outer mind, its
vital and physical do not like to pay the price. But, after all,
I am not trying to change the world all at once but only to
bring down centrally something into it it has not yet, a new
consciousness and power.

This transformation cannot be done individually or in a solitary
way only. No individual solitary transformation unconcerned
with the work for the earth (which means more than any individual transformation) would be either possible or useful. Also
no individual human being can by his own power alone work
out the transformation, nor is it the object of the yoga to create
an individual superman here and there. The object of the
yoga is to bring down the supramental consciousness on earth,
to fix it there, to create a new race with the principle of the
supramental consciousness governing the inner and outer
individual and collective life.

That force accepted by individual after individual according
to their preparation would establish the supramental consciousness in the physical world and so create a nucleus for its own
expansion.

*
**

It is first through the individuals that it [the supramental con-sciousness] becomes part of the earth-consciousness and after-wards it spreads from the first centres and takes up more and more of the global consciousness till it becomes an established force there.

All that is absurd. The descent of the supramental means only that the Power will be there in the earth-consciousness as a living force just as the thinking mental and higher mental are already there. But an animal cannot take advantage of the presence of the thinking mental Power or an undeveloped man of the presence of the higher mental Power — so too any-body will not be able to take advantage of the presence of the supramental Power. I have also often enough said that it will be at first for the few, not for the whole earth, — only there will be a growing influence of it on the earth-life.

It [the descent of the supermind into the earth-consciousness] would not necessarily be known by everybody. Besides, even if the descent were here one would have to be ready before one could get the final change.

Not in their entirety — for that [the transformation of the Cosmic Mind, Life and Matter] is not our business. It is our-selves that we have to transform and change the earth-conscious-ness by bringing in the supramental principle into the evolution there. Once there it will necessarily have a powerful influence in the whole earth-life — as mind has had through the evolu-tion of men, but much greater.

It is not possible for a force like the supramental to come down without making a large change in earth-conditions. It does not follow that all will become supramentalised and it is not necessary — but mind itself will be influenced as life has been influenced by the development of mind on earth.

Nothing permanent can be done without the real supramental Force. But the result of its descent would be that in human life intuition would become a greater and more developed force than it now is and the other intermediate powers between mind and supermind would become also more common and develop an organised action.

How do you know that it [our yoga] will have no effect on the ordinary people? It will inevitably increase their possibilities and even though all cannot rise to the highest, that will mean a great change for the earth.

It would on the contrary be impossible for them [the ordinary people] not to feel that a greater Light and Power had come on the earth.

It is not for considerations of gain or loss that the Divine Consciousness acts — that is a human standpoint necessary for human development. The Divine, as the Gita says, has nothing to gain and nothing that it has not, yet it puts forth its power of action in the manifestation. It is the earth-consciousness, not the supramental world that has to gain by the descent of the supramental principle — that is sufficient reason for it to descend. The supramental worlds remain as they are and are in no way affected by the descent.

"Opening from below"[1] means this — that the supramental force descending awakes a response from below in the earth-consciousness so that it is possible for a supramental activity to be formed in the material itself. All is involved as potentiality in the earth-consciousness, life, mind, supermind — but it is only when life force descended from the life plane into the material that active and conscious organised life was possible — so it was only when mind descended that the latent mind in Matter awoke and could be organised. The supramental descent must create the same kind of opening from below so that a supramental consciousness can be organised in the material.

It [the earth] contains all the potentialities which come out in the beings of earth and also much that is unexpressed.

Yes. The earth is the place of evolution in which all these forces meet and try to manifest and out of their working something has to develop. On the other planes (the mental, vital etc.) there is not the evolution — there each acts separately according to its own law.

[The earth-consciousness:] The consciousness of this Earth alone. There is a separate global consciousness of the earth (as of other worlds) which evolves with the evolution of life on the planet.

Yes all that is the earth-consciousness — mineral=matter, vegetable=the vital-physical creation, animal=the vital creation, man = the mental creation. Into the earth-consciousness so limi-

---

[1] "... it is only the very highest supramental Force descending from above and opening from below that can victoriously handle the physical Nature and annihilate its difficulties." Sri Aurobindo, *The Mother*, p. 2.

ted to mind, vital, matter has to come the supramental creation. Necessarily *at first* it cannot be in a great number — but even if it is only in a few at first, that does not mean that it will have no effect on the rest or will not change the whole balance of the earth-nature.

There is no reason why the vegetable, animal and human life should not evolve in the Truth and not in the Ignorance — if once the knowledge is there in the earth-plane.

It [the supermind] can act directly on everything if it is brought down into the material consciousness — at present in the arrangement of things here it is latent behind and acts through other media.

[Direct supramental action in the plants at present:] No, one can't say that. It is the vital force that works, but there is a sort of underlying Intuition in this Life-Force which is behind the whole action and that is what one might call a reflection or delegated Power at the back of which is latent supermind.

If spiritual and supramental were the same thing, as you say my readers imagine, then all the sages and devotees and yogis and sadhaks throughout the ages would have been supramental beings and all I have written about the supermind would be so much superfluous stuff, useless and otiose. Anybody who had spiritual experiences would then be a supramental being; the Ashram would be chock-full of supramental beings and every other Ashram in India also. Spiritual experiences can fix themselves in the inner consciousness and alter it, transform it, if you like; one can realise the Divine everywhere, the Self in all and all in the Self, the universal Shakti doing all things; one can feel merged in the Cosmic Self or full of ecstatic bhakti or Ananda. But one may and usually does still go on in the outer parts of Nature thinking with the intellect or at best the intuitive mind, willing with a mental will, feeling joy and sorrow on the vital surface, undergoing physical afflictions and suffering from the struggle of life in the body with death and disease. The change then only will be that the inner self will watch all that without getting disturbed or bewildered, with a perfect equality, taking it as an inevitable part of Nature, inevitable at least so long as one does not withdraw to the Self out of Nature. That is not the transformation I envisage. It is quite another power of knowledge, another kind of will, another luminous nature of emotion and aesthesis, another constitution of the physical consciousness that must come in by the supramental change.

The spiritual realisation can be had on any plane by contact with the Divine (who is everywhere) or by perception of the Self within, which is pure and untouched by the outer movements. The supermind is something transcendent — a dynamic Truth-Consciousness which is not there yet, something to be brought down from above.

It is only the supramental that is all-knowledge. All below that from overmind to Matter is Ignorance — an Ignorance growing from level to level towards the full knowledge. Below supermind there may be knowledge but it is not all-knowledge.

I have not said that everything is falsehood except the supramental Truth. I said that there was no complete Truth below the supramental. In the overmind the Truth of supermind which is whole and harmonious enters into a separation into parts, many truths fronting each other and moved each to fulfil itself, to make a world of its own or else to prevail or take its share in worlds made of a combination of various separated Truths and Truth-forces. Lower down in the scale, the fragmentation becomes more and more pronounced, so as to admit of positive error, falsehood, ignorance, finally inconscience like that of Matter. This world here has come out of the Inconscience and developed the Mind which is an instrument of Ignorance trying to reach out to the Truth through much limitation, conflict, confusion and error. To get back to overmind, if one can do it completely, which is not easy for physical beings, is to stand on the borders of the supramental Truth with the hope of entry there.

There can be no mental rule or definition. One has first to live in the Divine and attain to the Truth — the will and awareness of the Truth will organize the life.

It is in the inactive Brahman that one merges, if one seeks Laya or Moksha. One can dwell in the Personal Divine, but one does not merge in him. As for the Supreme Divine, he holds in himself the world-existence and it is in his consciousness that it moves, so by entering into the Supreme one rises above subjection to Nature, but one does not disappear from all consciousness of world-existence.

The general Divine Will in the universe is for the progressive manifestation in the universe. But that is the general will — it admits the withdrawal of individual souls who are not ready to persevere in the world.

It is not immortality of the body, but the consciousness of immortality *in* the body that can come with the descent of overmind into Matter or even into the physical mind or with the touch of the modified supramental Light on the physical mind-consciousness. These are preliminary openings, but they are not the supramental fulfilment in Matter.

If the supramental is decreed, nothing can prevent it; but all things are worked out here through a play of forces, and an unfavourable atmosphere or conditions can delay even when they cannot prevent. Even when a thing is destined, it does not present itself as a certitude in the consciousness here (overmind-mind-vital-physical) till the play of forces has been worked out up to a certain point at which the descent not only is, but appears as inevitable.

The supramental change is the ultimate stage of siddhi and it is not likely to come so soon; but there are many levels between the normal mind and the supermind and it is easy to mistake an ascent into one of them or a descent of their consciousness or influence for a supramental change.

It is quite impossible to ascend to the real Ananda *plane* (except in a profound trance), until after the supramental consciousness has been entered, realised and possessed; but it is quite possible and normal to feel some form of Ananda *consciousness* on any level. This consciousness wherever it is felt is a derivation from the Ananda plane, but it is very much diminished in power and modified to suit the lesser power of receptivity of the inferior levels.

I presume it is the development of the Truth-Power and the Ananda-Power in the overmind consciousness that is being prepared. The transcendent Ananda in itself could descend only after the complete supramentalisation of the being and would mean a stupendous change in the earth-consciousness. It is the divine Truth in the overmind and the divine Ananda in the overmind that can now prepare their manifestation and it is that which is being indicated in these experiences.

It is the supermind we have to bring down, manifest, realise — anything higher than that is impossible at this stage of the evolution except as a reflection in the consciousness or a power delegated and modified in its descent.

I do not know what Mahatma Gandhi means by complete realisation.[1] If he means a realisation with nothing more to realise, no farther development possible, then I agree — I have myself spoken of farther divine progression, an infinite development. But the question is not that: the question is whether the Ignorance can be transcended, whether a complete essential realisation turning the consciousness from darkness to light, from an instrument of the Ignorance seeking for Knowledge into an instrument or rather a manifestation of Knowledge proceeding to greater Knowledge, Light enlarging, heightening into greater Light, is or is not possible. My view is that this conversion is not only possible, but inevitable in the spiritual evolution of the being here. The embodiment of life has nothing to do with it. This embodiment is not of life, but of consciousness and its energy of which life is only one phase or force. As life has developed mind, and the embodiment has modified itself to suit this development (mind is precisely the main instrument of ignorance seeking for knowledge), so mind can develop supermind which is in its nature knowledge not seeking for itself, but manifesting itself by its own automatic power, and the embodiment can again modify itself or be modified from above so as to suit this development. Faith is a necessary means for arriving at realisation, because we are ignorant and do not yet know that which we are seeking to realise; faith is indeed knowledge giving the ignorance an intimation of itself previous to its own manifestation, it is the gleam sent before by the yet unrisen Sun. When the Sun shall rise, there will be no longer any need of the gleam. The supramental knowledge supports itself. It does not need to be supported by faith; it lives by its own certitude. You may say that farther progression, farther development will need faith. No, for the farther development will proceed on a basis of Knowledge, not of Ignorance. We shall walk in the light of Knowledge towards its own wider vistas of self-fulfilment.

---

[1] These observations are apropos of the following statement in an article by Mahatma Gandhi submitted by a sadhak to Sri Aurobindo for his opinion:

"I hold that a complete realisation is impossible in this embodied life. Nor is it neces-

An evolution from the Inconscient need not be a painful one if there is no resistance; it can be a deliberately slow and beautiful efflorescence of the Divine. One ought to be able to see how beautiful outward Nature can be and usually is, although it is itself apparently "inconscient". Why should the growth of consciousness in inward Nature be attended by so much ugliness and evil spoiling the beauty of the outward creation? Because of a perversity born from the Ignorance, which came in with Life and increased in Mind — that is the Falsehood, the Evil that was born because of the starkness of the Inconscient's sleep separating its action from the luminosity of the secret Conscient that is all the time within it. But it need not have been so except for the overriding Will of the Supreme which meant that the possibilities of perversion by inconscience and ignorance should be manifested in order to be eliminated through being given their chance, since all possibility has to manifest somewhere: once it is eliminated, the Divine Manifestation in Matter will be greater than it otherwise could be, because it will combine all the possibilities involved in this difficult creation and not some of them as in an easier and less strenuous creation might naturally happen.

"From beauty to greater beauty, from joy to intenser joy, by an especial adjustment of the senses" — yes, that would be the normal course of a divine manifestation, however gradual, in Matter. "Discordant sound and offensive odour" are creations of a disharmony between consciousness and Nature and do not exist in themselves; they would not be present to a liberated and harmonised consciousness, for they would be foreign to its being, nor would they afflict a rightly developing harmonised soul and Nature. Even the "belching volcano, crashing thunderstorm and whirling typhoon" are in themselves grandiose and beautiful things and only harmful or terrible to a consciousness unable to meet or deal with them or make a pact with the spirits of Wind and Fire. You are assuming that the manifestation from the Inconscient must be what it is now and here and that no other kind of world of Matter was possible, but the harmony of material Nature in itself shows that it need not necessarily be a dis-

sary. A living immovable faith is all that is required for reaching the full spiritual height attainable by human beings."

cordant, evil, furiously perturbed and painful creation — the psychic being, if allowed to manifest from the first in Life and Mind and lead the evolution instead of being relegated behind the veil, would have been the principle of a harmony ever out-flowing: everyone who has felt the psychic at work within him, free of the vital intervention, can at once see that this would be its effect because of its unerring perception, true choice, harmonic action. If it has not been so, it is because the Dark Powers have made Life a claimant instead of an instrument. The reality of the Hostiles and the nature of their role and trend of their endea-vour cannot be doubted by anyone who has had his inner vision unsealed and made their unpleasant acquaintance.

It is not to be denied, no spiritual experience will deny that this is an unideal and unsatisfactory world, strongly marked with the stamp of inadequacy, suffering, evil. Indeed this perception is in a way the starting-point of the spiritual urge — except for the few to whom the greater experience comes spontaneously without being forced to it by the strong or overwhelming, the afflicting and detaching sense of the Shadow overhanging the whole range of this manifested existence. But still the question remains whe-ther this is indeed, as is contended, the essential character of all manifestation or so long at least as there is a physical world it must be of this nature, so that the desire of birth, the will to manifest or create has to be regarded as the original sin and withdrawal from birth or manifestation as the sole possible way of salvation. For those who perceive it so or with some kindred look — and these have been the majority — there are well-known ways of issue, a straight-cut to spiritual deliverance. But equally it may not be so but only seem so to our ignorance or to a partial knowledge — the imperfection, the evil, the suffering may be a besetting circumstance or a dolorous passage, but not the very condition of manifestation, not the very essence of birth in Nature. And if so, the highest wisdom will lie not in escape, but in the urge towards a victory here, in a consenting association with the Will behind the world, in a discovery of the spiritual gate to perfection which will be at the same time an opening for the entire descent of the Divine Light, Knowledge, Power, Beatitude.

All spiritual experience affirms that there is a Permanent above the transience of this manifested world we live in and this limited consciousness in whose narrow borders we grope and struggle and that its characters are infinity, self-existence, freedom, absolute Light, absolute Beatitude. Is there then an unbridgeable gulf between that which is beyond and that which is here or are they two perpetual opposites and only by leaving this adventure in Time behind, by overleaping the gulf can men reach the Eternal? That is what seems to be at the end of one line of experience which has been followed to its rigorous conclusion by Buddhism and a little less rigorously by a certain type of Monistic spirituality which admits some connection of the world with the Divine, but still opposes them in the last resort to each other as truth and illusion. But there is also this other and indubitable experience that the Divine is here in everything as well as above and behind everything, that all is in That and is That when we go back from its appearance to its Reality. It is a significant and illumining fact that the Knower of Brahman even moving and acting in this world, even bearing all its shocks, can live in some absolute peace, light and beatitude of the Divine. There is then here something other than that mere trenchant opposition — there is a mystery, a problem which one would think must admit of some less desperate solution. This spiritual possibility points beyond itself and brings a ray of hope into the darkness of our fallen existence.

And at once a first question arises — is this world an unchanging succession of the same phenomena always or is there in it an evolutionary urge, an evolutionary fact, a ladder of ascension somewhere from an original apparent Inconscience to a more and more developed consciousness, from each development still ascending, emerging on highest heights not yet within our normal reach? If so, what is the sense, the fundamental principle, the logical issue of that progression? Everything seems to point to such a progression as a fact — to a spiritual and not merely a physical evolution. Here too there is a justifying line of spiritual experience in which we discover that the Inconscient from which all starts is apparent only, for in it there is an involved Consciousness with endless possibilities, a consciousness not limited but cosmic and infinite, a concealed and self-imprisoned Divine, imprisoned in Matter but with every potentiality held in its secret depths. Out of this apparent Inconscience each potentiality is revealed in its turn, first organised Matter concealing the indwelling Spirit, then Life emerging in the plant and associated in the animal with a growing Mind, then Mind itself evolved and organised in Man. This evolution, this spiritual progression — does it stop short here in the imperfect mental being called Man? Or is the secret of it simply a succession of rebirths whose only purpose of issue is to labour towards the point at which it can learn its own futility, renounce itself and take its leap into some original unborn Existence or Non-Existence? There is at least the possibility, there comes at a certain point the certitude, that there is a far greater consciousness than what we call Mind, and that by ascending the ladder still farther we can find a point at which the hold of the material Inconscience, the vital and mental Ignorance ceases; a principle of consciousness becomes capable of manifestation which liberates not partially, not imperfectly, but radically and wholly this imprisoned Divine. In this vision each stage of evolution appears as due to the descent of a higher and higher Power of consciousness, raising the terrestrial level, creating a new stratum, but the highest yet remain to descend and it is by their descent that the riddle of terrestrial existence will receive its solution and not only the soul but Nature herself find her deliverance. This is the Truth which has been seen in flashes, in more and more entirety of its terms by the line of seers whom the Tantra would call the hero-seekers and the divine-seekers and which may now be nearing the point of readiness for its full revelation and experience. Then whatever be the heavy weight of strife and suffering and darkness in the world, yet if there is this as its high result awaiting us, all that has gone before may not be counted too great a price by the strong and adventurous for the glory that is to come. At any rate the shadow lifts; there is a Divine Light that leans over the world and is not only a far-off incommunicable Lustre.

It is true that the problem still remains why all this that yet

is should have been necessary — these crude beginnings, this long
and stormy passage — why should the heavy and tedious price
be demanded, why should evil and suffering ever have been
there. For to the how of the fall into the Ignorance as opposed
to the why, the effective cause, there is a substantial agreement
in all spiritual experience. It is the division, the separation, the
principle of isolation from the Permanent and One that brought
it about; it is because the ego set up for itself in the world emphasising its own desire and self-affirmation in preference to its
unity with the Divine and its oneness with all; it is because instead of the one supreme Force, Wisdom, Light determining the
harmony of all forces each Idea, Force, Form of things was
allowed to work itself out as far as it could in the mass of infinite
possibilities by its separate will and inevitably in the end by conflict with others. Division, ego, the imperfect consciousness
and groping and struggle of a separate self-affirmation are the
efficient cause of the suffering and ignorance of this world.
Once consciousnesses separated from the one consciousness,
they fell inevitably into Ignorance and the last result of Ignorance
was Inconscience; from a dark immense Inconscient this material world arises and out of it a soul that by evolution is struggling
into consciousness, attracted towards the hidden Light, ascending but still blindly towards the lost Divinity from which it came.

But why should this have happened at all? One common
way of putting the question and answering it ought to be eliminated from the first, — the human way and its ethical revolt
and reprobation, its emotional outcry. For it is not, as some
religions suppose, a supra-cosmic, arbitrary, personal Deity
himself altogether uninvolved in the fall who has imposed evil
and suffering on creatures made capriciously by his fiat. The
Divine we know is an Infinite Being in whose infinite manifestation these things have come — it is the Divine itself that is here,
behind us, pervading the manifestation, supporting the world
with its oneness; it is the Divine that is in us upholding itself the
burden of the fall and its dark consequence. If above It stands
for ever in its perfect Light, Bliss and Peace, It is also here; its
Light, Bliss and Peace are secretly here supporting all; in ourselves there is a spirit, a central presence greater than the series

of surface personalities which, like the supreme Divine itself, is
not overborne by the fate they endure. If we find out this Divine
within us, if we know ourselves as this spirit which is of one
essence and being with the Divine, that is our gate of deliverance
and in it we can remain ourselves even in the midst of this world's
disharmonies, luminous, blissful and free. That much is the age-
old testimony of spiritual experience.

But still what is the purpose and origin of the disharmony
— why came this division and ego, this world of painful evolution? Why must evil and sorrow enter into the divine Good,
Bliss and Peace? It is hard to answer to the human intelligence
on its own level, for the consciousness to which the origin of this
phenomenon belongs and to which it stands as it were automatically justified in a supra-intellectual knowledge, is a cosmic and
not an individualised human intelligence; it sees in larger spaces,
it has another vision and cognition, other terms of consciousness
than human reason and feeling. To the human mind one might
answer that while in itself the Infinite might be free from those
perturbations, yet once manifestation began infinite possibility
also began and among the infinite possibilities which it is the
function of the universal manifestation to work out, the negation,
the apparent effective negation — with all its consequences —
of the Power, Light, Peace, Bliss was very evidently one. If it is
asked why even if possible it should have been accepted, the
answer nearest to the Cosmic Truth which the human intelligence can make is that in the relations or in the transition of the
Divine in the Oneness to the Divine in the Many, this ominous
possible became at a certain point an inevitable. For once it
appears it acquires for the Soul descending into evolutionary
manifestation an irresistible attraction which creates the inevitability — an attraction which in human terms on the terrestrial
level might be interpreted as the call of the unknown, the joy of
danger and difficulty and adventure, the will to attempt the impossible, to work out the incalculable, the will to create the new
and the uncreated with one's own self and life as the material,
the fascination of contradictories and their difficult harmonisation — these things translated into another supraphysical, superhuman consciousness, higher and wider than the mental, were

the temptation that led to the fall. For to the original being of light on the verge of the descent the one thing unknown was the depths of the abyss, the possibilities of the Divine in the Ignorance and Inconscience. On the other side from the Divine Oneness a vast acquiescence, compassionate, consenting, helpful, a supreme knowledge that this thing must be, that having appeared it must be worked out, that its appearance is in a certain sense part of an incalculable infinite wisdom, that if the plunge into Night was inevitable the emergence into a new unprecedented Day was also a certitude, and that only so could a certain manifestation of the Supreme Truth be effected — by a working out with its phenomenal opposites as the starting-point of the evolution, as the condition laid down for a transforming emergence. In this acquiescence was embraced too the will of the great Sacrifice, the descent of the Divine itself into the Inconsience to take up the burden of the Ignorance and its consequences, to intervene as the Avatar and the Vibhuti walking between the double sign of the Cross and the Victory towards the fulfilment and deliverance. A too imaged rendering of the inexpressible Truth? But without images how to present to the intellect a mystery far beyond it? It is only when one has crossed the barrier of the limited intelligence and shared in the cosmic experience and the knowledge which sees things from identity that the supreme realities which lie behind these images — images corresponding to the terrestrial fact — assume their divine forms and are felt as simple, natural, implied in the essence of things. It is by entering into that greater consciousness alone that one can grasp the inevitability of its self-creation and its purpose.

This is indeed only the Truth of the manifestation as it presents itself to the consciousness when it stands on the border line between Eternity and the descent into Time where the relation between the One and the Many in the evolution is self-determined, a zone where all that is to be is implied but not yet in action. But the liberated consciousness can rise higher where the problem exists no longer and from there see it in the light of a supreme identity where all is predetermined in the automatic self-existent truth of things and self-justified to an absolute consciousness and wisdom and absolute Delight which is behind all

creation and non-creation and the affirmation and negation are
both seen with the eyes of the ineffable Reality that delivers and
reconciles them. But that knowledge is not expressible to the
human mind; its language of light is too undecipherable, the
light itself too bright for a consciousness accustomed to the
stress and obscurity of the cosmic riddle and entangled in it to
follow the clue or to grasp its secret. In any case, it is only when
we rise in the spirit beyond the zone of the darkness and the
struggle that we enter into the full significance of it and there is a
deliverance of the soul from its enigma. To rise to that height
of liberation is the true way out and the only means of the indubitable knowledge.

But the liberation and transcendence need not necessarily
impose a disappearance, a sheer dissolving out from the manifestation; it can prepare a liberation into action of the highest
Knowledge and an intensity of Power that can transform the
world and fulfil the evolutionary urge. It is an ascent from
which there is no longer a fall but a winged or self-sustained
descent of light, force and Ananda.

It is what is inherent in force of being that manifests as becoming; but what the manifestation shall be, its terms, its
balance of energies, its arrangement of principles depends on the
consciousness which acts in the creative force, on the power of
consciousness which Being delivers from itself for manifestation.
It is in the nature of Being to be able to grade and vary its powers
of consciousness and determine according to the grade and
variation its world or its degree and scope of self-revelation.
The manifested creation is limited by the power to which it belongs and sees and lives according to it and can only see more,
live more powerfully, change its world by opening or moving
towards or making descend a greater power of consciousness
that was above it. This is what is happening in the evolution of
consciousness in our world, a world of inanimate matter producing under the stress of this necessity a power of life, a power
of mind which bring into it new forms of creation and still labour-
ing to produce, to make descend into it some supramental power.
It is further an operation of creative force which moves between
two poles of consciousness. On one side there is a secret con-

sciousness within and above which contains in it all potentialities — there eternally manifest, here awaiting delivery — of light, peace, power and bliss. On the other side there is another, outward on the surface and below, that starts from the apparent opposite of unconsciousness, inertia, blind stress, possibility of suffering and grows by receiving into itself higher and higher powers which make it always re-create its manifestation in larger terms, each new creation of this kind bringing out something of the inner potentiality, making it more and more possible to bring down the Perfection that waits above. As long as the outward personality we call ourselves is centred in the lower powers of consciousness, the riddle of its own existence, its purpose, its necessity is to it an insoluble enigma; if something of the truth is at all conveyed to this outward mental man, he but imperfectly grasps it and perhaps misinterprets and misuses and mislives it. His true staff of walking is made more of a fire of faith than any ascertained and indubitable light of knowledge. It is only by rising toward a higher consciousness beyond the mental line and therefore superconscient now to him that he can emerge from his inability and his ignorance. His full liberation and enlightenment will come when he crosses the line into the light of a new superconscient existence. That is the transcendence which was the object of aspiration of the mystics and the spiritual seekers.

But in itself this would change nothing in the creation here, the evasion of a liberated soul from the world makes to that world no difference. But this crossing of the line if turned not only to an ascending but to a descending purpose would mean the transformation of the line from what it now is, a lid, a barrier, into a passage for the higher powers of consciousness of the Being now above it. It would mean a new creation on earth, a bringing in of the ultimate powers which would reverse the conditions here, in as much as that would produce a creation raised into the full flood of spiritual and supramental light in place of one emerging into a half-light of mind out of a darkness of material inconscience. It is only in such a full flood of the realised spirit that the embodied being could know, in the sense of all that was involved in it, the meaning and temporary necessity of

his descent into the darkness and its conditions and at the same
time dissolve them by a luminous transmutation into a manifestation here of the revealed and no longer of the veiled and
disguised or apparently deformed Divine.

I suppose you have not read my *Riddle of this World*,[1] but it is a
similar solution I put there. X's way of putting it is a trifle too
"Vedantic-Theistic" — in my view it is a transaction between
the One and the Many. In the beginning it was you (not the
human you who is now complaining but the central being) which
accepted or even invited the adventure of the Ignorance; sorrow
and struggle are a necessary consequence of the plunge into the
Inconscience and the evolutionary emergence out of it. The explanation is that it had an object, the eventual play of the Divine
Consciousness and Ananda not in its original transcendence but
under conditions for which the plunge into the Inconscience was
necessary. It is fundamentally a cosmic problem and can be
understood only from the cosmic consciousness. If you want a
solution which will be agreeable to the human mind and feelings,
I am afraid there is none. No doubt if human beings had made
the universe, they would have done much better; but they were
not there to be consulted when they were made. Only your central being was there and that was much nearer in its temerarious
foolhardiness to Vivekananda's or X's than to the repining
prudence of your murmuring and trembling human mentality
of the present moment — otherwise it would never have come
down into the adventure. Or perhaps it did not realise what it was
in for? It is the same with the wallowers under their cross. Even
now they wallow because something in them likes the wallowing
and bear the cross because something in them chooses to suffer.
So? —

The European type of monism is usually pantheistic and weaves

---

[1] This was the title given to the preceding long letter when it was first published in
November 1933, along with some other letters, in a book bearing the same title.

the universe and the Divine so intimately together that they can hardly be separated. But what explanation of the evil and misery can there be there? The Indian view is that the Divine is the inmost substance of the universe, but he is also outside it, transcendent; good and evil, happiness and misery are only phenomena of cosmic experience due to a division and a diminution of consciousness in the manifestation but are not part of the essence or of the undivided whole-consciousness either of the Divine or of our own spiritual being.

The involution is of the Divine in the Inconscience and it is done by the interposition of intermediate planes (overmind etc., mind, vital — then the plunge into the Inconscient which is the origin of matter). But all that is not a process answering to the evolution in the inverse sense — for there is no need for that, but a gradation of consciousness which is intended to make the evolution upwards possible.

There are three powers of the cosmos to which all things are subject — creation, preservation and destruction; whatever is created lasts for a time, then begins to crumble down. The taking away of the Force of destruction implies a creation that will not be destroyed but last and develop always. In the Ignorance destruction is necessary for progress — in the Knowledge, the Truth-creation, the law is that of a constant unfolding without any Pralaya.

[Great catastrophic upheavals when the supermind descends:] There need not be. There will necessarily be great changes but they are not bound to be catastrophic. When there is a strong pressure from overmind forces for change, then there are likely to be catastrophes because of the resistance and clash of forces. The supramental has a greater — in its fullness a complete

mastery of things and power of harmonisation which can overcome resistance by other means than dramatic struggle and
violence.

Yes, there has been some progress in that respect [the psychic
change] and all progress in the psychic or spiritual consciousness of the sadhaks makes the descent more easy. But the main
cause is that the overmind principle which is the immediate secret
support of the present earth-nature with all its limitations is more
and more undergoing the pressure of the supramental and letting
through a greater Light and Power. For so long as the overmind
intervenes (the principle of overmind being a play of forces, each
trying to realise itself as the Truth) the law of struggle remains
and with it the opportunity for the adverse Forces.

As far as I can see, once the supramental is established in Matter,
the transformation will be possible under much less troublesome
conditions than now are there. These bad conditions are due to
the fact that the Ignorance is in possession and the hostile Powers
an established authority, as it were, who do not care to give up
their hold and there is no full force of Light established in the
earth-consciousness which would not only meet but outweigh
their full force of darkness.

The fallacy of the argument lies in the premiss laid down in the
beginning that even after supramentalisation difficulties and
attacks will continue. In the supramental consciousness such
attacks are not possible — the coexistence of supramental and
the lower darkness in the same being and body is not possible.
It is precisely for that reason that the supramentalisation of the
body consciousness is laid down as the condition of the successful transformation. If attacks continue and can come in success-

fully, it means that the body consciousness is not yet supra-mentalised.

The descent of the supramental can hasten things, but it is not going to act as a patent medicine or change everything in the twinkle of an eye.

It is the darkest nights that prepare the greatest dawns — and it is so because it is into the deepest inconscience of material life that we have to bring, not an intermediate glimmer, but the full play of the divine Light.

1. 2. 34 It is supposed to be always a year of manifestation. 2. 3. 45 is the year of power — when the thing manifested gets full force. 4. 5. 67 is the year of complete realisation.

INTEGRAL YOGA AND OTHER PATHS

Integral Yoga and Other Paths

I DO not agree with the view that the world is an illusion, *mithyā*. The Brahman is here as well as in the supracosmic Absolute. The thing to be overcome is the Ignorance which makes us blind and prevents us from realising Brahman in the world as well as beyond it and the true nature of existence.

*
* *

The Shankara knowledge is, as your Guru pointed out, only one side of the Truth; it is the knowledge of the Supreme as realised by the spiritual Mind through the static silence of the pure Existence. It was because he went by this side only that Shankara was unable to accept or explain the origin of the universe except as illusion, a creation of Maya. Unless one realises the Supreme on the dynamic as well as the static side, one cannot experience the true origin of things and the equal reality of the active Brahman. The Shakti or Power of the Eternal becomes then a power of illusion only and the world becomes incomprehensible, a mystery of cosmic madness, an eternal delirium of the Eternal. Whatever verbal or ideative logic one may bring to support it, this way of seeing the universe explains nothing; it only erects a mental formula of the inexplicable. It is only if you approach the Supreme through his double aspect of Sat and Chit-Shakti, double but inseparable, that the total truth of things can become manifest to the inner experience. This other side was developed by the Shakta Tantriks. The two together, the Vedantic and the Tantric truth unified, can arrive at the integral knowledge.

But philosophically this is what your Guru's teaching comes to and it is obviously a completer truth and a wider knowledge than that given by the Shankara formula. It is already indicated in the Gita's teaching of the Purushottama and the Parashakti (Adya Shakti) who become the Jiva and uphold the universe. It is evident that Purushottama and Parashakti are both eternal and are inseparable and one in being; the Parashakti manifests the universe, manifests too the Divine in the universe as the Ishwara and Herself appears at His side as the Ishwari Shakti. Or, we may say, it is the Supreme Conscious Power of the Supreme that manifests or puts forth itself as Ishwara Ishwari, Atma Atma-shakti, Purusha Prakriti, Jiva Jagat. That is the truth in its completeness as far as the mind can formulate it. In the supermind these questions do not even arise: for it is the mind that creates the problem by creating oppositions between aspects of the Divine which are not really opposed to each other but are one and inseparable.

This supramental knowledge has not yet been attained, because the supermind itself has not been attained, but the reflection of it in intuitive spiritual consciousness is there and that was what was evidently realised in experience by your Guru and what he was expressing in mental terms in the quoted passage. It is possible to go towards the knowledge by beginning with the experience of dissolution in the One, but on condition that you do not stop there, taking it as the highest Truth, but proceed to realise the same One as the supreme Mother, the Consciousness-Force of the Eternal. If, on the other hand, you approach through the Supreme Mother, she will give you the liberation in the silent One also as well as the realisation of the dynamic One, and from that it is easier to arrive at the Truth in which both are one and inseparable. At the same time, the gulf created by mind between the Supreme and His manifestation is bridged, and there is no longer a fissure in the truth which makes all incomprehensible. If in the light of this you examine what your Guru taught, you will see that it is the same thing in less metaphysical language.

As for Adesh, people speak of Adesh without making the necessary distinctions, but these distinctions have to be made. The Divine speaks to us in many ways and it is not always the imperative Adesh that comes. When it does, it is clear and irresistible, the mind has to obey and there is no question possible, even if what comes is contrary to the preconceived ideas of the mental intelligence. It was such an Adesh that I had when I came away to Pondicherry. But more often what is said is an intimation or even less, a mere indication, which the mind may not follow because it is not impressed with its imperative necessity. It is something offered but not imposed, perhaps something not even offered but only suggested from the Truth above.

If Shankara's conception of the undifferentiated pure Consciousness as the Brahman is your view of it, then it is not the path of this yoga that you should choose; for here the realisation of pure Consciousness and Being is only a first step and not the goal. But an inner creative urge from within can have no place in an undifferentiated Consciousness — all action and creation must necessarily be foreign to it.

I do not base my yoga on the insufficient ground that the Self (not soul) is eternally free. That affirmation leads to nothing beyond itself, or, if used as a starting-point, it could equally well lead to the conclusion that action and creation have no significance or value. The question is not that but of the meaning of creation, whether there is a Supreme who is not merely a pure undifferentiated Consciousness and Being, but the source and support also of the dynamic energy of creation and whether the cosmic existence has for It a significance and a value. That is a question which cannot be settled by metaphysical logic which deals in words and ideas, but by a spiritual experience which goes beyond Mind and enters into spiritual realities. Each mind is satisfied with its own reasoning, but for spiritual purposes that satisfaction has no validity, except as an indication of how far and on what line each one is prepared to go in the field of spiritual experience. If your reasoning leads you towards the Shankara idea of the Supreme, that might be an indication that the Vedanta Adwaita (Mayavada) is your way of advance.

This yoga accepts the value of cosmic existence and holds it to be a reality; its object is to enter into a higher Truth-Consciousness or Divine supramental Consciousness in which action and creation are the expression not of ignorance and imperfection, but of the Truth, the Light, the Divine Ananda. But for that, surrender of the mortal mind, life and body to that Higher Consciousness is indispensable, since it is too difficult for the mortal human being to pass by its own effort beyond mind to a supramental Consciousness in which the dynamism is no longer mental but of quite another power. Only those who can accept the call to such a change should enter into this yoga.

I don't know that I can help you very much with an answer to your friend's questions. I can only state my own position with regard to these matters.

1. SHANKARA'S EXPLANATION OF THE UNIVERSE

It is rather difficult to say nowadays what really was Shankara's philosophy: there are numberless exponents and none of them agrees with any of the others. I have read accounts given by some scores of his exegetes and each followed his own line. We are even told by some that he was no Mayavadin at all, although he has always been famed as the greatest exponent of the theory of Maya, but rather, the greatest Realist in philosophical history. One eminent follower of Shankara even declared that my philosophy and Shankara's were identical, a statement which rather took my breath away. One used to think that Shankara's philosophy was this that the Supreme Reality is a spaceless and timeless Absolute (Parabrahman) which is beyond all feature or quality, beyond all action or creation, and that the world is a creation of Maya, not absolutely unreal, but real only in time and while one lives in time; once we get into a knowledge of the Reality, we perceive that Maya and the world and all in it have no abiding or true existence. It is, if not non-existent, yet false, *jaganmithyā*; it is a mistake of the consciousness, it is and it is not; it is an irrational and inexplicable mystery in its origin, though we can see its process or at least how it keeps itself imposed on the consciousness. Brahman is seen in Maya as Ishwara upholding the works of Maya and the apparently individual soul is really nothing but Brahman itself. In the end, however, all this seems to be a myth of Maya, *mithyā*, and not anything really true. If that is Shankara's philosophy, it is to me unacceptable and incredible, however brilliantly ingenious it may be and however boldly and incisively reasoned; it does not satisfy my reason and it does not agree with my experience.

I don't know exactly what is meant by this *yuktivāda*. If it is meant that it is merely for the sake of arguing down opponents, then this part of the philosophy has no fundamental validity; Shankara's theory destroys itself. Either he meant it as a sufficient explanation of the universe or he did not. If he did, it is no use dismissing it as Yuktivada. I can understand that thoroughgoing Mayavadin's declaration that the whole question is illegitimate, because Maya and the world do not really exist; in fact, the problem how the world came to existence is only a part of Maya, is like Maya unreal and does not truly arise; but if an explanation is to be given, it must be a real, valid and satisfying explanation. If there are two planes and in putting the question we are confusing the two planes, that argument can only be of value if both planes have some kind of existence and the reasoning and explanation are true in the lower plane but cease to have any meaning for a consciousness which has passed out of it.

2. ADWAITA

People are apt to speak of the Adwaita as if it were identical with Mayavada monism, just as they speak of Vedanta as if it were identical with Adwaita only; that is not the case. There are several forms of Indian philosophy which base themselves upon the One Reality, but they admit also the reality of the world, the reality of the Many, the reality of the differences of the Many as well as the sameness of the One (*bhedābheda*). But the Many exist in the One and by the One, the differences are variations in manifestation of that which is fundamentally ever the same. This we actually see as the universal law of existence where oneness is always the basis with an endless multiplicity and difference in the oneness; as, for instance, there is one mankind but many kinds of man, one thing called leaf or flower but many forms, patterns, colours of leaf and flower. Through this we can look back into one of the fundamental secrets of existence, the secret which is contained in the one Reality itself. The oneness of the Infinite is not something limited, fettered to its unity; it is capable of an infinite multiplicity. The Supreme Reality is an Absolute not limited by either oneness or multiplicity but simultaneously capable of both; for both are its aspects, although the oneness is fundamental and the multiplicity depends upon the oneness.

There is possible a realistic as well as an illusionist Adwaita. The philosophy of *The Life Divine* is such a realistic Adwaita. The world is a manifestation of the Real and therefore is itself real. The reality is the infinite and eternal Divine, infinite and eternal Being, Consciousness-Force and Bliss. This Divine by his power has created the world or rather manifested it in his own infinite Being. But here in the material world or at its basis he has hidden himself in what seem to be his opposites, Non-Being, Inconscience and Insentience. This is what we nowadays call the Inconscient which seems to have created the material universe by its inconscient Energy, but this is only an appearance, for we find in the end that all the dispositions of the world can only have been arranged by the working of a supreme secret Intelligence. The Being which is hidden in what seems to be an inconscient void emerges in the world first in Matter, then in Life, then in Mind and finally as the Spirit. The apparently inconscient Energy which creates is in fact the Consciousness-Force of the Divine and its aspect of consciousness, secret in Matter, begins to emerge in Life, finds something more of itself in Mind and finds its true self in a spiritual consciousness and finally a supramental Consciousness through which we become aware of the Reality, enter into it and unite ourselves with it. This is what we call evolution which is an evolution of Consciousness and an evolution of the Spirit in things and only outwardly an evolution of species. Thus also, the delight of existence emerges from the original insentience, first in the contrary forms of pleasure and pain, and then has to find itself in the bliss of the Spirit or, as it is called in the Upanishads, the bliss of the Brahman. That is the central idea in the explanation of the universe put forward in *The Life Divine*.

3. NIRGUNA AND SAGUNA

In a realistic Adwaita there is no need to regard the Saguna as a creation from the Nirguna or even secondary or subordinate to it: both are equal aspects of the one Reality, its position of silent status and rest and its position of action and dynamic force; a silence of eternal rest and peace supports an eternal action and movement. The one Reality, the Divine Being, is bound by neither, since it is in no way limited; it possesses both. There is no incompatibility between the two, as there is none between the Many and the One, the sameness and the difference. They are all eternal aspects of the universe which could not exist if either of them were eliminated, and it is reasonable to suppose that they both came from the Reality which has manifested the universe and are both real. We can only get rid of the apparent contradiction — which is not really a contradiction but only a natural concomitance — by treating one or the other as an illusion. But it is hardly reasonable to suppose that the eternal Reality allows the existence of an eternal illusion with which it has nothing to do or that it supports and enforces on being a vain cosmic illusion and has no power for any other and real action. The force of the Divine is always there in silence as in action, inactive in silence, active in the manifestation. It is hardly possible to suppose that the Divine Reality has no power or force or that its only power is to create a universal falsehood, a cosmic lie — *mithyā*.

COMPOUNDS AND DISINTEGRATION

No doubt, all compounds, being not integral things in themselves but integrations, can disintegrate. Also it is true of life, though not a physical compound, that it has a curve of birth or integration and, after it reaches a certain point, of disintegration, decay and death. But these ideas or this rule of existence cannot be safely applied to things in themselves. The soul is not a compound but an integer, a thing in itself; it does not disintegrate, but at most enters into manifestation and goes out of manifestation. That is true even of forms other than constructed physical or constructed life-forms; they do not disintegrate but appear and disappear or at most fade out of manifestation. Mind itself as opposed to particular thoughts is something essential and permanent; it is a power of the Divine Consciousness. So is life, as opposed to constructed living bodies; so I think is what we call material energy which is really the force of essential substance in motion, a power of the Spirit. Thoughts, lives, material objects are formations of these energies, constructed or simply manifested according to the habit of the play of the particular energy. As for the elements, what is the pure natural condition of an element? According to modern Science, what used to be called elements turn out to be compounds and the pure natural condition, if any, must be a condition of pure energy; it is that pure condition into which compounds including what we call elements must go when they pass by disintegration into Nirvana.

5. NIRVANA

What then is Nirvana? In orthodox Buddhism it does mean a disintegration, not of the soul — for that does not exist — but of a mental compound or stream of associations or *samskāras* which we mistake for ourself. In illusionist Vedanta it means, not a disintegration but a disappearance of a false and unreal individual self into the one real Self or Brahman; it is the idea and experience of individuality that so disappears and ceases, — we may say a false light that is extinguished (*nirvāṇa*) in the true Light. In spiritual experience it is sometimes the loss of all sense of individuality in a boundless cosmic consciousness; what was the individual remains only as a centre or a channel for the flow of a cosmic consciousness and a cosmic force and action. Or it may be the experience of the loss of individuality in a transcendent being and consciousness in which the sense of cosmos as well as the individual disappears. Or again, it may be in a transcendence which is aware of and supports the cosmic action. But what do we mean by the individual? What we usually call by that name is a natural ego, a device of Nature which holds together her action in the mind and body. This ego has to be extinguished, otherwise there is no complete liberation possible; but the individual self or soul is not this ego. The individual soul is the spiritual being which is sometimes described as an eternal portion of the Divine, but can also be described as the Divine himself supporting his manifestation as the Many. This is the true spiritual individual which appears in its complete truth when we get rid of the ego and our false separative sense of individuality, realise our oneness with the transcendent and cosmic Divine and with all beings. It is this which makes possible the Divine Life. Nirvana is a step towards it; the disappearance of the false separative individuality is a necessary condition for our realising and living in our true eternal being, living divinely in the Divine. But this we can do in the world and in life.

6. REBIRTH

If evolution is a truth and is not only a physical evolution of species, but an evolution of consciousness, it must be a spiritual and not only a physical fact. In that case, it is the individual who evolves and grows into a more and more developed and perfect consciousness and obviously that cannot be done in the course of a brief single human life. If there is the evolution of a conscious individual, then there must be rebirth. Rebirth is a logical necessity and a spiritual fact of which we can have the experience. Proofs of rebirth, sometimes of an overwhelmingly convincing nature, are not lacking, but as yet they have not been carefully registered and brought together.

7. EVOLUTION

In my explanation of the universe I have put forward this cardinal fact of a spiritual evolution as the meaning of our existence here. It is a series of ascents from the physical being and consciousness to the vital, the being dominated by the life-self, thence to the mental being realised in the fully developed man and thence into the perfect consciousness which is beyond the mental, into the supramental Consciousness and the supramental being, the Truth-Consciousness which is the integral consciousness of the spiritual being. Mind cannot be our last conscious expression because mind is fundamentally an ignorance seeking for knowledge; it is only the supramental Truth-Consciousness that can bring us the true and whole Self-Knowledge and world-Knowledge; it is through that only that we can get to our true being and the fulfilment of our spiritual evolution.

*
**

The sentence[1] is rather loose in expression. It does not mean that Maya is Brahman's freedom, but "the doctrine of Maya simply comes to this that Brahman is free from the circumstances through which He expresses Himself." This limited play is not He, for He is illimitable; it is only a conditioned (partial) manifestation, but He is not bound by the conditions (circumstances) as the play is bound. The world is a figure of something of Himself which He has put forth into it, but He is more than that figure. The world is not unreal or illusory, but our present seeing or consciousness of it is ignorant, and therefore the world *as seen by us* can be described as an illusion. So far the Maya idea is true. But if we see the world as it really is, a partial and developing manifestation of Brahman, then it can no longer be described as an illusion, but rather as a Lila. He is still more than His Lila, but He is in it and it is in Him; it is not an illusion.

About Nirvana:

When I wrote in the *Arya*,[2] I was setting forth an overmind view of things to the mind and putting it in mental terms, that was why I had sometimes to use logic. For in such a work — mediating between the intellect and the supra-intellectual — logic has a place, though it cannot have the chief place it occupies in purely mental philosophies. The Mayavadin himself labours to establish his point of view or his experience by a rigorous logical reasoning. Only, when it comes to an explanation of Maya, he, like the scientist dealing with Nature, can do no more than arrange and organise his ideas of the process of this universal mystification; he cannot explain how or why his illusionary mystifying Maya came into existence. He can only say, "Well, but it is there."

Of course, it is there. But the question is, first, what is it? Is it really an illusionary Power and nothing else, or is the Mayavadin's idea of it a mistaken first view, a mental imperfect

---

[1] "Maya means nothing more than the freedom of Brahman from the circumstances through which he expresses himself." Sri Aurobindo, *The Yoga and its Objects* (1968 Edition), p. 39.

[2] A philosophical journal conducted by Sri Aurobindo during the years 1914-21.

reading, even perhaps itself an illusion? And next, "Is illusion the sole or the highest Power which the Divine Consciousness or Superconsciousness possesses?" The Absolute is an absolute Truth free from Maya, otherwise liberation would not be possible. Has then the supreme and absolute Truth no other active Power than a power of falsehood and with it, no doubt, for the two go together, a power of dissolving or disowning the falsehood, — which is yet there for ever? I suggested that this sounded a little queer. But queer or not, if it is so, it is so — for, as you point out, the Ineffable cannot be subjected to the laws of logic. But who is to decide whether it is so? You will say, those who get there. But get where? To the Perfect and the Highest, *pūrṇam param*. Is the Mayavadin's featureless Brahman that Perfect, that Complete — is it the very Highest? Is there not or can there not be a higher than that highest, *parātparam*? That is not a question of logic, it is a question of spiritual fact, of a supreme and complete experience. The solution of the matter must rest not upon logic, but upon a growing, ever heightening, widening spiritual experience — an experience which must of course include or have passed through that of Nirvana and Maya, otherwise it would not be complete and would have no decisive value.

Now to reach Nirvana was the first radical result of my own yoga. It threw me suddenly into a condition above and without thought, unstained by any mental or vital movement; there was no ego, no real world — only when one looked through the immobile senses, something perceived or bore upon its sheer silence a world of empty forms, materialised shadows without true substance. There was no One or many even, only just absolutely That, featureless, relationless, sheer, indescribable, unthinkable, absolute, yet supremely real and solely real. This was no mental realisation nor something glimpsed somewhere above, — no abstraction, — it was positive, the only positive reality, — although not a spatial physical world, pervading, occupying or rather flooding and drowning this semblance of a physical world, leaving no room or space for any reality but itself, allowing nothing else to seem at all actual, positive or substantial. I cannot say there was anything exhilarating or rapturous in the experience, as it then came to me, — (the ineffable Ananda I had years afterwards), — but what it brought was an inexpressible Peace, a stupendous silence, an infinity of release and freedom. I lived in that Nirvana day and night before it began to admit other things into itself or modify itself at all, and the inner heart of experience, a constant memory of it and its power to return remained until in the end it began to disappear into a greater Superconsciousness from above. But meanwhile realisation added itself to realisation and fused itself with this original experience. At an early stage the aspect of an illusionary world gave place to one in which illusion[1] is only a small surface phenomenon with an immense Divine Reality behind it and a supreme Divine Reality above it and an intense Divine Reality in the heart of everything that had seemed at first only a cinematic shape or shadow. And this was no reimprisonment in the senses, no diminution or fall from supreme experience, it came rather as a constant heightening and widening of the Truth; it was the spirit that saw objects, not the senses, and the Peace, the Silence, the freedom in Infinity remained always, with the world or all worlds only as a continuous incident in the timeless eternity of the Divine.

Now, that is the whole trouble in my approach to Mayavada. Nirvana in my liberated consciousness turned out to be the beginning of my realisation, a first step towards the complete thing, not the sole true attainment possible or even a culminating finale. It came unasked, unsought for, though quite welcome. I had no least idea about it before, no aspiration towards it, in fact my aspiration was towards just the opposite, spiritual power to help the world and to do my work in it, yet it came — without even a "May I come in" or a "By your leave". It just happened and settled in as if for all eternity or as if it had been really there always. And then it slowly grew into something not less but greater than its first self. How then could I accept Mayavada or persuade myself to pit against the Truth imposed on me from above the logic of Shankara?

---

[1] In fact it is not an illusion in the sense of an imposition of something baseless and unreal on the consciousness, but a misinterpretation by the conscious mind and sense and a falsifying misuse of manifested existence.

But I do not insist on everybody passing through my experience or following the Truth that is its consequence. I have no objection to anybody accepting Mayavada as his soul's truth or his mind's truth or their way out of the cosmic difficulty. I object to it only if somebody tries to push it down my throat or the world's throat as the sole possible, satisfying and all-comprehensive explanation of things. For it is not that at all. There are many other possible explanations; it is not at all satisfactory, for in the end it explains nothing; and it is — and must be unless it departs from its own logic — all-exclusive, not in the least all-comprehensive. But that does not matter. A theory may be wrong or at least one-sided and imperfect and yet extremely practical and useful. This has been amply shown by the history of Science. In fact, a theory whether philosophical or scientific, is nothing else than a support for the mind, a practical device to help it to deal with its object, a staff to uphold it and make it walk more confidently and get along on its difficult journey. The very exclusiveness and one-sidedness of the Mayavada make it a strong staff or a forceful stimulus for a spiritual endeavour which means to be one-sided, radical and exclusive. It supports the effort of the Mind to get away from itself and from Life by a short cut into superconscience. Or rather it is the Purusha in Mind that wants to get away from the limitations of Mind and Life into the superconscient Infinite. Theoretically, the way for that is for the mind to deny all its perceptions and all the preoccupations of the vital and see and treat them as illusions. Practically, when the mind draws back from itself, it enters easily into a relationless peace in which nothing matters, — for in its absoluteness there are no mental or vital values, — and from which the mind can rapidly move towards that great short cut to the superconscient, mindless trance, *suṣupti*. In proportion to the thoroughness of that movement all the perceptions it had once accepted become unreal to it — illusion, Maya. It is on its road towards immergence.

Mayavada therefore with its sole stress on Nirvana, quite apart from its defects as a mental theory of things, serves a great spiritual end and, as a path, can lead very high and far. Even, if the Mind were the last word and there were nothing beyond it

except the pure Spirit, I would not be averse to accepting it as
the only way out. For what the mind with its perceptions and the
vital with its desires have made of life in this world, is a very
bad mess, and if there were nothing better to be hoped for, the
shortest cut to an exit would be the best. But my experience is
that there is something beyond Mind; Mind is not the last word
here of the Spirit. Mind is an ignorance-consciousness and its
perceptions cannot be anything else than either false, mixed
or imperfect — even when true, a partial reflection of the Truth
and not the very body of Truth herself. But there is a Truth-
Consciousness, not static only and self-introspective, but also
dynamic and creative, and I prefer to get at that and see what
it says about things and can do rather than take the short cut
away from things offered as its own end by the Ignorance.

Still, I would have no objection if your attraction towards
Nirvana were not merely a mood of the mind and vital but an
indication of the mind's true road and the soul's issue. But it
seems to me that it is only the vital recoiling from its own disappointed desires in an extreme dissatisfaction, not the soul
leaping gladly to its true path. This Vairagya is itself a vital
movement; vital Vairagya is the reverse side of vital desire —
though the mind of course is there to give reasons and say ditto.
Even this Vairagya, if it is one-pointed and exclusive, can lead or
point towards Nirvana. But you have many sides to your personality or rather many personalities in you; it is indeed their discordant movements each getting in the way of the other, as
happens when they are expressed through the external mind, that
have stood much in the way of your sadhana. There is the vital
personality which was turned towards success and enjoyment and
got it and wanted to go on with it but could not get the rest of the
being to follow. There is the vital personality that wanted enjoyment of a deeper kind and suggested to the other that it could
very well give up these unsatisfactory things if it got an equivalent
in some faeryland of a higher joy. There is the psycho-vital personality that is the Vaishnava within you and wanted the Divine
Krishna and bhakti and Ananda. There is the personality which
is the poet and musician and a seeker of beauty through these
things. There is the mental-vital personality which, when it saw

the vital standing in the way, insisted on a grim struggle of Tapasya, and it is no doubt that also which approves Vairagya and Nirvana. There is the physical-mental personality which is the Russellite, extrovert, doubter. There is another mental-emotional personality all whose ideas are for belief in the Divine, yoga, bhakti, Guruvada. There is the psychic being also which has pushed you into the sadhana and is waiting for its hour of emergence.

What are you going to do with all these people? If you want Nirvana, you have either to expel them or stifle them or beat them into coma. All authorities assure us that the exclusive Nirvana business is a most difficult job (*duḥkham dehavadbhiḥ*, says the Gita), and your own attempt at suppressing the others was not encouraging, — according to your own account it left you as dry and desperate as a sucked orange, no juice left anywhere. If the desert is your way to the promised land, that does not matter. But — well, if it is not, then there is another way — it is what we call the integration, the harmonisation of the being. That cannot be done from outside, it cannot be done by the mind and vital being — they are sure to bungle their affair. It can be done only from within by the soul, the Spirit which is the centraliser, itself the centre of these radii. In all of them there is a truth that can harmonise with the true truth of the others. For there is a truth in Nirvana — Nirvana is nothing but the peace and freedom of the Spirit which can exist in itself, be there world or no world, world-order or world-disorder. Bhakti and the heart's call for the Divine have a truth — it is the truth of the divine Love and Ananda. The will for Tapasya has in it a truth — it is the truth of the Spirit's mastery over its members. The musician and poet stand for a truth, it is the truth of the expression of the Spirit through beauty. There is a truth behind the mental affirmer; even there is a truth behind the mental doubter, the Russellian, though far behind him — the truth of the denial of false forms. Even behind the two vital personalities there is a truth, the truth of the possession of the inner and outer worlds not by the ego but by the Divine. That is the harmonisation for which our yoga stands — but it cannot be achieved by any outward arrangement, it can only be achieved by going inside and looking, willing and acting from the psychic and from the spiritual centre. For the truth of the being is there and the secret of Harmony also is there.

One may be aware of the essential static self without relation to the play of the cosmos. Again one may be aware of the universal static self omnipresent in everything without being progressively awake to the movement of the dynamic *viśva-prakṛti*. The first realisation of the Self or Brahman is often a realisation of something that separates itself from all form, name, action, movement, exists in itself only, regarding the cosmos as only a mass of cinematographic shapes unsubstantial and empty of reality. That was my own first complete realisation of the Nirvana in the Self. That does not mean a wall between Self and Brahman, but a scission between the essential self-existence and the manifested world.

I believe according to the Adwaitins God is only the reflection of Brahman in Maya — just as Brahman is seen outwardly as the world which has only a practical not a real reality, so subjectively Brahman is seen as God, Bhagavan, Ishwara, and that also would be a practical not a real reality — which is and can be only the relationless Brahman all by itself in a worldless eternity. At least that is what I have read — I don't know whether Shankara himself says that. One is always being told by modern Adwaitins that Shankara did not mean what people say he meant — so one has to be careful in attributing any opinion to him.

They want to show that Shankara was not so savagely illusionist as he is represented — that he gave a certain temporary reality to the world, admitted Shakti etc. But these (supposing he made them) are concessions inconsistent with the logic of his own philosophy which is that only the Brahman exists and the rest is ignorance and illusion. The rest has only a temporary and therefore an illusory reality in Maya. He further maintained that Brahman could not be reached by works. If that was not his philosophy, I should like to know what was his philosophy. At any rate that was how his philosophy has been understood by people. Now that the general turn is away from the rigorous Illusionism, many of the Adwaitins seem to want to hedge and make Shankara hedge with them.

Vivekananda accepted Shankara's philosophy with modifications, the chief of them being Daridra-Narayan-Seva which is a mixture of Buddhist compassion and modern philanthropy.

Of course Shankara must have meant Mayavada. It is hardly possible that everybody should have misunderstood his ideas (which were not in the least veiled or enigmatic) till his modern apologists discovered what they really were.

Shankara surely stands or falls by the Mayavada. Even the *Bhaja-Govindam* poem is Mayavadic in spirit. I am not well-acquainted with these other writings — so it is difficult for me to say anything about that side of the question.

Chittashuddhi belongs to Rajayoga. In the pure Adwaita the method is rather to detach oneself by *vicāra* and *viveka* and realise "I am not the mind, not the life, etc. etc." In that case, no *śuddhi* would be necessary — the self would separate from the nature good or bad and regard it as a machinery which having no more the support of the *ātman* would fall away of itself along with the body. Of course *cittaśuddhi* can be resorted to also, but for cessation of the *cittavṛtti*, not for their better dynamism as an instrument of the Divine. Shankara insists that all karma must fall off before one can be liberated — the soul must realise itself as *akartā*, there is no solution in or by works in the pure Yoga of

Knowledge. So how could Shankara recognise dynamism? Even if he recognises *cittaśuddhi* as necessary, it must be as a preparation for getting rid of karma, not for anything else.

The essential "I" sense disappears when there is the stable realisation of the one universal Self in all and that remains at all moments in all conditions under any circumstances. Usually this comes first in the Purusha consciousness and the extension to the Prakriti movements is not immediate. But even if there are "I" movements in the Prakriti reactions, the Purusha within observes them as the continued running of an old mechanism and does not feel them as his own. Most Vedantists stop there, because they do think that those reactions will fall away from one at death and all will disappear into the One. But for a change of the nature it is necessary that the experience and seeing of the Purusha should spread to all the parts, mind, vital, physical, subconscient. Then the ego movements of Prakriti can also disappear gradually from one field after another till none is left. For this a perfect *samatā* even in the cells of the body and in every vibration of the being is necessary — *samam hi brahma*. One is then quite free from it in works also. The individual remains but that is not the small separative ego, but a form and power of the Universal which feels itself one with all beings, an acting centre and instrument of the Universal Transcendent, full of the Ananda of the presence and the action but not thinking or moving independently or acting for its own sake. That cannot be called egoism. The Divine can be called an ego only if he is a separate Person limited as in the Christian idea of God by his separateness (though even there esoteric Christianity abolishes the limitation). An I which is not separate in that way is no I at all.

I doubt whether the condition of which you speak is that of the realised Vedantin — except of course the loss of the sense of personality and the non-identification with desire and the movements of Prakriti. Still perhaps the condition of the *jaḍavat* Paramahamsa (like Jada Bharata) may resemble it. That theory of *prārabdha karma* goes farther than that — it assumes that even if there are vital movements, that is also only the continuance of the machine of Prakriti and will drop off at death. They may, perhaps. I don't base the gospel of the transformation of Nature on an impossibility of taking a static release as final — the static release is necessary, but I don't consider that to take it as final is the object of coming into world-existence. I hold that the static release is only a beginning, a first step in the Divine. If anyone is satisfied with the first step as all that is possible for him, I have no objection to his taking it like that.

Your objection is correct. The snake-rope image cannot be used to illustrate the non-existence of the world, it would only mean that our seeing of the world is not that of the world as it really is. The idea of complete illusion would better be illustrated by the juggler's rope-climbing trick where there is no rope and no climber, and yet one is persuaded that they are there.

The illusionist metaphors all fail when you drive them home — they are themselves an illusion. Identification with the body is an error, not an illusion. We are not the body, but the body is still something of ourselves. With realisation the erroneous identification ceases — in certain experiences the existence of the body is not felt at all. In the full realisation the body is within us, not we in it, it is an instrumental formation in our wider being, — our consciousness exceeds but also pervades it, — it can be dissolved without our ceasing to be the self. That is about all.

It is the Vedantic Adwaita experience of *laya*. It is only one phase of the experience, not the whole or the highest Truth of the Divine.

The impulse towards *laya* is a creation of the mind, it is not the sole possible destiny of the soul. When the mind tries to abolish its own Ignorance, it finds no escape from it except by *laya*, because it supposes that there is no higher principle of cosmic existence beyond itself — beyond itself is only the pure Spirit, the absolute impersonal Divine. Those who go through the heart (love, bhakti) do not accept *laya*, they believe in a state beyond of eternal companionship with the Divine or dwelling in the Divine without *laya*. All this quite apart from supramentalisation. What then becomes of your starting-point that *laya* is the inevitable destiny of the soul and it is only the personal descent of the Avatar that saves it from inevitable *laya*!

There were two points of error. (1) That the soul formerly had no other possibility once it reached the Divine than *laya*. There were other possibilities, e.g., passing into a higher plane, living in the Divine or in the presence of the Divine. Both imply the refusal of birth and leaving the Lila on earth. (2) That it was only for the sake of living with the incarnate Divine and by reason of this descent that the soul consented to give up *laya*. The capital point is the supramentalisation of the being which is the Divine intention in the evolution on earth and cannot fail to come; the descent or incarnation is only an instrumentation for bringing that about. Your statement therefore becomes wrong by incompleteness.

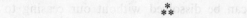

But they [the Mayavadic Vedantins] had no clear perception of these things [overmind, supermind, etc.] because they lived at the highest in the spiritualised higher mind, and for the rest could only receive things from even the overmind — they could not enter it except by deep samadhi (*suṣupti*). Prajna and Ishwara were for them Lord of the *suṣupti*.

II

In our yoga the Nirvana is the beginning of the higher Truth, as it is the passage from the Ignorance to the higher Truth. The Ignorance has to be extinguished in order that the Truth may manifest.

I don't think I have written, but I said once that souls which have passed into Nirvana may (not "must") return to complete the larger upward curve. I have written somewhere, I think, that for this yoga (it might also be added, in the natural complete order of the manifestation) the experience of Nirvana can only be a stage or passage to the complete realisation. I have said also that there are many doors by which one can pass into the realisation of the Absolute (Parabrahman), and Nirvana is one of them, but by no means the only one. You may remember Ramakrishna's saying that the Jivakoti can ascend the stairs, but not return, while the Ishwarakoti can ascend and descend at will. If that is so, the Jivakoti might be those who describe only the curve from Matter through Mind into the silent Brahman and the Ishwara-koti those who get to the integral Reality and can therefore combine the Ascent with the Descent and contain the "two ends" of existence in their single being.

The realisation of this yoga is not lower but higher than Nirvana or Nirvikalpa Samadhi.

If Buddha really combated and denied all Vedantic conceptions of the Self, then it can be no longer true that Buddha refrained from all metaphysical speculations or distinct pronouncements as to the nature of the ultimate Reality. The view you take of his conception of Nirvana seems to concur with the Mahayanist interpretation and its conception of the Permanent, *dhruvam*, which could be objected to as a later development like the opposite Nihilistic conception of the Shunyam. What Buddha very certainly taught was that the world is not-Self and that the individual has no true existence since what does exist in the world is a stream of impermanent consciousness from moment to moment and the individual person is fictitiously constituted by a bundle of *saṁskāras* and can be dissolved by dissolving the bundle. This is in conformity with the Vedantic Monistic view that there is no true separate individual. As to the other Vedantic view of the one Self, impersonal and universal and transcendent, it does not seem that Buddha made any distinct and unmistakable pronouncement on abstract and metaphysical questions; but if the world or all in the world is not-Self, *anātman*, there can be no more room for a universal Self, only at most for a transcendent Real Being. His conception of Nirvana was of something transcendent of the universe, but he did not define what it was because he was not concerned with any abstract metaphysical speculations about the Reality; he must have thought them unnecessary and irrelevant and any indulgence in them likely to divert from the true object. His explanation of things was psychological and not metaphysical and his methods were all psychological, — the breaking up of the false associations of consciousness which cause the continuance of desire and suffering, so getting rid of the stream of birth and death in a purely phenomenal (not unreal) world; the method of life by which this liberation could be effected was also a psychological method, the eightfold path developing right understanding and right action. His object was pragmatic and severely practical and so were his methods; metaphysical speculations would only draw the mind away from the one thing needful.

As to Buddha's attitude towards life, I do not quite see how "service to mankind" or any ideal of improvement of the world-existence can have been part of his aim, since to pass out of life into a transcendence was his object. His eightfold path was the means towards that end and not an aim in itself or indeed in any way an aim. Obviously, if right understanding and right action become the common rule of life, there would be a great improvement in the world, but for Buddha's purpose that could be an incidental result and not at all part of his central object. You say, "Buddha himself urged the necessity to serve mankind; his ideal was to achieve a consciousness of inner eternity and then be a source of radiant influence and action." But where and when did Buddha say these things, use these terms or express these ideas? "The service of mankind" sounds like a very modern and European conception; it reminds me of some European interpretations of the Gita as merely teaching the disinterested performance of duty or the pronouncement that the whole idea of the Gita is service. The exclusive stress or overstress on mankind or humanity is also European. Mahayanist Buddhism laid stress on compassion, fellow-feeling with all, *vasudhaiva kuṭumbakam*, just as the Gita speaks of the feeling of oneness with all beings and preoccupation with the good of all beings, *sarvabhūta hite ratāḥ*, but this does not mean humanity only, but all beings and *vasudhā* means all earth-life. Are there any sayings of Buddha which would justify the statement that the object or one object in attaining to Nirvana was to become a source of radiant influence and action? The consciousness of inner eternity may have that result, but can we really say that that was Buddha's ideal, the object which he held in view or for which he came?

There is no reason why the passage about Buddhism should be omitted. It gives one side of the Buddhistic teaching which is not much known or is usually ignored, for that teaching is by most rendered as Nirvana (Sunyavada) and a spiritual humanitarianism. The difficulty is that it is these sides that have been stressed especially in the modern interpretations of Buddhism and any strictures I may have passed were in view of these interpretations and that one-sided stress. I am aware of course of opposite tendencies in the Mahayana and the Japanese cult of Amitabha Buddha which is a cult of bhakti. It is now being said even of

Shankara that there was another side of his doctrine — but his followers have made him stand solely for the Great Illusion, the inferiority of bhakti, the uselessness of Karma — *jagan mithyā*.

Buddha, it must be remembered, refused always to discuss what was beyond the world. But from the little he said it would appear that he was aware of a Permanent beyond equivalent to the Vedantic Para-Brahman, but which he was quite unwilling to describe. The denial of anything beyond the world except a negative state of Nirvana was a later teaching, not Buddha's.

The Buddhist Nirvana and the Adwaitin's Moksha are the same thing. It corresponds to a realisation in which one does not feel oneself any longer as an individual with such a name or such a form, but an infinite eternal Self spaceless (even when in space), timeless (even when in time). Note that one can perfectly well do actions in that condition and it is not to be gained only by Samadhi.

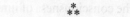

It [Nirvana of Buddha] is the same [as Brahma Nirvana of the Gita]. Only the Gita describes it as Nirvana in the Brahman while Buddha preferred not to give any name or say anything about that into which the Nirvana took place. Some later schools of Buddhists described it as Shunya, the equivalent of the Chinese Tao, described as the Nothing which is everything.

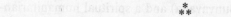

Buddhism is of many kinds and the entirely nihilistic kind is only one variety. Most Buddhism admits a Permanent as beyond the realm of Karma and Sanskaras. Even the Shunya of the Shunya-panthis is described like the Tao of Lao Tse as a Nothing which is All. So as a higher 'above mental' state is admitted which one tries to reach by a strong discipline of the consciousness, it may be called spirituality.

About the One [of the Buddhists] there are different versions. I just read somewhere that the Buddhist One is a Superbuddha from whom all Buddhas come — but it seemed to me a rehash of Buddhism in Vedantic terms born of a modern mind. The Permanent of Buddhism has always been supposed to be Supracosmic and Ineffable — that is why Buddha never tried to explain what it was; for, logically, how can one talk about the Ineffable? It has really nothing to do with the Cosmos which is a thing of Sanskaras and Karma.

The impressions in the approach to Infinity or the entry into it are not always quite the same; much depends on the way in which the mind approaches it. It is felt first by some as an infinity above, by others as an infinity around into which the mind disappears (as an energy) by losing its limits. Some feel not the absorption of the mind-energy into the infinite, but a falling entirely inactive; others feel it as a lapse or disappearance of energy into pure Existence. Some first feel the infinity as a vast existence into which all sinks or disappears, others, as you describe it, as an infinite ocean of Light above, others as an infinite ocean of Power above. If certain schools of Buddhists felt it in their experience as a limitless Shunya, the Vedantists, on the contrary, see it as a positive Self-Existence featureless and absolute. No doubt, the various experiences were erected into various philosophies, each putting its conception as definitive; but behind each conception there was such an experience. What you describe as a completely emptied mind-substance devoid of energy or light, completely inert, is the condition of neutral peace and empty stillness which is or can be a stage of the liberation. But it can afterwards feel itself filled with infinite existence, consciousness (carrying energy in it) and finally Ananda.

The passage[1] in *The Yoga and its Objects* is written from the point of view of the spiritualised mind approaching the supreme Truth directly, without passing through the supermind or disappearing into it. The mind spiritualises itself by shedding all its own activities and formations and reducing everything to a pure Existence, *sad-ātman*, from which all things and activities proceed and which supports everything. When it wants to go still beyond, it negates yet further and arrives at an *asat*, which is the negation of all this existence and yet something inconceivable to mind, speech or defining experience. It is the silent Unknowable, the Turiya or featureless and relationless Absolute of the monistic Vedantins, the Shunyam of the nihilistic Buddhists, the Tao or omnipresent and transcendent Nihil of the Chinese, the indefinable and ineffable Permanent of the Mahayana. Many Christian mystics also speak of the necessity of a complete ignorance in order to get the supreme experience and speak too of the divine Darkness — they mean the shedding of all mental knowledge, making a blank of the mind and engulfing it in the Unmanifest, the *param avyaktam*. All this is the mind's way of approaching the Supreme — for beyond the *avyaktam, tamasaḥ parastāt*, is the Supreme, the Purushottama of the Gita, the Para Purusha of the Upanishads. It is *ādityavarṇa* in contrast to the darkness of the Unmanifest; it is a metaphor, but not a mere metaphor, for it is a symbol also, a symbol visually seen by the *sūkṣma dṛṣṭi*, the subtle vision, and not merely a symbol, but, as one might say, a fact of spiritual experience. The sun in the yoga is the symbol of the supermind and the supermind is the first power of the Supreme which one meets across the border where the experience of spiritualised mind ceases and the unmodified divine Consciousness begins the domain of the supreme Nature, *parā prakṛti*. It is that Light of which the Vedic mystics got a glimpse and it is the opposite of the intervening darkness of the Christian mystics, for the supermind is all light and no darkness. To the mind the Supreme is *avyaktāt param avyaktam* but if we follow the line leading to the supermind, it is an increasing affirmation rather

----

[1] "For behind the *sad ātman* is the silence of the *asat* which the Buddhist Nihilists realised as the *śūnyam* and beyond that silence is the *parātpara puruṣa* (*puruṣo vareṇya ādityavarṇas tamasaḥ parastāt*)." Sri Aurobindo, *The Yoga and its Objects* (1968 Edition), pp. 12-13.

than an increasing negation through which we move.

Light is always seen in yoga with the inner eye, even with the outer eye, but there are many lights; all are not and all do not come from the supreme Light, *param jyotiḥ*.

The universe is only a partial manifestation and Brahman as its foundation is the Sat. But there is also that which is not manifested and beyond manifestation and is not contained in the basis of manifestation. The Buddhists and others got from that the conception of Asat as the ultimate thing.

Another meaning given is — Sat=the Eternal, Asat=the Temporary and Unreal.

The feeling of the Self as a vast peaceful Void, a liberation from existence as we know it, is one that one can always have, Buddhist or no Buddhist. It is the negative aspect of Nirvana — it is quite natural for the mind, if it follows the negative movement of withdrawal, to get that first, and if you lay hold on that and refuse to go farther, being satisfied with this liberated Non-Existence, then you will naturally philosophise like the Buddhists that Shunya is the eternal truth. Lao Tse is more perspicacious when he spoke of it as the Nothing that is All. Many of course have the positive experience of the Atman first, not as a void but as pure unrelated Existence like the Adwaitins (Shankara) or as the one Existent.

They [those who have the experience of Nirvana] do not feel as if they had any existence at all. In the Buddhistic Nirvana they feel as if there were no such thing at all, only an infinite zero without form. In the Adwaita Nirvana there is felt only one Vast Existence, no separate being is discernible anywhere. There are forms of course but they are only forms, not separate beings. Mind is silent, thought has ceased, — desires, passions, vital movements there are none. There is consciousness but only a formless elemental consciousness without limits. The body moves and acts, but the sense of the body is not there. Sometimes there is only the consciousness of pure existence, sometimes only pure consciousness, sometimes all that exists is only a ceaseless limitless Ananda. Whether all else is really dissolved or only covered up is a debatable point, but at any rate it is an experience as if of their dissolution.

The ego and its continuity, they [the Buddhists] say, are an illusion, the result of the continuous flowing of energies and ideas in a determined current. There is no real formation of an ego. As to the liberation, it is in order to get free from *duḥkha* etc., — it is a painful flow of energies and to get free from the pain they must break up their continuity. That is all right, but how it started, why it should end at all and how anybody is benefited by the liberation, since there is nobody there, only a mass of idea and action — these things are insoluble mysteries. But is there not the same difficulty with the Mayavadin also, since there is no Jiva really, only Brahman and Brahman is by nature free and unbound for ever? So how did the whole absurd affair of Maya come into existence and who is liberated? That is what the old sages said at last, "There is none bound, none freed, none seeking to be free". It was all a mistake (a rather long-standing one though). The Buddhists, I suppose, could say that also.

According to both Buddha and Shankara liberation means *laya* of the individual in some transcendent Permanence that is not individualised — so logically a belief in the individual soul must prevent liberation while the sense of misery in the world leads to the attempt to escape.

*
**

The phrase "to pass on"[1] shows that what is meant by them is an evolution not on earth but somewhere beyond, God knows where. In that case Nirvana would be a place or world on the way to other worlds and the soul evolves from one world to another — e.g. from earth to Nirvana and from Nirvana to some Beyond-Nirvana. This is an entirely European idea and it is most unlikely that it was held by the Buddhists. The Indian idea was that the evolution is here and even the Gods if they want to go beyond their godhead and get liberation have to come down on earth for the purpose. It is the Western spiritualists and others who think that the birth on earth is a stage of progress from some place inferior to earth and after once being born on earth one does not return but goes to some other world and remains there till one can progress to some other better world and so on and on.... Again, this "perfected social order on earth" is certainly not a Buddhist idea, the Buddhas never dreamed of it — their preoccupation was with helping men towards Nirvana, not towards a perfected order here. All that is a sheer contradiction of Buddhism.

Nirvana cannot be at once the ending of the Path with nothing beyond to explore and yet only a rest house or rather the beginning of the Higher Path with everything still to explore.... The reconciliation would be that it is the end of the lower Path through the lower Nature and the beginning of the Higher Evolution. In that case it would accord exactly with the teaching of our yoga.

How is this Absolute[2] different from the Absolute of the Vedanta? or this emancipation different from the Vedantic

---

[1] "The Great Ones... renounce their right to pass on to a still Higher Evolution and remain within the Cosmos for the good of all sentient beings.... It is these Bodhic Forces... which lead mankind...towards a perfected social order on Earth." *Tibetan Yoga and Secret Doctrines* by Dr. W. Y. Evans-Wentz.

[2] "Thus the Doctrine of Shunyata underlying the whole of the Prajna-Paramita, posits ... an Absolute as inherent in phenomena, for the Absolute is the source and support of the phenomena... and in the last analysis of things by the Bodhi-illuminated mind, freed of

Mukti? If it were so, there would never have been all this quarrel between Buddhism and the Vedantic schools. It must be a new-fangled version of Buddhism or else it was a later development in which Buddhism reduced itself back to Adwaita.

But, is this Higher Evolution really a Buddhistic idea or only a European version of what Nirvana might be?

There is no difference between such a description[1] and what is meant by soul, except that it is called "impersonal" — but evidently here impersonal is used as opposed to the thing dependent on name, body and form, what is called personality. Europeans especially, but also people without philosophic ideas would easily mistake this outward personality for the soul and then they would deny the name of soul to the unborn and endless entity. Do they then consider it as spirit or self — *ātman*? But the difficulty is that the old Buddhists rejected the conception of *ātman* also. So we are left entirely at sea. The Nihilistic Buddhistic teaching is plain and comprehensible that there is no soul, only a bundle of Sanskaras continuing or a stream of them renewing themselves without dissolution (Nirvana). But this Mahayanist affair seems a sort of loose and curt compromise with Vedanta.

There are elements in most yogas which enter into this one, so it is not surprising if there is something in Buddhism also. But such notions as a Higher Evolution beyond Nirvana seem to me not genuinely Buddhistic, unless of course there is some offshoot of Buddhism which developed something so interpreted by the

---

Ignorance, duality vanishes and there remains but the One in All, the All in One." *Ibid.*

[1] "An impersonal principle, this microcosmic representation of the macrocosmic persists throughout all existences, or states of conditioned being within the Sangsara.... But the impersonal consciousness principle is not to be in any way identified with the personality represented by a name, or bodily form or a Sangsaric mind... it is itself non-Sangsaric, being uncreated, unborn, unshaped, beyond human concept or definition, and therefore transcending time and space ... it is beginningless and endless." *Ibid.*

author. I never heard of it as part of Buddha's teachings — he always spoke of Nirvana as the goal and refused to discuss metaphysically what it might be.

*
**

The Jain philosophy is concerned with individual perfection. Our effort is quite different. We want to bring down the supermind as a new faculty. Just as the mind is now a permanent state of consciousness in humanity, so also we want to create a race in which the supermind will be a permanent state of consciousness.

III

It is not a fact that the Gita gives the whole base of Sri Aurobindo's message; for the Gita seems to admit the cessation of birth in the world as the ultimate aim or at least the ultimate culmination of yoga; it does not bring forward the idea of spiritual evolution or the idea of the higher planes and the supramental Truth-Consciousness and the bringing down of that consciousness as the means of the complete transformation of earthly life.

The idea of the supermind, the Truth-Consciousness is there in the Rig Veda according to Sri Aurobindo's interpretation and in one or two passages of the Upanishads, but in the Upanishads it is there only in seed in the conception of the being of knowledge, *vijñānamaya puruṣa*, exceeding the mental, vital and physical being; in the Rig Veda the idea is there but in principle only, it is not developed and even the principle of it has disappeared from the Hindu tradition.

It is these things among others that constitute the novelty of Sri Aurobindo's message as compared with the Hindu tradition — the idea that the world is not either a creation of Maya or only a play, *līlā*, of the Divine, or a cycle of births in the ignorance from which we have to escape, but a field of manifestation in which there is a progressive evolution of the soul and the nature in Matter and from Matter through Life and Mind to what is beyond Mind till it reaches the complete revelation of Sachchidananda in life. It is this that is the basis of the yoga and gives a new sense to life.

There is no real contradiction; the two passages[1] indicate in the Gita's system two different movements of its yoga, the complete surrender being the crowning movement. One has first to conquer the lower nature, deliver the self involved in the lower movement by means of the higher Self which rises into the divine nature; at the same time one offers all one's actions including the inner action of the yoga as a sacrifice to the Purushottama, the transcendent and immanent Divine. When one has risen into the higher Self, has the knowledge and is free, one makes the complete surrender to the Divine, abandoning all other dharmas, living only by the divine Consciousness, the divine Will and Force, the divine Ananda.

Our yoga is not identical with the yoga of the Gita although it contains all that is essential in the Gita's yoga. In our yoga we begin with the idea, the will, the aspiration of the complete surrender; but at the same time we have to reject the lower nature, deliver our consciousness from it, deliver the self involved in the lower nature by the self rising to freedom in the higher nature. If we do not do this double movement, we are in danger of making a tamasic and therefore unreal surrender, making no effort, no tapas and therefore no progress; or else we may make a rajasic surrender not to the Divine but to some self-made false idea or image of the Divine which masks our rajasic ego or something still worse.

This world is, as the Gita describes it, *anityamasukham*, so long as we live in the present world-consciousness; it is only by turn-

---

[1] "Deliver the self by means of the Self" (*Gita*, Ch. VI, 5); and "Abandon all dharmas" (*Ibid.*, Ch. XVIII, 66).

ing from that to the Divine and entering into the Divine Consciousness that one can possess, through the world also, the Eternal.

The language of the Gita in many matters seems sometimes contradictory because it admits two apparently opposite truths and tries to reconcile them. It admits the ideal of departure from *saṁsāra* into the Brahman as one possibility; also it affirms the possibility of living free in the Divine (in Me, it says) and acting in the world as the Jivanmukta. It is this latter kind of solution on which it lays the greatest emphasis. So Ramakrishna put the "divine souls" (Ishwarakoti) who can descend the ladder as well as ascend it higher than the Jivas (Jivakoti) who, once having ascended, have not the strength to descend again for divine work. The full truth is in the supramental consciousness and the power to work from there on life and Matter.

The Gita cannot be described as exclusively a gospel of love. What it sets forth is a yoga of knowledge, devotion and works based on a spiritual consciousness and realisation of oneness with the Divine and of the oneness of all beings in the Divine. Bhakti, devotion and love of God carrying with it unity with all beings and love for all beings is given a high place but always in connection with knowledge and works.

But note that the Gita was *not* meant by the writer to be an allegory — you can say, if you like, that now we should dismiss the ancient war element by interpreting it as if it were an allegory. The Gita is yoga, spiritual truth applied to the external life and action — but it may be *any* action and not necessarily an action *resembling* that of the Gita. The *principle* of the spiritual consciousness applied to action has to be kept — the particular example used by the Gita may be treated as a thing belonging to a past world.

The Gita does not speak expressly of the Divine Mother; it speaks always of surrender to the Purushottama — it mentions her only as the Para Prakriti who becomes the Jiva, that is, who manifests the Divine in the multiplicity and through whom all these worlds are created by the Supreme and he himself descends as the Avatar. The Gita follows the Vedantic tradition which leans entirely on the Ishwara aspect of the Divine and speaks little of the Divine Mother because its object is to draw back from world-nature and arrive at the supreme realisation beyond it; the Tantric tradition leans on the Shakti or Ishwari aspect and makes all depend on the Divine Mother because its object is to possess and dominate the world-nature and arrive at the supreme realisation through it. This yoga insists on both the aspects; the surrender to the Divine Mother is essential, for without it there is no fulfilment of the object of the yoga.

In regard to the Purushottama the Divine Mother is the supreme divine Consciousness and Power above the worlds, Adya Shakti; she carries the Supreme in herself and manifests the Divine in the worlds through the Akshara and Kshara. In regard to the Akshara she is the same Para Shakti holding the Purusha immobile in herself and also herself immobile in him at the back of all creation. In regard to the Kshara she is the mobile cosmic Energy manifesting all beings and forces.

*
**

I do not know that there is anything like a Purushottama consciousness which the human being can attain or realise *for himself*; for, in the Gita, the Purushottama is the Supreme Lord, the Supreme Being who is beyond the Immutable and the Mutable and contains both the One and the Many. Man, says the Gita, can attain the Brahmic consciousness, realise himself as an eternal portion of the Purushottama and live in the Purushottama. The Purushottama consciousness is the consciousness of the Supreme Being and man by loss of ego and realisation of his true essence can *live in* it.

In the spiritual thought of India during the time of the Rishis and even before, the Sankhya and Vedanta elements were always combined. The Sankhya account of the constitution of the being, (Purusha, Prakriti, the elements, Indriyas, Buddhi, etc.) was universally accepted and Kapila was mentioned with veneration everywhere. In the Gita he is mentioned among the great Vibhutis; Krishna says, "I am Kapila among the sages."

IV

Veda and Vedanta are one side of the One Truth; Tantra with its emphasis on Shakti is another; in this yoga all sides of the Truth are taken up, not in the systematic forms given them formerly but in their essence, and carried to the fullest and highest significance. But Vedanta deals more with the principles and essentials of the divine knowledge and therefore much of its spiritual knowledge and experience has been taken bodily into the *Arya*. Tantra deals more with forms and processes and organised powers — all these could not be taken as they were, for the integral yoga needs to develop its own forms and processes; but the ascent of the consciousness through the centres and other Tantric knowledge are there behind the process of transformation to which so much importance is given by me — also the truth that nothing can be done except through the force of the Mother.

The process of the Kundalini awakened rising through the centres as also the purification of the centres is a Tantric knowledge. In our yoga there is no willed process of the purification and opening of the centres, no raising up of the Kundalini by a set process either. Another method is used, but still there is the ascent of the consciousness from and through the different levels to join the higher consciousness above; there is the opening of

the centres and of the planes (mental, vital, physical) which
these centres command; there is also the descent which is the
main key of the spiritual transformation. Therefore, there is,
I have said, a Tantric knowledge behind the process of transformation in this yoga.

In our yoga there is no willed opening of the chakras, they open
of themselves by the descent of the Force. In the Tantric discipline they open from down upwards, the Muladhar first; in our
yoga, they open from up downward. But the ascent of the force
from the Muladhar does take place.

In the Tantra the centres are opened and Kundalini is awakened
by a special process, its action of ascent is felt through the spine.
Here it is a pressure of the Force from above that awakens it and
opens the centres. There is an ascension of the consciousness
going up till it joins the higher consciousness above. This
repeats itself (sometimes a descent also is felt) until all the centres
are open and the consciousness rises above the body. At a later
stage it remains above and widens out into the cosmic consciousness and the universal self. This is a usual course, but sometimes the process is more rapid and there is a sudden and
definite opening above.

The ascension and descent of the Force in this yoga accomplishes
itself in its own way without any necessary reproduction of the
details laid down in the Tantric books. Many become conscious
of the centres, but others simply feel the ascent or descent in a
general way or from level to level rather than from centre to
centre, that is, they feel the Force descending first to the head,
then to the heart, then to the navel and still below. It is not at
all necessary to become aware of the deities in the centres

according to the Tantric description, but some feel the Mother in the different centres. In these things our sadhana does not cleave to the knowledge given in the books, but only keeps to the central truth behind and realises it independently without any subjection to the old forms and symbols. The centres themselves have a different interpretation here from that given in the books of the Tantriks.

Yes, the object of our yoga is to establish direct contact with the Divine above and bring down the divine Consciousness from above into all the centres. Occult powers belonging to the mental, vital and subtle physical planes are not our object. One can have contact with various Divine Forces and Personalities on the way, but there is no need to establish them in the centres, though sometimes that happens automatically (as with the four Personalities of the Mother) for a time in the course of the sadhana. But it is not a rule to do so. Our yoga is meant to be plastic and to allow all necessary workings of the Divine Power according to the nature, but these in their details may vary with each individual.

Occultism is the knowledge and right use of the hidden forces of Nature.

Occult forces are the forces that can only be known by going behind the veil of apparent phenomena — especially the forces of the subtle physical and supraphysical planes.

Ordinarily, all the more inward and all the abnormal psychological experiences are called psychic. I use the word psychic for the soul as distinguished from the mind and vital. All movements and experiences of the soul would in that sense be called psychic, those which rise from or directly touch the psychic being; where mind and vital predominate, the experience would be called psychological (surface or occult). "Spiritual" has not a necessary connection with the Absolute. Of course the experience of the Absolute is spiritual. All contacts with self, the higher consciousness, the Divine above are spiritual. There are others that could not be so sharply classified or one set off against another.

The spiritual realisation is of primary importance and indispensable. I would consider it best to have the spiritual and psychic development first and have it with the same fullness before entering the occult regions. Those who enter the latter first may find their spiritual realisation much delayed — others fall into the mazy traps of the occult and do not come out in this life. Some no doubt can carry on both together, the occult and the spiritual, and make them help each other; but the process I suggest is the safer.

The governing factors for us must be the spirit and the psychic being united with the Divine — the occult laws and phenomena have to be known but only as an instrumentation, not as the governing principles. The occult is a vast field and complicated and not without its dangers. It need not be abandoned but it should not be given the first place.

An activity of the astral plane in contact with the astral forces attended by a leaving of the body is not a spiritual aim but belongs to the province of occultism. It is not a part of the aim of yoga. Also fasting is not permissible in the Ashram, as its practice is more often harmful than helpful to the spiritual endeavour.

This aim suggested to you seems to be part of a seeking for occult powers; such a seeking is looked on with disfavour for the most part by spiritual teachers in India, because it belongs to the inferior planes and usually pushes the seeker on a path which may lead him very far from the Divine. Especially, a contact with the forces and beings of the astral (or, as we term it, the vital) plane is attended with great dangers. The beings of this plane are often hostile to the true aim of spiritual life and establish contact with the seeker and offer him powers and occult experiences only in order that they may lead him away from the spiritual path or else that they may establish their own control over him or take possession of him for their own purpose. Often representing themselves as divine powers, they mislead, give erring suggestions and impulsions and pervert the inner life. Many are those who, attracted by these powers and beings of the vital plane, have ended in a definitive spiritual fall or in mental and physical perversion and disorder. One comes inevitably into contact with the vital plane and enters into it in the expansion of consciousness which results from an inner opening, but one ought never to put oneself into the hands of these beings and forces or allow oneself to be led by their suggestions and impulsions. This is one of the chief dangers of the spiritual life and to be on one's guard against it is a necessity for the seeker if he wishes to arrive at his goal. It is true that many supraphysical or supernormal powers come with the expansion of the consciousness in yoga; to rise out of the body consciousness, to act by subtle means on the supraphysical planes, etc. are natural activities for the yogi. But these powers are not sought after, they come naturally, and they have not the astral character. Also, they have to be used on purely spiritual lines, that is by the Divine Will and the Divine Force, as an instrument, but never as an instrumentation of the forces and beings of the vital plane. To seek their aid for such powers is a great error.

Prolonged fasting may lead to an excitation of the nervous being which often brings vivid imaginations and hallucinations that are taken for true experiences; such fasting is frequently suggested by the vital Entities, because it puts the consciousness into an unbalanced state which favours their designs. It is therefore discouraged here. The rule to be followed is that laid down by the Gita which says that "Yoga is not for one who eats too much or who does not eat" — a moderate use of food sufficient for the maintenance of health and strength of the body.

There is no brotherhood of the kind you describe in India. There are yogis who seek to acquire and practise occult powers but it is as individuals learning from an individual Master. Occult associations, lodges, brotherhoods for such a purpose as described by European occultists are not known in Asia.

As regards secrecy, a certain discretion or silence about the instructions of the Guru and one's own experiences is always advisable, but an absolute secrecy or making a mystery of these things is not. Once a Guru is chosen, nothing must be concealed from him. The suggestion of absolute secrecy is often a trick of the astral powers to prevent the seeking for enlightenment and succour.

All these "experiments" of yours are founded upon the vital nature and the mind in connection with it; working on this foundation, there is no security against falsehood and fundamental error. No amount of powers (small or great) developing can be a surety against wandering from the Truth; and, if you allow pride and arrogance and ostentation of power to creep in and hold you, you will surely fall into error and into the power of rajasic Maya and Avidya. Our object is not to get powers, but to ascend towards the divine Truth-Consciousness and bring its Truth down into the lower members. With the Truth all the necessary powers will come, not as one's own, but as the Divine's. The contact with the Truth cannot grow through rajasic mental and vital self-assertion, but only through psychic purity and surrender.

The *aṣṭasiddhis* as obtained in the ordinary yoga are vital powers or, as in the Rajayoga, mental siddhis. Usually they are uncertain in their application and precarious depending on the maintenance of the process by which they were attained.

The physical Nature does not mean the body alone but the phrase includes the transformation of the whole physical mind, vital, material nature — not by imposing siddhis on them, but by creating a new physical nature which is to be the habitation of the supramental being in a new evolution. I am not aware that this has been done by any Hathayogic or other process. Mental or vital occult power can only bring siddhis of the higher plane into the individual life — like the Sannyasi who could take any poison without harm, but he died of a poison after all when he forgot to observe the conditions of the siddhi. The working of the supramental power envisaged is not an influence on the physical giving it abnormal faculties but an entrance and permeation changing it wholly into a supramentalised physical. I did not learn the idea from Veda or Upanishad, and I do not know if there is anything of the kind there. What I received about the supermind was a direct, not a derived knowledge given to me; it was only afterwards that I found certain confirmatory revelations in the Upanishad and Veda.

There are many yogins of the Vedantic school who follow both siddhis and the final emancipation — they would say, I suppose, that they take the siddhis on the way to Nirvana. The harmonisation is in the supermind — the Divine Truth at once static and dynamic, a withdrawal and extinction of the Ignorance, a recreation in the Divine Knowledge.

I have not myself read the *Yoga-Vāsiṣṭha*, but from what I have read about it, it must be a book written by somebody with a remarkable occult knowledge.

V

It seems to me that these differences of valuation come from the mind laying stress on one side or another of the approach to the Divine or exalting one aspect of realisation over another. When there is the approach through the heart, through Love and Bhakti, the highest culmination is in a transcendent Ananda, an unspeakable Bliss or Beatitude of union with the Divine through Love. The school of Chaitanya laid especial

and indeed sole emphasis on this way and made this the whole
reality of Krishna consciousness. But the transcendent Ananda
is there at the origin and end of all existence and this is not and
cannot be the sole way to it. One can arrive at it through the
Vasudeva consciousness, which is a wider, more mentalised
approach — as in the method of the Gita where knowledge,
works, bhakti are all centred in Krishna, the One, the Supreme,
the All, and arrive through the cosmic consciousness to the luminous transcendence. There is the way too described in the
Taittiriya Upanishad, the Vedanta's Gospel of Bliss. These are
certainly wider methods, for they take up the whole existence
through all its parts and ways of being to the Divine. If less intense at their starting-point, a vaster and slower movement, there
is no reason to suppose that they are less intense on their summits
of arrival. It is the same transcendence to which all arrive,
either with a large movement gathering up everything spiritual
in us to take it there in a vast sublimation, or in a single intense
uplifting from one part, a single exaltation leaving all the rest
aside. But who shall say which is profounder of the two? Concentrated love has a profundity of its own which cannot be
measured; concentrated wisdom has a wider profundity, but
one cannot say that it is deeper.

Cosmic values are only reflections of the truth of the
Transcendence in a lesser truth of time experience which is
separative and sees diversely a thousand aspects of the One.
As one rises through the mind or any part of the manifested
being, any one or more of these aspects can become more and
more sublimated and tend towards its supreme transcendental
intensity, and whatever aspect is so experienced is declared by
the spiritualised mental consciousness to be the supreme thing.
But when one goes beyond mind, all tends not only to sublimate
but to fuse together until the separated aspects recover their
original unity, indivisible in the absoluteness of all made one.
Mind can conceive and have experience of existence without
consciousness or Ananda and this receives its utmost expression
in the inconscience attributed to Matter. So also it can conceive of Ananda or Love as a separate principle; it even feels
consciousness and existence losing themselves in a trance or

swoon of Love or Ananda. So, too, the limited personal loses itself in the illimitable Person, the lover in the supreme Beloved, or else the personal in the Impersonal — the lover feels himself immersed, losing himself in the transcendental reality of Love and Ananda. The personal and the impersonal are themselves posited and experienced by mind as separate realities and one or other is declared and seen as supreme, so that the personal can have *laya* in the Impersonal or, on the contrary, the impersonal disappears into the absolute reality of the supreme and divine Person — the impersonal in that view is only an attribute or power of the personal Divine. But at the summit of spiritual experience passing beyond mind one begins to feel the fusion of all these things into one. Consciousness, Existence, Ananda return to their indivisible unity, Sachchidananda. The personal and the impersonal become irrevocably one, so that to posit one as against the other appears as an act of ignorance. This tendency of unification is the basis of the supramental consciousness and experience; for cosmic or creative purposes the supermind can put forward one aspect prominently where that is needed but it is aware of all the rest behind it or contained in it and does not admit into its view any separation or opposition anywhere. For that reason a supramental creation would be a manifold harmony, not a separative process fragmenting or analysing the One into parts and setting these parts over against each other or else putting them contradictorily against each other and having afterwards to synthetise and piece them together in order to arrive at harmony or else to exclude one or all of the parts in order to realise the indivisible One.

You speak of the Vaishnava school emphasising the personal felicities, as in the classification of the Bhavas, and you say that these are short and quick feelings and lack in vastness or amplitude. No doubt, when they are first felt and as they are felt by the limited consciousness in its ordinary functioning and movement; but that is only because the emotional in man with this imperfect bodily instrument acts largely by spasms of intensity when it wants to sublimate and cannot maintain either the continuity or the extension or the sublimated paroxysm of these

things. But as the individual becomes cosmic (the universalising
of the individual without his losing his higher individuality as
a divine centre is one of the processes which leads towards the
supramental Truth), this disability begins to disappear. The
truth behind the *dāsya* or *madhura* or any other Bhava or fusion
of Bhavas becomes a vast and ample continuous state, — if,
by chance, they lose something of their briefer intensities by this
extension of themselves, they recover them a thousandfold in
the movement of the universalised individual towards the
Transcendence. There is an ever-enlarging experience which
takes up the elements of spiritual realisation, and in this uplifting
and transforming process they become other and greater things
than they were and more and more they take their place by
sublimation, first in the spiritual cosmic, then in the all-embracing
transcendent whole.

The difference of view between Shankara and Ramanuja
and on the other side Chaitanya about Krishna arises from
the turn of their experience. Krishna was only an aspect of
Vishnu to the others because that ecstatic form of love and
bhakti which had become associated with Krishna was not for
them the whole. The Gita, like Chaitanya, but from a different
viewpoint, regarded Krishna as the Divine himself. To Chaitanya he was Love and Ananda, and Love and Ananda being
for him the highest transcendental experience, so Krishna too
must be the Supreme. For the writer of the Gita, Krishna was
the source of Knowledge and Power as well as Love, the Destroyer, Preserver, Creator in one, so necessarily Vishnu was only
an aspect of this universal Divine. In the Mahabharata indeed
Krishna comes as an incarnation of Vishnu, but that can be
turned by taking it that it was through the Vishnu aspect as
his frontal appearance that he manifested; for that the greater
Godhead can manifest later than others is logical if we consider
the manifestation as progressive, — just as Vishnu is in the
Veda a younger Indra, Upendra, but gains upon his elder and
subsequently takes place above him in the Trimurti.

I cannot say much about the Vaishnava idea of the form
of Krishna. Form is the basic means of manifestation and
without it it may be said that the manifestation of anything is

not complete. Even if the Formless logically precedes Form, yet it is not illogical to assume that in the Formless, Form is inherent and already existent in a mystic latency, otherwise how could it be manifested? For, any other process would be the creation of the non-existent, not manifestation. If so, it would be equally logical to assume that there is an eternal form of Krishna, a spirit body. As for the highest Reality it is no doubt Absolute Existence, but is it only that? Absolute Existence as an abstraction may exclude everything else from itself and amount to a sort of very positive zero; but Absolute Existence as a reality who shall define and say what is or is not in its inconceivable depths, its illimitable Mystery? Mind can ordinarily conceive of the Absolute Existence only as a negation of its own concepts spatial, temporal or other. But it cannot tell what is at the basis of manifestation or what manifestation is or why there is any manifestation at all out of its positive zero — and the Vaishnavas, we must remember, do not admit this conception as the absolute and original truth of the Divine. It is therefore not rigidly impossible that what we conceive and perceive as spatial form may correspond to some power of the spaceless Absolute. I do not say all that as a definite statement of Truth, I am only pointing out that the Vaishnava position on its own ground is far from being logically or metaphysically untenable.

The Vaishnavites accept the world as a Lila, but the true Lila is elsewhere in the eternal Brindavan. All the religions which believe in the personal Godhead accept the universe as a reality, a Lila or a creation made by the Will of God, but temporal and not eternal. The aim is the eternal status above.

The idea of a temporary kingdom of heaven on earth is contained in the Puranas and conceived by some Vaishnava saints or poets; but it is a devotional idea, no philosophical base is given for the expectation. I think the Tantric overcoming of imperfections is an individual achievement, not collective.

You describe the rich human egoistic life you might have lived and you say "not altogether a wretched life, you will admit." On paper it sounds even very glowing and satisfactory, as you describe it. But there is no real or final satisfaction in it, except for those who are too common or trivial to seek anything else, and even they are not really satisfied or happy, — and in the end, it tires and palls. Sorrow and illness, clash and strife, disappointment, disillusionment and all kinds of human suffering come and beat its glow to pieces — and then decay and death. That is the vital egoistic life as man has found it throughout the ages, and yet it is that which this part of your vital regrets. How do you fail to see, when you lay so much stress on the desirability of a merely human consciousness, that suffering is its badge? When the vital resists the change from the human into the divine consciousness, what it is defending is its right to sorrow and suffering and all the rest of it, varied and relieved no doubt by some vital or mental pleasures and satisfactions, but very partially relieved by them and only for a time. In your own case, it was already beginning to pall on you and that was why you turned from it. No doubt, there were the joys of the intellect and of artistic creation, but a man cannot be an artist alone; there is the outer, quite human, lower vital part and, in all but a few, it is the most clamorous and insistent part. But what was dissatisfied in you? It was the soul within, first of all, and through it the higher mind and the higher vital. Why then find fault with the Divine for misleading you when it turned to the yoga or brought you here? It was simply answering to the demand of your own inner being and the higher parts of your nature. If you have so much difficulty and become restless, it is because you are still divided and something in your lower vital still regrets what it has lost or, as a price for its adhesion or a compensation — a price to be immeditely paid down to it — asks for something similar and equivalent in the spiritual life. It refuses to believe that there is a greater compensation, a larger vital life waiting for it, something positive in which there shall not be the old inadequacy and unrest and final dissatisfaction. The foolishness is not in the divine guidance, but in the irrational and obstinate resistance of this confused and obscure part of you to the demand, made not only by this yoga, but by all yoga — to the necessary conditions for the satisfaction of the aspiration of your own soul and higher nature.

The "human" vital consciousness has moved always between these two poles, the ordinary vital life which cannot satisfy and the recoil from it to the ascetic solution. India has gone fully through that seesaw, Europe is beginning once more after a full trial to feel the failure of the mere vital egoistic life. The traditional yogas — to which you appeal — are founded upon the movement between these two poles. On one side are Shankara and Buddha and most go, if not by the same road, yet in that direction; on the other are Vaishnava or Tantric lines which try to combine asceticism with some sublimation of the vital impulse. And where did these lines end? They fell back to the other pole, to a vital invasion, even corruption˙and a loss of their spirit. At the present day the general movement is towards an attempt at reconciliation, and you have alluded sometimes to some of the protagonists of this attempt and asked me my opinion about them, yours being unfavourable. But these men are not mere charlatans, and if there is anything wrong with them (on which I do not pronounce), it can only be because they are unable to resist the magnetic pull of this lower pole of the egoistic vital desire-nature. And if they are unable to resist, it is because they have not found the true force which will not only neutralise that pull and prevent deterioration and downward lapse, but transform and utilise and satisfy in their own deeper truth, instead of destroying or throwing away, the life-force and the embodiment in Matter; for, that can only be done by the supermind power and by no other.

You appeal to the Vaishnava-Tantric traditions; to Chaitanya, Ramprasad, Ramakrishna. I know something about them and, if I did not try to repeat them, it is because I do not find in them the solution, the reconciliation I am seeking. Your

quotation from Ramprasad does not assist me in the least
— and it does not support your thesis either. Ramprasad is not
speaking of an embodied, but of a bodiless and invisible Divine
— or visible only in a subtle form to the inner experience. When
he speaks of maintaining his claim or case against the Mother
until she lifts him into her lap, he is not speaking of any outer
vital or physical contact, but of an inner psychic experience;
precisely, he is protesting against her keeping him in the external
vital and physical nature and insists on her taking him on the
psycho-spiritual plane into spiritual union with her.

All that is very good and very beautiful, but it is not enough:
the union has indeed to be realised in the inner psycho-spiritual
experience first, because without that nothing sound or lasting
can be done; but also there must be a realisation of the Divine
in the outer consciousness and life, in the vital and physical
planes on their own essential lines. It is that which, without
your mind understanding it or how it is to be done, you are asking
for, and I too; only I see the necessity of a vital transformation,
while you seem to think and to demand that it should be done
without any radical transformation, leaving the vital as it is.
In the beginning, before I discovered the secret of the supermind, I myself tried to seek the reconciliation through an association of the spiritual consciousness with the vital, but my
experience and all experience show that this leads to nothing
definite and final, — it ends where it began, midway between
the two poles of human nature. An association is not enough,
a transformation is indispensable.

The tradition of later Vaishnava Bhakti is an attempt to sublimate the vital impulses through love by turning human love
towards the Divine. It made a strong and intense effort and
had many rich and beautiful experiences; but its weakness was
just there, that it remained valid only as an inner experience
turned towards the inner Divine, but it stopped at that point.
Chaitanya's *prema* was nothing but a psychic divine love with
a strong sublimated vital manifestation. But the moment
Vaishnavism before or after him made an attempt at greater
externalisation, we know what happened — a vitalistic deterioration, much corruption and decline. You cannot appeal to

Chaitanya's example as against psychic or divine love; his was not something merely vital-human; in its essence, though not in its form, it was very much the first step in the transformation, which we ask of the sadhaks, to make their love psychic and use the vital not for its own sake, but as an expression of the soul's realisation. It is the first step and perhaps for some it may be sufficient, for we are not asking everybody to become supramental; but for any full manifestation on the physical plane the supramental is indispensable.

In the later Vaishnava tradition the sadhana takes the form of an application of human vital love in all its principal turns to the Divine; *viraha*, *abhimāna*, even complete separation (like the departure of Krishna to Mathura) are made prominent elements of this yoga. But all that was only meant — in the sadhana itself, not in the Vaishnava poems — as a passage of which the end is *milana* or complete union; but the stress laid on the untoward elements by some would almost seem to make strife, separation, *abhimāna*, the whole means, if not the very object of this kind of *prema-yoga*. Again, this method was only applied to the inner, not to a physically embodied Divine and had a reference to certain states and reactions of the inner consciousness in its seeking after the Divine. In the relations with the embodied Divine Manifestation, or, I may add, of the disciple with the Guru, such things might rise as a result of human imperfection, but they were not made part of the theory of the relations. I do not think they formed a regular and authorised part of the relations of the bhaktas to the Guru. On the contrary, the relation of the disciple to the Guru in the Guruvada is supposed always to be that of worship, respect, a complete happy confidence, an unquestioning acceptance of the guidance. The application of the unchanged vital relations to the embodied Divine may lead and has led to movements which are not conducive to the progress of the yoga.

Ramakrishna's yoga was also turned only to an inner realisation of the inner Divine, — nothing less, but also nothing more. I believe Ramakrishna's sentence about the claim of the sadhak on the Divine for whom he has sacrificed everything was the assertion of an inner and not an outer claim, on the inner rather than on any physically embodied Divine: it was a claim for the full spiritual union, the God-lover seeking the Divine, but the Divine also giving himself and meeting the God-lover. There can be no objection to that; such a claim all seekers of the Divine have; but as to the modalities of this divine meeting, it does not carry us much farther. In any case, my object is a realisation on the physical plane and I cannot consent merely to repeat Ramakrishna. I seem to remember too that for a long time he was withdrawn into himself, all his life was not spent with his disciples. He got his siddhi first in retirement and when he came out and received everyone, well, a few years of it wore out his body. To that, I suppose, he had no objection; for he even pronounced a theory, when Keshav Chandra was dying, that spiritual experience ought to wear out the body. But at the same time, when asked why he got illness in the throat, he answered that it was the sins of his disciples which they threw upon him and he had to swallow. Not being satisfied, as he was, with an inner liberation alone, I cannot accept these ideas or these results, for that does not sound to me like a successful meeting of the Divine and the sadhak on the physical plane, however successful it might have been for the inner life. Krishna did great things and was very clearly a manifestation of the Divine. But I remember a passage of the Mahabharata in which he complains of the unquiet life his followers and adorers gave him, their constant demands, reproaches, their throwing of their unregenerate vital nature upon him. And in the Gita he speaks of this human world as a transient and sorrowful affair and, in spite of his gospel of divine action, seems almost to admit that to leave it is after all the best solution. The traditions of the past are very great in their own place, in the past, but I do not see why we should merely repeat them and not go farther. In the spiritual development of the consciousness upon earth the great past ought to be followed by a greater future.

There is the rub that you seem all to ignore entirely — the difficulties of the physical embodiment and the divine realisation on the physical plane. For most it seems to be a simple alternative, either the Divine comes down in full power and the thing is done, no difficulty, no necessary condition, no law or process, only miracle and magic, or else, well, this cannot be the Divine. Again you all (or almost all) insist on the Divine becoming human, remaining in the human consciousness and you protest against any attempt to make the human Divine. On the other hand, there is an outcry of disappointment, bewilderment, distrust, perhaps indignation if there are human difficulties, if there is strain in the body, a swaying struggle with adverse forces, obstacles, checks, illness and some begin to say, "Oh, there is nothing Divine here!" — as if one could remain vitally and physically in the untransformed individual human consciousness, in unchanged contact with it, satisfy its demands, and yet be immune under all circumstances and in all conditions against strain and struggle and illness. If I want to divinise the human consciousness, to bring down the supramental, the Truth-Consciousness, the Light, the Force into the physical to transform it, to create there a great fullness of Truth and Light and Power and Bliss and Love, the response is repulsion or fear or unwillingness — or a doubt whether it is possible. On one side there is the claim that illness and the rest should be impossible, on the other a violent rejection of the only condition under which these things can become impossible. I know that this is the natural inconsistency of the human vital mind wanting two inconsistent and incompatible things together; but that is one reason why it is necessary to transform the human and put something a little more luminous in its place.

But is the Divine then something so terrible, horrible or repellent that the idea of its entry into the physical, its divinising of the human should create this shrinking, refusal, revolt or fear? I can understand that the unregenerate vital attached to its own petty sufferings and pleasures, to the brief ignorant drama of life, should shrink from what will change it. But why should a God-lover, a God-seeker, a sadhak fear the divinisation of the consciousness? Why should he object to become one in nature with what he seeks, why should he recoil from *sādṛśya-mukti*? Behind this fear there are usually two causes: first, there is the feeling of the vital that it will have to cease to be obscure, crude, muddy, egoistic, unrefined (spiritually), full of stimulating desires and small pleasures and interesting sufferings (for it shrinks even from the Ananda which will replace this); next there is some vague ignorant idea of the mind, due, I suppose, to the ascetic tradition, that the divine nature is something cold, bare, empty, austere, aloof, without the glorious riches of the egoistic human vital life. As if there were not a divine vital and as if that divine vital is not itself and, when it gets the means to manifest, will not make the life on earth also infinitely more full of beauty, love, radiance, warmth, fire, intensity and divine passion and capacity for bliss than the present impotent, suffering, pettily and transiently excited and soon tired vitality of the still so imperfect human creation.

But you will say that it is not the Divine from which you recoil, rather you accept and ask for it (provided that it is not too divine), but what you object to is the supramental — grand, aloof, incomprehensible, unapproachable, a sort of austere Nirakar Brahman. The supramental so described is a bogey created by this part of your vital mind in order to frighten itself and justify its attitude. Behind this strange description there seems to be an idea that the supramental is a new version of the Vedantic featureless and incommunicable Parabrahman, vast, grand, cold, empty, remote, devastating, overwhelming; it is not quite that, of course, since it can come down, but for all practical purposes it is just as bad! It is curious that you admit your ignorance of what the supramental can be, and yet you in these moods not only pronounce categorically what it is like, but reject emphatically my experience about it as of no practical validity or not valid for anybody but myself! I have not insisted, I have answered only casually because I am not asking you now to be non-human and divine, much less to be supramental; but as you are always returning to this point when you have these attacks and making it the pivot — or at least a main support — of your depression, I am obliged to answer. The supramental is *not* grand, aloof, cold and austere; it is not something opposed to or inconsistent with a full vital and physical manifestation; on the contrary, it carries in it the only possibility of the full fullness of the vital force and the physical life on earth. It is because it is so, because it was so revealed to me and for no other reason that I have followed after it and persevered till I came into contact with it and was able to draw down some power of it and its influence. I am concerned with the earth, not with worlds beyond for their own sake; it is a terrestrial realisation that I seek and not a flight to distant summits. All other yogas regard this life as an illusion or a passing phase; the supramental yoga alone regards it as a thing created by the Divine for a progressive manifestation and takes the fulfilment of the life and the body for its object. The supramental is simply the Truth-Consciousness and what it brings in its descent is the full truth of life, the full truth of consciousness in Matter. One has indeed to rise to high summits to reach it, but the more one rises, the more one can bring down below. No doubt, life and body have not to remain the ignorant, imperfect, impotent things they are now; but why should a change to fuller life-power, fuller body-power be considered something aloof, cold and undesirable? The utmost Ananda the body and life are now capable of is a brief excitement of the vital mind or the nerves or the cells which is limited, imperfect and soon passes: with the supramental change all the cells, nerves, vital forces, embodied mental forces can become filled with a thousandfold Ananda, capable of an intensity of bliss which passes description and which need not fade away. How aloof, repellent and undesirable! The supramental love means an intense unity of soul with soul, mind with mind, life with life, and an entire flooding of the body consciousness with the physical experience of oneness, the presence of the Beloved in every part, in every cell of the body. Is that too something aloof and grand but undesirable? With the supramental change, the very thing on which you insist, the possibility of the free physical meeting of the embodied Divine with the sadhak without conflict of forces and without undesirable reactions becomes possible, assured and free. That too is, I suppose, something aloof and undesirable? I could go on — for pages, but this is enough for the moment.

The supramental is something in which the basis is absolute calm and however intense a Divine Love there is in it, it does not disturb the calm but increases its depth. Chaitanya's expe-

rience was not that of supermind, but of Love and Ananda
brought from above into the vital — the response of the vital is
an extreme passion and exultation of Godward love and Ananda
the result of which are these *vikāras*. Chaitanya claimed this
supremacy for the Radha experience because Ananda is higher
than the experiences of the spiritual mind, Ananda being, according to the Upanishads, the supreme plane of experience. But
this is a logical conclusion which cannot be accepted wholly —
one must pass through the supermind to arrive to the highest
Ananda, and in the supermind there is an unification and harmonisation of all the divine Powers (Knowledge etc. as well as Love
and Ananda). Different sadhaks emphasise one aspect or other
as the highest, but it is this union of all that must be the true basis
of the highest realisation and experience.

It is not necessary to repeat past forms [of Bhakti Yoga] — to
bring out the Bhakti of the psychic being and give it whatever
forms come naturally in the development is the proper way for
our sadhana.

It is not I only who have done what the Vedic Rishis did not
do. Chaitanya and others developed an intensity of Bhakti which
is absent in the Veda and many other instances can be given.
Why should the past be the limit of spiritual experience?

Well, I don't suppose the new race can be created by or according to logic or that any race has been. But why should the
idea of the creation of a new race be illogical?... As for the past
seers, they don't trouble me. If going beyond the experiences of
past seers and sages is so shocking, each new seer or sage in turn
has done that shocking thing — Buddha, Shankara, Chaitanya,
etc. all did that wicked act. If not, what was the necessity of
their starting new philosophies, religions, schools of yoga? If

they were merely verifying and meekly repeating the lives and experiences of past seers and sages without bringing the world some new thing, why all that stir and pother? Of course, you may say, they were simply explaining the old truth but in the right way — but this would mean that nobody had explained or understood it rightly before — which is again "giving the lie etc." Or you may say that all the new sages (they were not among X's cherished past ones in their day), e.g., Shankara, Ramanuja, Madhva were each merely repeating the same blessed thing as all the past seers and sages had repeated with an unwearied monotony before them. Well, well, but why repeat it in such a way that each "gives the lie" to the others? Truly, this shocked reverence for the past is a wonderful and fearful thing! After all, the Divine is infinite and the unrolling of the Truth may be an infinite process or at least, if not quite so much, yet with some room for new discovery and new statement, even perhaps new achievement, not a thing in a nutshell cracked and its contents exhausted once for all by the first seer or sage, while the others must religiously crack the same nutshell all over again, each tremblingly fearful not to give the lie to the "past" seers and sages.

Sri Krishna never set out to arrive at any physical transformation, so anything of the kind could not be expected in his case.

Neither Buddha nor Shankara nor Ramakrishna had any idea of transforming the body. Their aim was spiritual mukti and nothing else. Krishna taught Arjuna to be liberated in works, but he never spoke of any physical transformation.

I do not know that we can take this [Yudhisthira entering the heavenly kingdom in the Himalayas with his mortal body] as a historical fact. *Svarga* is not somewhere in the Himalayas, it is another world in another plane of consciousness and substance. Whatever the story may mean, therefore, it has nothing to do with the question of physical transformation on earth.

Ramakrishna himself never thought of transformation or tried
for it. All he wanted was bhakti for the Mother and along with
that he received whatever knowledge she gave him and did whatever she made him do. He was intuitive and psychic from the
beginning and only became more and more so as he went on.
There was no need in him for the transformation which we seek;
for although he spoke of the divine man (Ishwarakoti) coming
down the stairs as well as ascending, he had not the idea of a
new consciousness and a new race and the divine manifestation
in the earth-nature.

Whatever may have happened to Chaitanya or Ramalingam,
whatever physical transformation they may have gone through
is quite irrelevant to the aim of the supramentalisation of the
body. Their new body was either a non-physical or subtle
physical body not adapted for life on the earth. If it were not so,
they would not have disappeared. The object of supramentalisation is a body fitted to embody and express the physical consciousness on earth so long as one remains in the physical life.
It is a step in the spiritual evolution on the earth, not a step in
the passage towards a supraphysical world. The supramentalisation is the most difficult part of the change arrived at by the
supramental yoga, and all depends on whether a sufficient
change can be achieved in the consciousness at present to make
such a step possible, but the nature of the step is different from
that aimed at by other yogas. There is not therefore much utility
in these discussions — one has first of all to supramentalise
sufficiently the mind and vital and physical consciousness
generally — afterwards one can think of supramentalisation of
the body. The psychic and spiritual transformation must come
first, only afterwards would it be practical or useful to discuss
the supramentalisation of the whole being down to the body.

By divine realisation is meant the spiritual realisation — the
realisation of Self, Bhagwan or Brahman on the mental-spiritual

plane or else the overmental plane. That is a thing (at any rate the mental-spiritual) which thousands have done. So it is obviously easier to do than the supramental. Also nobody can have the supramental realisation who has not had the spiritual. ... It is true that neither can be got in an effective way unless the whole being is turned towards it — unless there is a real and very serious spirit and dynamic reality of sadhana... It is true that I want the supramental not for myself but for the earth and souls born on the earth, and certainly therefore I cannot object if anybody wants the supramental. But there are the conditions. He must.want the divine Will first and the soul's surrender and spiritual realisation (through works, bhakti, knowledge, self-perfection) on the way...

The central sincerity is the first thing and sufficient for an aspiration to be entertained — a total sincerity is needed for the aspiration to be fulfilled...

There are different statuses (*avasthā*) of the Divine Consciousness. There are also different statuses of transformation. First is the psychic transformation, in which all is in contact with the Divine through the individual psychic consciousness. Next is the spiritual transformation in which all is merged in the Divine in the cosmic consciousness. Third is the supramental transformation in which all becomes supramentalised in the divine gnostic consciousness. It is only with the last that there can begin the *complete* transformation of mind, life and body — in my sense of completeness.

You are mistaken in two respects. First, the endeavour towards this achievement is not new and some yogis have achieved it, I believe — but not in the way I want it. They achieved it as a personal siddhi maintained by yoga-siddhi — not a dharma of the nature. Secondly, the supramental transformation is not the same as the spiritual-mental. It is a change of mind, life and body which the mental or overmental-spiritual cannot achieve. All whom you mention were spirituals, but in different ways. Krishna's mind for instance was overmentalised, Ramakrishna's intuitive, Chaitanya's spiritual-psychic, Buddha's illumined higher mental. I don't know about B.G. — he seems to have been brilliant but rather chaotic. All that is different from the supramental. Then take the vital of the Paramhansas. It is said that their vital behaves either like a child (Ramakrishna) or like a madman or like a demon or like something inert (cf. Jadabharata). Well, there is nothing supramental in all that.

One can be a fit instrument of the Divine in any of the transformations. The question is, an instrument for what?

The Paramhansa is a particular grade of realisation, there are others supposed to be lower or higher. I have no objection to them in their own place. But I must remind you that in my yoga all vital movements must come under the influence of the psychic and of the spiritual calm, knowledge, peace. If they conflict with the psychic or the spiritual control, they upset the balance and prevent the forming of the base of transformation. If unbalance is good for other paths, that is the business of those who follow them. It does not suit mine.

I do not know that any except a very few great yogis have really changed their outer nature. In all the Ashrams I have seen people were just as others except for certain specific moral controls put on certain kinds of outer action (food, sex etc.), but the general nature was the human nature (as in the story of Narad and Janaka). It is even a theory of the old yogas that the *prārabdha karma* and therefore necessarily the permanent elements of the external character do not change — only one gets the inner realisation and separates oneself from it so that it drops off at death like a soiled robe and leaves the spirit free to enter into Nirvana. Our object is a spiritual change and not merely an ethical control, but this can only come first by a spiritual rejection from within and then by a supramental descent from above.

I don't know of any [Vedic Rishis] that have taken birth this time.

According to the Puranic stories there must have been many
Rishis who were far from being *jitendriya jitakrodha*. But also
there are many yogis who are satisfied with having the inner
experience of the Self but allow movements of a rajasic or tamasic
nature on the surface, holding that these will fall off with the
body.

*
**

Wonderful! The realisation of the Self which includes the
liberation from ego, the consciousness of the One in all, the established and consummated transcendence out of the universal
Ignorance, the fixity of the consciousness in the union with the
Highest, the Infinite and Eternal is not anything worth doing or
recommending to anybody — is "not a very difficult stage"!

Nothing new! Why should there be anything new? The
object of spiritual seeking is to find out what is eternally true, not
what is new in Time.

From where did you get this singular attitude towards the
old yogas and yogis? Is the wisdom of the Vedanta and Tantra
a small and trifling thing? Have then the sadhaks of the Ashram
attained to self-realisation and are they liberated Jivanmuktas,
free from ego and ignorance? If not, why then do you say, "it is
not a very difficult stage", "their goal is not high", "is it such a
long process?"

I have said that this yoga is "new" because it aims at the
integrality of the Divine in this world and not only beyond it
and at a supramental realisation. But how does that justify a
superior contempt for the spiritual realisation which is as much
the aim of this yoga as of any other?

As for the depreciation of the old yogas as something quite easy,
unimportant and worthless and the depreciation of Buddha,
Yajnavalkya and other great spiritual figures of the past, is it
not evidently absurd on the face of it?

Why should Mother dislike Yoga of Knowledge? The realisation of self and of the cosmic being (without which the realisation of self is incomplete) are essential steps in our yoga; it is the end of other yogas, but it is, as it were, the beginning of ours, that is to say, the point where its own characteristic realisations commence.

VI

By transformation I do not mean some change of the nature — I do not mean, for instance, sainthood or ethical perfection or yogic siddhis (like the Tantrik's) or a transcendental (*cinmaya*) body. I use transformation in a special sense, a change of consciousness radical and complete and of a certain specific kind which is so conceived as to bring about a strong and assured step forward in the spiritual evolution of the being of a greater and higher kind and of a larger sweep and completeness than what took place when a mentalised being first appeared in a vital and material animal world. If anything short of that takes place or at least if a real beginning is not made on that basis, a fundamental progress towards this fulfilment, then my object is not accomplished. A partial realisation, something mixed and inconclusive, does not meet the demand I make on life and yoga.

Light of realisation is not the same thing as Descent. Realisation by itself does not necessarily transform the being as a whole; it may bring only an opening or heightening or widening of the consciousness at the top so as to realise something in the Purusha part without any radical change in the parts of Prakriti. One may have some light of realisation at the spiritual summit of the consciousness but the parts below remain what they were. I have seen any number of instances of that. There must be a descent of the light not merely into the mind or part of it but into all the being down to the physical and below before a real transformation can take place. A light in the mind may spiritualise or otherwise change the mind or part of it in one way or another, but it need not change the vital nature; a light in the vital may purify and enlarge the vital movements or else silence and immobilise the vital being, but leave the body and the physical consciousness as it was, or even leave it inert or shake its balance. And the descent of Light is not enough, it must be the descent of the whole higher consciousness, its Peace, Power, Knowledge, Love, Ananda. Moreover, the descent may be enough to liberate, but not to perfect, or it may be enough to make a great change in the inner being, while the outer remains an imperfect instrument, clumsy, sick or unexpressive. Finally, transformation effected by the sadhana cannot be complete unless it is a supramentalisation of the being. Psychicisation is not enough, it is only a beginning; spiritualisation and the descent of the higher consciousness is not enough, it is only a middle term; the ultimate achievement needs the action of the supramental Consciousness and Force. Something less than that may very well be considered enough by the individual, but it is not enough for the earth-consciousness to take the definitive stride forward it must take at one time or another.

I have never said that my yoga was something brand new in all its elements. I have called it the integral yoga and that means that it takes up the essence and many processes of the old yogas — its newness is in its aim, standpoint and the totality of its method. In the earlier stages which is all I deal with in books like the "Riddle" or the "Lights" or in the new book to be published[1] there is nothing in it that distinguishes it from the old yogas except the aim underlying its comprehensiveness, the spirit in its movements and the ultimate significance it keeps before it — also the scheme of its psychology and its workings: but as that was not and could not be developed systematically or schematically in these letters, it has not been grasped by those who are not already acquainted with it by mental familiarity or some amount of practice. The detail or method of the later stages of the yoga which go into little known or untrodden regions, I have not made public and I do not at present intend to do so.

I know very well also that there have been seemingly allied ideals and anticipations — the perfectibility of the race, certain Tantric sadhanas, the effort after a complete physical siddhi by certain schools of yoga, etc., etc. I have alluded to these things

---

[1] *Bases of Yoga.*

myself and have put forth the view that the spiritual past of the race has been a preparation of Nature not merely for attaining the Divine beyond the world, but also for this very step forward which the evolution of the earth-consciousness has still to make. I do not therefore care in the least — even though these ideals were, up to some extent parallel, yet not identical with mine — whether this yoga and its aim and method are accepted as new or not; that is in itself a trifling matter. That it should be recognised as true in itself by those who can accept or practise it and should make itself true by achievement is the one thing important; it does not matter if it is called new or a repetition or revival of the old which was forgotten. I laid emphasis on it as new in a letter to certain sadhaks so as to explain to them that a repetition of the aim and idea of the old yogas was not enough in my eyes, that I was putting forward a thing to be achieved that has not yet been achieved, not yet clearly visualised, even though it is the natural but still secret outcome of all the past spiritual endeavour.

It is new as compared with the old yogas:

1. Because it aims not at a departure out of world and life into Heaven or Nirvana, but at a change of life and existence, not as something subordinate or incidental, but as a distinct and central object. If there is a descent in other yogas, yet it is only an incident on the way or resulting from the ascent — the ascent is the real thing. Here the ascent is the first step, but it is a means for the descent. It is the descent of the new consciousness attained by the ascent that is the stamp and seal of the sadhana. Even the Tantra and Vaishnavism end in the release from life; here the object is the divine fulfilment of life.

2. Because the object sought after is not an individual achievement of divine realisation for the sake of the individual, but something to be gained for the earth-consciousness here, a cosmic, not solely a supra-cosmic achievement. The thing to be gained also is the bringing in of a Power of Conciousness (the supramental) not yet organised or active directly in earth-nature,

even in the spiritual life, but yet to be organised and made directly active.

3. Because a method has been preconized for achieving this purpose which is as total and integral as the aim set before it, viz., the total and integral change of the consciousness and nature, taking up old methods but only as a part action and present aid to others that are distinctive. I have not found this method (as a whole) or anything like it professed or realised in the old yogas. If I had, I should not have wasted my time in hewing out a road and in thirty years of search and inner creation when I could have hastened home safely to my goal in an easy canter over paths already blazed out, laid down, perfectly mapped, macadamised, made secure and public. Our yoga is not a retreading of old walks, but a spiritual adventure.

I meant by it the descent of the supramental consciousness upon earth; all truths below the supramental (even that of the highest spiritual on the mental plane, which is the highest that has yet manifested) are either partial or relative or otherwise deficient and unable to transform the earthly life; they can only at most modify and influence it. The supermind is the vast Truth-Consciousness of which the ancient seers spoke; there have been glimpses of it till now, sometimes an indirect influence or pressure, but it has not been brought down into the consciousness of the earth and fixed there. To so bring it down is the aim of our yoga.

But it is better not to enter into sterile intellectual discussions. The intellectual mind cannot even realise what the supermind is; what use, then, can there be in allowing it to discuss what it does not know? It is not by reasoning but by constant experience, growth of consciousness and widening into the Light that one can reach those higher levels of consciousness above the intellect from which one can begin to look up to the Divine Gnosis. Those levels are not yet the supermind, but they can receive something of its knowledge.

The Vedic Rishis never attained to the supermind for the earth or perhaps did not even make the attempt. They tried to rise individually to the supramental plane, but they did not bring it down and make it a permanent part of the earth-consciousness. Even there are verses of the Upanishad in which it is hinted that it is impossible to pass through the gates of the Sun (the symbol of the supermind) and yet retain an earthly body. It was because of this failure that the spiritual effort of India culminated in Mayavada. Our yoga is a double movement of ascent and descent; one rises to higher and higher levels of consciousness, but at the same time one brings down their power not only into mind and life, but in the end even into the body. And the highest of these levels, the one at which it aims is the supermind. Only when that can be brought down is a divine transformation possible in the earth-consciousness.

I can't say whether any of them [the Vedic Rishis] attained the supramental plane, but the ascent to it was their object. *Svar* is evidently the illumined regions of Mind, between the supramental and the human intelligence formed by the rays of the Sun. According to the Upanishads those who ascend into the rays of the Sun return, but those who ascend into the Sun itself do not come back. That is because the ascent to supermind was envisaged, but the descent and organisation of the supermind here (as apart from the descent of the Rays) was not. We need not bother about the rebirth of the Rishis — they will come along if they are needed, I suppose.

It is quite possible that the *śloka* refers to a going up into higher worlds of felicity and light and this can be called a liberation or release. In later times the idea was strong that from all these higher worlds return is inevitable and it is only the release from all cosmic existence that gives *mukti*. The Vedic Rishis seem to have looked to an ascent into a luminous world or state above the falsehood and ignorance. In the Upanishad the sun is the symbol of the supramental Truth and it is said that those who pass into it may return but those who pass through the gates of the sun itself do not; possibly this means that an ascent into the supermind itself above the golden lid of overmind was the definitive liberation. The Veda speaks of the Truth hidden by a Truth where the Sun looses his horses from his car and there all the myriad rays are drawn together into one and that was considered the goal. The Isha Upanishad also speaks of the golden lid hiding the face of the Truth by removing which the Law of the Truth is seen, and the highest knowledge in which the one Purusha is known (*so'hamasmi*) is described as the '*kalyāṇatama*' form of the Sun. All this seems to refer to the supramental states of which the Sun is the symbol.

The Vedic Rishis were mystics of the ancient type who everywhere, in India, Greece, Egypt and elsewhere, held the secret truths and methods of which they were in possession as very sacred and secret things, not to be disclosed to the unfit who would misunderstand, misapply, misuse and degrade the knowledge. Their writings were therefore so couched as only to be intelligible in their secret meaning to the initiated, *niṇyā vacāṁsi nivacanāni kavaye*[1] — secret words that carry their significance only to the seer. They were equipped with an apparent meaning exoteric and religious for the people, esoteric, occult and spiritual for the initiates. That the people should not find out the real Truth was their intention; they wanted them only to know the outward truths for which they were fit.

The fundamental difference is in the teaching that there is a dynamic divine Truth (the supermind) and that into the present world of Ignorance that Truth can descend, create a new Truth-Consciousness and divinise Life. The old yogas go straight from

[1] *Rig Veda*, IV. 3. 16.

mind to the absolute Divine, regard all dynamic existence as
Ignorance, Illusion or Lila; when you enter the static and immutable Divine Truth, they say, you pass out of cosmic existence.

This yoga aims at the conscious union with the Divine in the
supermind and the transformation of the nature. The ordinary
yogas go straight from Mind into some featureless condition of
the cosmic silence and through it try to disappear upward into the
Highest. The object of this yoga is to transcend Mind and enter
into the Divine Truth of Sachchidananda which is not only
static but dynamic and raise the whole being into that truth.

Divine union, yes — but for the ascetic schools it was union with
the featureless Brahman, the Unknowable beyond existence or,
if with the Ishwara, still it was the Ishwara in a supracosmic
consciousness. From that point of view Patanjali's aphorism[1] is
sound enough. When he says yoga, he means the process of
yoga, the object which has to be kept in view in the process —
for by the cessation of *cittavṛtti* one gets into *samādhi* and
samādhi is the only way of unity solely and completely with the
Brahman beyond existence.

In the former yogas it was the experience of the Spirit which
is always free and one with the Divine that was sought. The
nature had to change only enough to prevent its being an obstacle
to that knowledge and experience. The complete change down
to the physical was only sought for by a few and then more as
a "siddhi" than anything else, not as the manifestation of a new
Nature in the earth-consciousness.

---

[1] *Yogaścittavṛttinirodhaḥ.*

There are many planes above man's mind, — the supramental is not the only one, and on all of them the Self can be realised, — for they are all spiritual planes.

Mind, vital and physical are inextricably mixed together only on the surface consciousness — the inner mind, inner vital, inner physical are separated from each other. Those who seek the Self by the old yogas separate themselves from mind, life and body and realise the self of it all as different from these things. It is perfectly easy to separate mind, vital and physical from each other without the aid of supermind. It is done by the ordinary yogas. The difference between this and the old yogas is not that they are incompetent and cannot do these things — they can do this perfectly well — but that they proceed from realisation of Self to Nirvana or some Heaven and abandon life, while this does not abandon life. The supramental is necessary for the transformation of terrestrial life and being, not for reaching the Self. One must realise Self first, only afterwards can one realise the supermind.

One can feel the experiences of any sadhana as a part of this one.

The realisation of the Spirit comes long before the development of overmind or supermind; hundreds of sadhaks in all times have had the realisation of the Atman in the higher mental planes, *buddheḥ paratah*, but the supramental realisation was not theirs. One can get *partial* realisations of the Self or Spirit or the Divine on any plane, mental, vital, physical even, and when one rises above the ordinary mental plane of man into a higher and larger mind, the Self begins to appear in all its conscious wideness.

It is by full entry into this wideness of the Self that cessation of mental activity becomes possible; one gets the inner Silence. After that this inner Silence can remain even when there is activity of any kind; the being remains silent within, the action goes on in the instruments, and one receives all the necessary initiations and execution of action whether mental, vital or physical from a higher source without the fundamental peace and calm of the Spirit being troubled.

The overmind and supermind states are something yet higher than this; but before one can understand them, one must first have the self-realisation, the full action of the spiritualised mind and heart, the psychic awakening, the liberation of the imprisoned consciousness, the purification and entire opening of the Adhar. Do not think now of those ultimate things (overmind, supermind), but get first these foundations in the liberated nature.

Spiritualisation means the descent of the higher peace, force, light, knowledge, purity, Ananda, etc., which belong to any of the higher planes from Higher Mind to overmind, for in any of these the Self can be realised. It brings about a subjective transformation; the instrumental Nature is only so far transformed that it becomes an instrument for the Cosmic Divine to get some work done, but the self within remains calm and free and united with the Divine. But this is an incomplete individual transformation — the full transformation of the instrumental Nature can only come when the supramental change takes place. Till then the nature remains full of many imperfections, but the Self in the higher planes does not mind them, as it is itself free and unaffected. The inner being down to the inner physical can also become free and unaffected. The overmind is subject to limitations in the working of the effective Knowledge, limitations in the working of the Power, subject to a partial and limited Truth, etc. It is only in the supermind that the full Truth-Consciousness comes into being.

Living in the true consciousness is living in a consciousness in which one is spiritually in union with the Divine in one way or another. But it does not follow that by so living one will have the complete, exact and infallible truth about all actions, all things and all persons.

The Divine can be realised on any plane according to the capacity of that plane, as the Divine is everywhere. The yogis and saints realise the Divine on the spiritualised mind plane; that does not mean they become supramental.

Because he is a great man does it follow that everything he thinks or says is right? or because he lives in the light does it follow that his light is absolute and complete? The "Truth-Consciousness" is a phrase I use for the supermind. X is not in the supermind. He may be and is in a true Consciousness, but that is a different matter.

Perhaps you are of the opinion of X, "The Divine is here, how can he descend from anywhere?" The Divine may be here, but if he has covered here his Light with darkness of Ignorance and his Ananda with suffering, that, I should think, makes a big difference to the plane and, even if one enters into that sealed Light etc., it makes a difference to the consciousness but very little to the Energy at work in this plane which remains of a dark or mixed character.

The Divine Force can act on any plane — it is not limited to the supramental Force. The supramental is only one aspect of the power of the Divine.

The sadhak of integral yoga who stops short at the Impersonal is no longer a sadhak of integral yoga. Impersonal realisation is the realisation of the silent Self, of the pure Existence, Consciousness and Bliss in itself without any perception of an Existent, Conscient, Blissful. It leads therefore to Nirvana. In the integral knowledge the realisation of the Self and of the impersonal Sachchidananda is only a step, though a very important

step, or part of the integral knowledge. It is a beginning, not an
end of the highest realisation.

These feelings are the usual attitude of the physical consciousness left to itself towards the Divine — a complete Agnosticism
and inability to experience.

The knowledge of the impersonal Divine by itself does not
affect the material facts of earth or at least need not. It only
produces a subjective change in the being itself and, if it is complete, a new vision and attitude towards all things immaterial
or material. But the complete knowledge of the Divine can produce a change in material things, for it sets a Force working
which ends by acting even upon these material things that seem
to the physical consciousness so absolute, invincible and unchangeable.

Why cannot one love or experience [the Cosmic and the Transcendent Divine] concretely? Many have done it. And why
assume that He is immobile, silent and aloof ? The Cosmic
Divine can be as close to one as one's own self and the Transcendent as intimate as the closest friend or lover. It is only in the
physical consciousness that there is some difficulty in realising it.

The Jain realisation of an individual godhead is all right so
far as it goes — its defect is that it is too individual and isolated.

I never heard of silence descending in other yogas — the mind
goes into silence. Since however I have been writing of ascent
and descent, I have been told from several quarters that there is
nothing new in this yoga — so I am wondering whether people
were not getting ascents and descents without knowing it! or
at least without noticing the process. It is like the rising above
the head and taking the station there — which I and others have
experienced in this yoga. When I spoke of it first, people stared

and thought I was talking nonsense. Wideness must have been
felt in the old yogas because otherwise one could not feel the
universe in oneself or be free from the body consciousness or
unite with the Anantam Brahman. But generally as in Tantric
yoga one speaks of the consciousness rising to the Brahmarandhra, top of the head, as the summit. Rajayoga of course lays
stress on Samadhi as the means of the highest experience. But
obviously if one has not the *brāhmī sthiti* in the waking state,
there is no completeness in the realisation. The Gita distinctly
speaks of being *samāhita* (which is equivalent to being in Samadhi) and the *brāhmī sthiti* as a waking state in which one lives
and does all actions.

* *
*

So I have always thought. I explain this absence of the descent
experiences myself by the old yogas having been mainly confined
to the psycho-spiritual-occult range of experience — in which the
higher experiences come into the still mind or the concentrated
heart by a sort of filtration or reflection — the field of this experience being from the Brahmarandhra downward. People went
above this only in Samadhi or in a condition of static *mukti* without any dynamic descent. All that was dynamic took place in
the region of the spiritualised mental and vital-physical consciousness. In this yoga the consciousness (after the lower field
has been prepared by a certain amount of psycho-spiritual-
occult experience) is drawn upwards above the Brahmarandhra
to ranges above belonging to the spiritual consciousness proper
and instead of merely receiving from there has to live there and
from there change the lower consciousness altogether. For there
is a dynamism proper to the spiritual consciousness whose nature
is Light, Power, Ananda, Peace, Knowledge, infinite Wideness
and that must be possessed and descend into the whole being.
Otherwise one can get *mukti* but not perfection or transformation
(except a relative psycho-spiritual change.) But if I say that, there
will be a general howl against the unpardonable presumption of
claiming to have a knowledge not possessed by the ancient saints
and sages and pretending to transcend them. In that connection
I may say that in the Upanishads (notably the Taittiriya) there

are some indications of these higher planes and their nature and the possibility of gathering up the whole consciousness and rising into them. But this was forgotten afterwards and people spoke only of the buddhi as the highest thing with the Purusha or Self just above, but there was no clear idea of these higher planes. Ergo, ascent possibly to unknown and ineffable heavenly regions in Samadhi, but no descent possible — therefore no resource, no possibility of transformation here, only escape from life and *mukti* in Goloka, Brahmaloka, Shivaloka or the Absolute.

It happens that people may get the descent without noticing that it is a descent because they feel the result only. The ordinary yoga does not go beyond the spiritual mind — people feel at the top of the head the joining with the Brahman, but they are not aware of a consciousness above the head. In the same way in the ordinary yoga one feels the ascent of the awakened lower consciousness (Kundalini) to the Brahmarandhra where the Prakriti joins the Brahman-consciousness, but they do not feel the descent. Some may have had these things, but I don't know that they understood their nature, principle or place in a complete sadhana. At least I never heard of these things from others before I found them out in my own experience. The reason is that the old yogins when they went above the spiritual mind passed into Samadhi, which means that they made no attempt to be conscious in these higher planes — their aim being to pass away into the Superconscient and not to bring the Superconscient into the waking consciousness, which is that of my yoga.

In the Veda there is no idea or experience of a personal emanation or incarnation of any of the Vedic gods. When the Rishis speak of Indra or Agni or Soma in men, they are speaking of the god in his cosmic presence, power or function. This is evident from the very language when they speak of Agni as the immortal in mortals, the immortal Light in men, the inner Warrior, the

Guest in human beings. It is the same with Indra or Soma. The building of the gods in man means a creation of the divine Powers, — Indra the Power of the Light, Soma the Power of the Ananda, — in the human nature.

No doubt, the Rishis felt the actual presence of the gods above, near, around or in them, but this was a common experience of all, not special and personal, not an emanation or incarnation. One may see or feel the presence of the Divine or a divine Power above the head or in the heart or in any or all the centres, feel the presence, see the form living there; one may be governed in all one's actions, thoughts and feelings by it; one may lose one's separate personality in it, may identify and merge. But all that does not constitute an incarnation or emanation of the Divine or of the Power. These things are universal experiences to which any yogin may arrive; to reach this condition with relation to the Divine is indeed a common object of yoga.

An incarnation is something more, something special and individual to the individual being. It is the substitution of the Person of a divine being for the human person and an infiltration of it into all the movements so that there is a dynamic personal change in all of them and in the whole nature; not merely a change of the character of the consciousness or general surrender into its hands, but a subtle intimate personal change. Even when there is an incarnation from the birth, the human elements have to be taken up, but when there is a descent, there is a total conscious substitution.

This is a long, subtle and persistent process. The incarnating Person first overshadows as an influence, then enters into the centres one after the other sometimes in the same form, sometimes in different forms, then takes up all the nature and its actions. What you describe does not correspond to this process; it seems to be an endeavour to build the gods in yourself in the Vedic sense and the Vedic manner. That can bring, if it succeeds, their powers and a sense of their presence; it cannot bring about an incarnation. An incarnation is destined, is chosen for you; the human person cannot choose or create an incarnation for himself by his own personal will. To attempt it is to invite a spiritual disaster.

One thing must be said — that an incarnation is not the object of this yoga; it is only a condition or means towards the object. The one and the only aim we have before us is to bring down the supramental Consciousness and the supramental Truth into the world; the Truth and nothing but the Truth is our aim, and if we cannot embody this Truth, a hundred incarnations do not matter. But to bring down the true supramental, to escape from all mental mixture is not an easy matter. The mere descent of the suns into the centres, even of all the seven suns into all the seven centres is only the seed; it is not the thing itself done and finished. One may feel the descent of the suns, one may have the attempt, the beginning of an incarnation, and yet in the end one may fail, if there is a flaw in the nature or a failure to pass through all the ordeals and satisfy all the hard conditions of the perfect spiritual success. Not only the whole mental, vital and physical nature of the ignorant human being has to be overcome and transformed, but also the three states of mental consciousness which intervene between the human and the supramental and like all mind are capable of admitting great and capital errors. Till then there may be descents of the supramental influence, light, power, Ananda, but the supramental Truth cannot be possessed, organised, put in possession of the whole nature. One must not think before that that one possesses the supermind, for that is a delusion which would prevent the fulfilment.

One thing more. The more intense the experiences that come, the higher the forces that descend, the greater become the possibilities of deviation and error. For the very intensity and the very height of the force excites and aggrandises the movements of the lower nature and raises up in it all opposing elements in their full force, but often in the disguise of truth, wearing a mask of plausible justification. There is needed a great patience, calm, sobriety, balance, an impersonal detachment and sincerity free from all taint of ego or personal human desire. There must be no attachment to any idea of one's own, to any experience, to any kind of imagination, mental building or vital demand; the light of discrimination must always play to detect those things, however fair or plausible they may seem. Otherwise, the Truth will have no chance of establishing itself in its purity in the nature.

The methods described in the account are the well-established methods of Jnana Yoga — (1) one-pointed concentration followed by thought-suspension, (2) the method of distinguishing or finding out the true self by separating it from mind, life, body and coming to the pure 'I' behind; this also can disappear into the impersonal Self. The usual result is a merging in the Atman or Brahman — which is what one would suppose is meant by the Overself, for it is that which is the real Overself. This Brahman or Atman is everywhere, all is in it, it is in all, but it is in all not as an individual being in each but is the same in all — as the Ether is in all. When the merging in the Overself is complete, there is no ego, no distinguishable I, nor any formed separative person or personality. All is an indivisible and undistinguishable Oneness either free from all formation or carrying all formations in it without being affected; one can realise it in either way. There is a realisation in which all things are moving in the one Self and this Self is there stable in all beings; there is another more complete and thorough-going in which not only is it so but all are vividly realised as the Self, the Brahman, the Divine. In the former, it is possible to dismiss all beings as creations of Maya, leaving the one Self alone as true — in the other it is easier to regard them as real manifestations of the Self, not as illusions. But one can also regard all beings as souls, independent realities in an eternal Nature dependent on the one Divine. These are the characteristic realisations of the Overself familiar to the Vedanta. But on the other hand, you say that this Overself is realised as lodged in the heart-centre, and it is described as something concealed which when it manifests appears as the real Thinker, source of all action but now guiding thought and action in the Truth. Now the first description applies to the Purusha in the heart, described by the Gita as Ishwara situated in the heart and by the Upanishads as the Purusha Antaratma; the second could apply also to the mental Purusha, *manomayaḥ prāṇaśarira netā* of the Upanishads, the mental Being or Purusha who leads the life and the body. So your question is one which on the data given relates to and accepts all these experiences, but they are strung together without any sufficient distinction or gradation being made or thought necessary between the various aspects of the one Being. There are a thousand ways of approaching and realising the Divine and each way has its own experiences which have their own truth and stand really on a basis one in essence but complex in aspects, common to all but not expressed in the same way by all. There is not much use in discussing these variations; the important thing is to follow one's own way well and thoroughly. In this yoga, one can realise the psychic being as a portion of the Divine seated in the heart with the Divine supporting it there — this psychic being takes charge of the sadhana and turns the whole being to the Truth, the Divine, with results in the mind, the vital and the physical consciousness which I need not go into here — that is the first transformation. We realise next the one Self, Brahman, Divine, first *above* the body, life, mind and not only within the heart supporting them — above and free and unattached as the static Self in all and dynamic too as the active Divine Being and Power, Ishwara-Shakti, containing the world and pervading it as well as transcending it, manifesting all cosmic aspects. But what is most important for us is that it manifests as a transcending Light, Knowledge, Power, Purity, Peace, Ananda of which we become aware and which descends into the being and progressively replaces the ordinary consciousness itself by its own movements — that is the second transformation. We realise also the consciousness itself as moving upward, ascending through many planes, physical, vital, mental, overmental to the supramental and Ananda planes. This is nothing new; it is stated in the Taittiriya Upanishad that there are five Purushas, the physical, the vital, the mental, the Truth Purusha (supramental) and the Bliss Purusha; it says that one has to draw the physical self into the vital self, the vital into the mental, the mental into the Truth self, the Truth self into the Bliss self and so attain perfection. But in this yoga we become aware not only of this taking up but of a pouring down of the power of the higher Self, so that there comes in the possibility of a descent of the supramental Self and Nature to dominate and change our present nature and turn it from nature of Ignorance into nature of Truth-Knowledge (and through the supramental into nature of Ananda) — this is the third or supramental transformation. It does not always go in this order, for with many the spiritual descent begins first in an imperfect way before the psychic is in front and in charge, but the psychic development has to be attained before a perfect and unhampered spiritual descent can take place, and the last or supramental change is impossible so long as the two first have not become full and complete. That's the whole matter put as briefly as possible.

What you demand of me would mean a volume, not a letter — especially as these are matters of which people know a great deal less than nothing and would either understand nothing or misunderstand everything. Some day, I suppose, I shall write something but the supramental won't bear talking of now. Something about the spiritual transformation might be possible and I may finish the letter on that point.

I do not want to go further into the question of M's realisation. As I have said, comparisons are of no use; each path has its own aim and direction and method, and the truth of each one does not invalidate the truth of the other. The Divine (or if you like, the Self) has many aspects and can be realised in many ways — to dwell upon these differences is irrelevant and without use.

"Transformation" is a word that I have brought in myself (like "supermind") to express certain spiritual concepts and spiritual facts of the integral yoga. People are now taking them up and using them in senses which have nothing to do with the significance which I put into them. Purification of the nature by the "influence" of the Spirit is not what I mean by transformation; purification is only part of a psychic change or a psycho-spiritual change — the word besides has many senses and is very often given a moral or ethical meaning which is foreign to my purpose. What I mean by the spiritual transformation is something dynamic (not merely liberation of the

Self or realisation of the One which can very well be attained
without any descent). It is a putting on of the spiritual consciousness, dynamic as well as static, in every part of the being down
to the subconscient. That cannot be done by the influence of the
Self leaving the consciousness fundamentally as it is with only
purification, enlightenment of the mind and heart and quiescence
of the vital. It means a bringing down of the Divine Consciousness static and dynamic into all these parts and the entire replace-
ment of the present consciousness by that. This we find unveiled
and unmixed above mind, life and body. It is a matter of the
undeniable experience of many that this can descend and it is my
experience that nothing short of its *full* descent can thoroughly
remove the veil and mixture and effect the full spiritual transformation. No metaphysical or logical reasoning in the void as
to what the Atman "must" do or can do or needs or needs not to
do is relevant here or of any value. I may add that transformation is not the central object of other paths as it is of this yoga
— only so much purification and change is demanded by them as
will lead to liberation and the beyond-life. The influence of the
Atman can no doubt do that — a full descent of a new consciousness into the whole nature from top to bottom to transform life
here is not needed at all for the spiritual escape from life.

The heart spoken of by the Upanishads corresponds with the
physical cardiac centre; it is the *hṛtpadma* of the Tantriks. As
a subtle centre, *cakra*, it is supposed to have its apex on the spine
and to broaden out in front. Exactly where in this area one or
another feels it does not matter much; to feel it there and be
guided by it is the main thing. I cannot say what M has realised —
but what is described as the Self is certainly this Purusha Antaratma but concerned here rather with Mukti and a liberated action
than with transformation of the nature. What the psychic
realisation does bring is a psychic change of the nature purifying
it and turning it altogether towards the Divine. After that or
along with it comes the realisation of the cosmic Self. It is these
two things that the old yogas encompassed and through them

they passed to Moksha, Nirvana or the departure into some kind of celestial transcendence. The yoga practised here includes both liberation and transcendence, but it takes liberation or even a certain Nirvana, if that comes, as a first step and not as the last step of its siddhi. Whatever exit to or towards the Transcendent it achieves is an ascent accompanied by a descent of the power, light, consciousness that has been achieved and it is by such descents that is achieved the spiritual and supramental transformation here. This does not seem to be admitted in M's thought; he considers the Descent as superfluous and logically impossible. "The Divine is here, from where will He descend?" is his argument. But the Divine is everywhere, he is above as well as within, he has many habitats, many strings to his bow of Power, there are many levels of his dynamic Consciousness and each has its own light and force. He is not confined to his position in the heart or to the single word of the psycho-spiritual realisation. He has also his supramental station above the heart-centre and mind-centre and can descend from there if he wills to do so.

I think Ramatirtha's realisations were more mental than anything else. He had opening of the higher mind and a realisation there of the cosmic Self, but I find no evidence of a transformed mind and vital; that transformation is not a result or object of the Yoga of Knowledge. The realisation of the Yoga of Knowledge is when one feels that one lives in the wideness of something silent, featureless and universal (called the Self) and all else is seen as only forms and names; the Self is real, nothing else. The realisation of "*my* self in other forms" is a part of this or a step towards it, but in the full realisation the "my" should drop so that there is only *the* one Self or rather only the Brahman. For the Self is merely a subjective aspect of the Brahman, just as the Ishwara is its objective aspect. That is the Vedantic "Knowledge". Its result is peace, silence, liberation. As for the active Prakriti, (mind, vital, body,) that Yoga of Knowledge does not make it its aim to transform them — that would be no use as the idea is that if the liberation has come, it will all drop off at death.

The only change wanted is to get rid of the idea of ego and realise as true only the supreme Self, the Brahman.

I have not read R's writings nor am I at all acquainted with his personality or what may be the level of his experience. The words you quote from him could be expressions either of a simple faith or of a pantheistic experience; evidently, if they are used or intended to establish the thesis that the Divine is everywhere and is all and therefore all is good, being Divine, they are very insufficient for that purpose. But as an experience, it is a very common thing to have this feeling or realisation in the Vedantic sadhana — in fact without it there would be no Vedantic sadhana. I have had it myself on various levels of consciousness and in numerous forms and I have met scores of people who have had it very genuinely — not as an intellectual theory or perception, but as a spiritual reality which was too concrete for them to deny whatever paradoxes it may entail for the ordinary intelligence.

Of course it does not mean that all here is good or that in the estimation of values a brothel is as good as an Ashram, but it does mean that all are part of one manifestation and that in the inner heart of the harlot as in the inner heart of the sage or saint there is the Divine. Again his experience is that there is One Force working in the world both in its good and in its evil — one Cosmic Force; it works both in the success (or failure) of the Ashram and in the success (or failure) of the brothel. Things are done in this world by the use of the force, although the use made is according to the nature of the user, one uses it for the works of Light, another for the works of Darkness, yet another for a mixture. I don't think any Vedantin (except perhaps some modernised ones) would maintain that all is good here — the orthodox Vedantic idea is that all is here an inextricable mixture of good and evil, a play of the Ignorance and therefore a play of the dualities. The Christian missionaries, I suppose, hold that all that God does is morally good, so they are shocked by the Taoist priests aiding the work of the brothel by their rites. But do not the Christian priests invoke the aid of God for the destruction of men in battle and did not some of them sing Te Deums over a victory won by the massacre of men and the starvation of women and children? The Taoist who believes only in the Impersonal Tao is more consistent and the Vedantin who believes that the Supreme is beyond good and evil, but that the Cosmic Force the Supreme has put out here works through the dualities, therefore through both good and evil, joy and suffering, has a theory which at least accounts for the double fact of the experience of the Supreme which is All Light, All Bliss and All Beauty and a world of mixed light and darkness, joy and suffering, what is fair and what is ugly. He says that the dualities come by a separative Ignorance and so long as you accept this separative Ignorance, you cannot get rid of that, but it is possible to draw back from it in experience and to have the realisation of the Divine in all and the Divine everywhere and then you begin to realise the Light, Bliss and Beauty behind all and this is the one thing to do. Also you begin to realise the one Force and you can use it or let it use you for the growth of the Light in you and others — no longer for the satisfaction of the ego and for the works of the ignorance and darkness.

As to the dilemma about the cruelty of things, I do not know what answer R would give. One answer might be that the Divine within is felt through the psychic being and the nature of the psychic being is that of the Divine Light, Harmony, Love, but it is covered by the mental and separative vital ego from which strife, hate, cruelty naturally come. It is therefore natural to feel in the kindness the touch of the Divine, while the cruelty is felt as a disguise or perversion in Nature, although that would not prevent the man who has the realisation from feeling and meeting the Divine behind the disguise. I have known even instances in which the perception of the Divine in all accompanied by an intense experience of universal love or a wide experience of an inner harmony had an extraordinary effect in making all around kind and helpful, even the most coarse and hard and cruel. Perhaps it is some such experience which is at the base of R's statement about the kindness. As for the Divine working, the experience of the Vedantin's realisation is that behind the confused mixture of good and evil something is working that he realises as the Divine and in his own life he can look back and see what each step, happy or unhappy, meant for his progress and how it led towards the growth of his spirit. Naturally this comes fully as the realisation progresses; before that he had to walk by faith and may have often felt his faith fail and yielded to grief, doubt and despair for a time.

As for my writings, I don't know if there is any that would clear up the difficulty. You would find mostly the statement of the Vedantic experience, for it is that through which I passed and, though now I have passed to something beyond, it seems to me the most thorough-going and radical preparation for whatever is beyond, though I do not say that it is indispensable to pass through it. But whatever the solution, it seems to me that the Vedantin is right in insisting that one must, to arrive at it, admit the two facts, the prevalence of evil and suffering here and the experience of that which is free from these things — and it is only by the progressive experience that one can get a solution — whether through reconciliation, a conquering descent or an escape. If we start from the basis taken as an axiom that the prevalence of suffering and evil in the present and in the hard, outward fact of things, disproves of itself all that has been experienced by sages and mystics of the other side, the realisable Divine, then no solution seems possible.

No, certainly I did not mean that the Vedantin who sees a greater working behind the appearances of the world is living in a different world from this material one — if I had meant that, all that I had written would be without point or sense. I meant a Vedantin who lives in this world with all its suffering and ignorance and ugliness and evil and has had a full measure of these things, betrayal and abandonment by friends, failure of outward objects and desires in life, attack and persecution, accumulated illnesses, constant difficulty, struggles, stumblings in his yoga. It is not that he lives in a different world, but he has a different way of meeting its ordeals, blows and dangers. He takes them as the nature of this world and the result of the ego-consciousness in which it lives. He tries therefore to grow into another consciousness in which he feels what is behind the outward appearance, and as he grows into that larger consciousness he begins to feel more and more a working behind which is helping him to grow in the spirit and leading him toward mastery and freedom from ego and ignorance and he sees that all has been used for that purpose. Till he reaches this consciousness with its larger knowledge of things, he has to walk by faith and his faith may sometimes fail him, but it returns and carries him through all the difficulties. Everybody is not bound to accept this faith and this consciousness, but there is something great and true behind it for the spiritual life.

One thing I feel I must say in connection with your remark about the soul of India and X's observation about "this stress on this-worldliness to the exclusion of other-worldliness". I do not quite understand in what connection his remark was made or what he meant by this-worldliness, but I feel it necessary to state my own position in the matter. My own life and my yoga have always been, since my coming to India, both this-worldly and other-worldly without any exclusiveness on either side. All human interests are, I suppose, this-worldly and most of them have entered into my mental field and some, like politics, into my life, but at the same time, since I set foot on the Indian soil on the Apollo Bunder in Bombay, I began to have spiritual experiences, but these were not divorced from this world but had an inner and infinite bearing on it, such as a feeling of the Infinite pervading material space and the Immanent inhabiting material objects and bodies. At the same time I found myself entering supraphysical worlds and planes with influences and an effect from them upon the material plane, so I could make no sharp divorce or irreconcilable opposition between what I have called the two ends of existence and all that lies between them. For me all is Brahman and I find the Divine everywhere. Everyone has the right to throw away this-worldliness and choose other-worldliness only, and if he finds peace by that choice he is greatly blessed.

I, personally, have not found it necessary to do this in order to have peace. In my yoga also I found myself moved to include both worlds in my purview — the spiritual and the material — and to try to establish the Divine Consciousness and the Divine Power in men's hearts and earthly life, not for a personal salvation only but for a life divine here. This seems to me as spiritual an aim as any and the fact of this life taking up earthly pursuits and earthly things into its scope cannot, I believe, tarnish its spirituality or alter its Indian character. This at least has always been my view and experience of the reality and nature of the world and things and the Divine: it seemed to me as nearly as possible the integral truth about them and I have therefore spoken of the pursuit of it as the integral yoga. Everyone is, of course, free to reject and disbelieve in this kind of integrality or to believe in the spiritual necessity of an entire other-worldliness altogether, but that would make the exercise of my yoga impossible. My yoga can include indeed a full experience of the other worlds, the plane of the Supreme Spirit and the other planes in between and their possible effects upon our life and the material world; but it will be quite possible to insist only on the realisation of the Supreme Being or Ishwara even in one aspect, Shiva, Krishna as Lord of the world and Master of ourselves and our works or else the Universal Sachchidananda, and attain to the essential results of this yoga and afterwards to proceed from them to the integral results if one accepted the ideal of the divine life and this material world conquered by the Spirit. It is this view and experience of things and of the truth of existence that enabled me to write *The Life Divine* and *Savitri*. The realisation of the Supreme, the Ishwara, is certainly the essential thing; but to approach Him with love and devotion and *bhakti*, to serve Him with one's works and to know Him, not necessarily by the intellectual cognition, but in a spiritual experience, is also essential in the path of the integral yoga. If you accept K's insistence that this and no other must be *your* path, it is this you have to attain and realise, then any exclusive other-worldliness cannot be *your* way. I believe that you are quite capable of attaining this and realising the Divine and I have never been able to share your constantly recurring doubts about your capacity and their persistent recurrence is not a valid ground for believing that they can never be overcome. Such a persistent recurrence has been a feature in the sadhana of many who have finally emerged and reached the goal; even the sadhana of very great yogis has not been exempt from such violent and constant recurrences, they have sometimes been special objects of such persistent assaults, as I have indeed indicated in *Savitri* in more places than one, and that was indeed founded on my own experience. In the nature of these recurrences there is usually a constant return of the same adverse experiences, the same adverse resistance, thoughts destructive of all belief and faith and confidence in the future of the sadhana, frustrating doubts of what one has known as the truth, urgings to abandonment of the yoga or to other disastrous counsels of *déchéance*. The course taken by the attacks is not indeed the same for all, but still they have strong family resemblance. One can eventually overcome if one begins to realise the nature and source of these assaults and acquires the faculty of observing them, bearing, without being involved or absorbed into their gulf, finally becoming the witness of their phenomena and understanding them and refusing the mind's sanction even when the vital is still tossed in the whirl and the most outward physical mind still reflects the adverse suggestions. In the end, these attacks lose their power and fall away from the nature; the recurrence becomes feeble or has no power to last: even, if the detachment is strong enough, they can be cut out very soon or at once. The strongest attitude to take is to regard these things as what they really are: incursions of dark forces from outside taking advantage of certain openings in the physical mind or the vital part, but not a real part of oneself or spontaneous creation in one's own nature. To create a confusion and darkness in the physical mind and to throw into it or awake in it mistaken ideas, dark thoughts, false impressions is a favourite method of these assailants, and if they can get the support of this mind from over-confidence in its own correctness or the natural rightness of its impressions and inferences, then they can have a field-day until the true mind reasserts itself and blows the clouds away. Another device of theirs is to awake some hurt or rankling sense of grievance in the lower vital parts and keep them hurt or rankling as long as possible. In that case one has to discover these openings in one's nature and learn to close them permanently to such attacks or to throw out the intruders at once or as soon as possible. The recurrence is no proof of a fundamental incapacity; if one takes the right inner attitude, it can and will be overcome. One must have faith in the Master of our life and works, even if for a long time He conceals Himself, and then in His own right time He will reveal His Presence.

You have always believed in Guruvada: I would ask you then to put your faith in the Guru and the guidance and rely on the Ishwara for the fulfilment, to have faith in my abiding love and affection, in the affection and divine goodwill and loving kindness of the Mother, stand firm against all attacks and go forward perseveringly towards the spiritual Goal and the all-fulfilling and all-satisfying touch of the All-Blissful, the Ishwara.

I send you the promised letter today; you will see that it is less a reply to the exact terms of your letter than a "defence of the gospel of divinisation of life" against the strictures and the incomprehensions of the mentality (or more often the vitality) that either misunderstands or shrinks from it — or perhaps misunderstands because it shrinks, and shrinks too because it misunderstands both my method and my object. It is not a complete defence, but only raises or answers a main point here and there. The rest will come hereafter.

But all language is open to misunderstanding; so I had better in sending on the letter make or try to make certain things clear.

Although I have laid stress on things divine in answer to an excessive (because contrary) insistence on things human, it must not be understood that I reject everything human, — human love or worship or any helpful form of human approach as part of the yoga. I have never done so, otherwise the Ashram could not be in existence. The sadhaks who enter the yoga are human beings and if they were not allowed a human approach at the beginning and long after, they would not be able to start the yoga or would not be able to continue it. The discussion arises only because the word "human" is used in practice, not only as identical with the human vital (and the outward mind), but with certain forms of human vital ego-nature. But the human vital has many other things in it and is full of excellent material. All that is asked by the yoga is that this material should be utilised in the right way and with the right spiritual attitude and also, that the human approach to the Divine should not be constantly turned into a human revolt and reproach against it. And that too we ask only for the success of the approach itself and of the human being who is making it.

Divinisation itself does not mean the destruction of the human elements; it means taking them up, showing them the way to their own perfection, raising them by purification and perfection to their full power and Ananda and that means the raising of the whole of earthly life to its full power and Ananda.

If there were not a resistance in vital human nature, a pressure of forces adverse to the change, forces which delight in imperfection and even in perversion, this change would effect itself without difficulty by a natural and painless flowering — as, for example, your own powers of poetry and music have flowered out here with rapidity and ease under the light and rain of a spiritual and psychic influence — because everything in you desired that change and your vital was willing to recognise imperfections, to throw away any wrong attitude — e.g., the desire for mere fame, and to be dedicated and perfect. Divinisation of life means, in fact, a greater art of life; for the present art of life produced by ego and ignorance is something comparatively mean, crude and imperfect (like the lower forms of art, music and literature which are yet more attractive to the ordinary human mind and vital), and it is by a spiritual and psychic opening and refinement that it has to reach its true perfection. This can only be done by its being steeped in the divine Light and Flame in which its material will be stripped of all heavy dross and turned into the true metal.

Unfortunately, there *is* the resistance, a very obscure and obstinate resistance. That necessitates a negative element in the yoga, an element of rejection of things that stand in the way and of pressure upon those forms that are crude and useless to dis-

appear, on those that are useful but imperfect or have been
perverted to retain or to recover their true movement. To the
vital this pressure is painful, first, because it is obscure and does
not understand and, secondly, because there are parts of it that
want to be left to their crude motions and not to change. That is
why the intervention of a psychic attitude is so helpful. For the
psychic has the happy confidence, the ready understanding and
response, the spontaneous surrender; it knows that the touch
of the Guru is meant to help and not to hurt, or, like Radha in
the poem, that whatever the Beloved does is meant to lead to the
Divine Rapture.

At the same time, it is not from the negative part of the
movement that you have to judge the yoga, but from its positive
side; for the negative part is temporary and transitional and will
disappear, the positive alone counts for the ideal and for the
future. If you take conditions which belong to the negative side
and to a transitional movement as the law of the future and the
indication of the character of the yoga, you will commit a serious
misjudgment, a grave mistake. This yoga is not a rejection of
life or of closeness and intimacy between the Divine and the
sadhaks. Its ideal aims at the greatest closeness and unity on the
physical as well as the other planes, at the most divine largeness
and fullness and joy of life.

Sri Aurobindo has no remarks[1] to make on Huxley's comments
with which he is in entire agreement. But in the phrase "to its
heights we can always reach", very obviously "we" does not
refer to humanity in general but to those who have a sufficiently
developed inner spiritual life. It is probable that Sri Aurobindo

---

[1] These remarks were dictated by Sri Aurobindo apropos of the phrase "to its heights
we can always reach" occurring in the following passage in *The Life Divine* quoted and commented upon by Aldous Huxley in his book, *The Perennial Philosophy* (1946 Edition), p. 74:

"The touch of Earth is always reinvigorating to the son of Earth, even when he seeks a
supraphysical Knowledge. It may even be said that the supraphysical can only be really mastered in its fullness — to its heights we can always reach — when we keep our feet firmly on the
physical. 'Earth is His footing,' says the Upanishad whenever it images the Self that manifests in the universe." (American Edition, p. 13.)

was thinking of his own experience. After three years of spiritual effort with only minor results he was shown by a yogi the way to silence his mind. This he succeeded in doing entirely in two or three days by following the method shown. There was an entire silence of thought and feeling and all the ordinary movements of consciousness except the perception and recognition of things around without any accompanying concept or other reaction. The sense of ego disappeared and the movements of the ordinary life as well as speech and action were carried on by some habitual activity of Prakriti alone which was not felt as belonging to oneself. But the perception which remained saw all things as utterly unreal; this sense of unreality was overwhelming and universal. Only some undefinable Reality was perceived as true which was beyond space and time and unconnected with any cosmic activity, but yet was met wherever one turned. This condition remained unimpaired for several months and even when the sense of unreality disappeared and there was a return to participation in the world-consciousness, the inner peace and freedom which resulted from this realisation remained permanently behind all surface movements and the essence of the realisation itself was not lost. At the same time an experience intervened: something else than himself took up his dynamic activity and spoke and acted through him but without any personal thought or initiative. What this was remained unknown until Sri Aurobindo came to realise the dynamic side of the Brahman, the Ishwara, and felt himself moved by that in all his sadhana and action. These realisations and others which followed upon them, such as that of the Self in all and all in the Self and all as the Self, the Divine in all and all in the Divine, are the heights to which Sri Aurobindo refers and to which he says we can always rise; for they presented to him no long or obstinate difficulty. The only real difficulty which took decades of spiritual effort to work out towards completeness was to apply the spiritual knowledge utterly to the world and to the surface psychological and outer life and to effect its transformation both on the higher levels of Nature and on the ordinary mental, vital and physical levels down to the subconscience and the basic Inconscience and up to the supreme Truth-Consciousness or supermind in which alone the dynamic transformation could be entirely integral and absolute.

***

I do not gather from these extracts[1] the true nature of the transformation spoken of here. It seems to be something mental and moral with the love of God and a certain kind of union in separateness brought about by this divine love as the spiritualising element.

Love of God and union in separateness through that love and a transformation of the nature by realising certain mental, ethical, emotional — perhaps even physical possibilities (for the Vaishnavas speak of a new *cinmaya* body) is the principle of Vaishnava yoga. So there is nothing here that was not already present in that line of Asiatic mysticism which looks to a Personal Deity and insists on the eternal pre-existence and survival of the individual being. A spiritual raising of the nature to its highest possibilities is a part of the Tantric discipline — so that too is not absent from Indian yoga. The writer seems, like most European writers, to know only Illusionism and Buddhism and to accept them as the whole wisdom of Asia (sagesse asiatique); but even there he misinterprets their idea and their experience. Adwaita even in its extreme form does not aim at the extinction of existence, the adoption of nothingness, the end of the being and destruction of the essence. Only a certain kind of Nihilistic Buddhism aims at that and even so, that Nothingness, Shunya, is described on another side of it as the Permanent. What these disciplines aim at is a passing from Time to Eternity, a putting off of the finite and putting on of the Infinite, a casting off of the bonds of ego and its results, desire, suffering, a falsified existence, in order to live in the true Self. These descriptions of the Christian writer betray an entire ignorance of the realisation which he decries, its infinity, freedom, surpassing peace, the ecstasy of the Brahmananda. It is an extinction of the limited individual personality but a liberation into cosmic and then into transcendent consciousness — an extinction of thought and life

---

[1] From *La Defense de l'Occident* by Henri Massis.

but a liberation into an unlimited consciousness and knowledge and being. The personality is extinguished but in something greater than itself, not in something less nor in mere "Néant". If it be said that that negates earthly life, so does the Christian ideal, for the Christian ideal aims at the attainment of a celestial existence beyond the earth existence (beyond this single earth life, for reincarnation is not admitted), which is only a vale of sorrows and a passing ordeal. It insists on the preservation of the spiritual personality, but so do Vaishnavism and Shaivism and other "Asiatic" ideals. The writer's ignorance of the many-sidedness of Asiatic wisdom deprives this depreciation of it of all value.

The phrases which struck you as resembling superficially at least our ideal of transformation are of a general character and could be adopted without hesitation by almost any spiritual discipline, even Illusionism would be willing to include it as a stage or experience on the way. All depends on the content you put into the words, what actual change in the consciousness and life they are intended to cover. If the transformation be "from sin to sainthood" by the union of the soul with God "in an intellectual light full of love" — which is the most definite description of it in these extracts, — then it is not at all identical, but rather very far from what I mean by transformation. For the transformation I aim at is not from sin to sainthood, but from the lower nature of the Ignorance to the Divine Nature of Light, Peace, Truth, Divine Power and Bliss beyond the Ignorance. It journeys towards a supreme self-existent good and leaves behind it the limited struggling human conception of sin and virtue; it is not an intellectual light that is the sun of its aspiration but a spiritual supra-intellectual supramental light; it is not sainthood that is its culmination but divine consciousness — or if you like, soul-hood, spirit-hood, conscious self-hood, divine-hood. There is therefore between these two kinds or two degrees of transformation an immense difference.

I. "C'est un abandon héroïque où l'âme parvient au sommet de l'activité libre, où la personne se transforme, où ses facultés sont épurées, déifiées par la grâce, sans que son essence soit detruite."

What is meant by free activity? With us the freedom consists in freedom from the darkness, limitation, error, suffering, transience of the ignorant lower Nature, but also in a total surrender to the Divine. Free action is the action of the Divine in us and through us; no other action can be free. That seems to be accepted in II and III; but this perception, this conception is as old as spiritual knowledge itself — it is not peculiar to Catholicism. What again is meant by the purification and deification of the faculties by Grace? If it is an ethical purification, that goes a very small way and does not bring deification. Again, if the deification is limited by the intellectual light, it must be a rather petty affair at the best. There was a similar aim in ancient Indian spirituality, but it had a larger sweep and a higher height than that. No spiritual discipline aims at purification or deification by the destruction of the essence — there can be no such thing, the very phrase is meaningless and self-contradictory. The essence of the being is indestructible. Even the most rigid Adwaita discipline does not aim at any such destruction; its object is the purest purity of the essential self. Transformation aims at this essential purity of the pure Spirit, but it asks also for the purity and divinity of the supreme Nature; it is not the essence of being but the accidents of our undeveloped imperfect nature that are destroyed and replaced by the manifestation of the divine Nature. The monistic Adwaita aims at the disappearance of the ego, not of the essence of the person; it arrives at this disappearance by identity with the One, by dissolution of the Nature-constructed ego into the reality of the eternal Self, for that, it says, not ego, is the essence of the person — *so'ham, tat tvam asi.* In our idea of transformation also there is the destruction of the ego, its dissolution into the cosmic and the divine consciousness, but by that destruction we recover the true or spiritual person which is an eternal portion of the Divine.

II. "La contemplation du Chrétien est inséparable de l'état de Grâce[1] et de la vie divine. S'il doit s'anéantir, c'est encore sa personnalité qui triomphe en se laissant arracher à tout ce qui n'est pas

---

[1] Grace is not a conception peculiar to the Christian spiritual idea — it is there in Vaishnavism, Shaivism, the Shakta religion, — it is as old as the Upanishads.

elle, en brisant tous les liens qui l'unissent à son individu de chair, afin que le Dieu vivant puisse s'en saisir, l'assumer, l'habiter."

III. "Liberté consiste d'abord à subordonner ce qui est inférieur dans sa nature à ce qui lui est supérieur."

These passages can be taken in the above sense and as approximating to our ideal; but the confusion here is in the use of the word "personality". Personality is a temporary formation and to eternise it would be to eternise ignorance and limitation. The true "I" is not the mental ego or the present personality which is only a mask, but the eternal "I" which assumes various personalities in various lives. The Christian and European conception of a single life on earth tends to bring about this error by making our present personality appear as if it were our whole self.... Again, it is not merely the bodily individuality to which ignorance ties us, but the mental individuality and vital individuality also. All these ties have to be broken, the imperfect forms of mind and life transcended, mind transformed into something beyond mind, life into divine life, if the transformation is to be real and not merely a new shaping or heightening of the lights of the Ignorance.

IV. "Cette solitude de l'âme (de l'ascète asiatique) ... n'est pas le vrai loisir spirituel, la solitude active où s'opère la transformation du péché en sainteté par l'union de l'âme avec Dieu dans une lumière intellectuelle toute pleine d'amour."

I have commented already on this description of the transformation to be effected and have to add only one more reserve. The solitude of the self in the Divine has no doubt to be active as well as passive and static; but none who has not arrived at the silence and motionless solitude of the eternal Self can have the free and integral activity of the higher divine Nature. For the action is based on the silence and by the silence it is free.

V. "... la vie chrétienne — mystique, progressive — qui est un enrichissement, un élargissement infini de la personne humaine."

This is not our idea of transformation — for the human person is the mental being limited by life and body. An enrichment and enlargement of it cannot go beyond the extreme limit of that formula, it can only widen and adorn its present poverty and narrowness. It cannot ascend out of the mental ignorance into a greater Truth and Light or bring that down in any fullness into earthly nature, which is the aim of transformation as we conceive it.

VI. "Pour l'asiatique la personnalité est la chute de l'homme; pour le chrétien, c'est le dessein même de Dieu, le principe de l'union, le sommet naturel de la création, qu'il appelle tout entière à la Grâce."

The personality of this single life in man is a formation in the Ignorance, therefore a fall; it cannot be the summit of the being. We do not admit that it is the summit of the natural creation either, but say there are higher summits to which we have to climb and reveal their powers in earthly nature. The natural creation is an evolution of the hidden Divine Consciousness in Nature which is limited and disguised at first by the Ignorance. It has still to climb out of the Ignorance — therefore to get beyond the human person into the divine person. It is in this spiritual evolution that the Plan Divine (dessein de Dieu) manifests its central and significant line and calls all creation to the crowning Grace.

You will see, therefore, that the resemblance of the transformation here to our ideal is only on the surface, in the words, but not in the content of the words which is much narrower and of another order. So far as there is agreement and coincidence, it is because there is contained in them what is common (a certain conversion of the consciousness) to all spiritual disciplines; for all, in the East or in the West, have a common core of experience — it is in their developments, range, turn to this or that aspect or else their will towards the totality of the Truth that they differ.

*
**

There is no connection between the Christian conception (of the Kingdom of Heaven) and the idea of the supramental descent. The Christian conception supposes a state of things brought about by religious emotion and moral purification; but these things are no more capable of changing the world, whatever value they may have for the individual, than mental idealism or any other power yet called upon for the purpose. The Christian proposes to substitute the sattwic religious ego for the rajasic and tamasic ego, but although this can be done as an individual achievement, it has never succeeded and will never succeed in accomplishing itself in the mass. It has no higher spiritual or psychological knowledge behind it and ignores the foundation of human character and the source of the difficulty — the duality of mind, life and body. Unless there is a descent of a new Power of Consciousness, not subject to the dualities but still dynamic which will provide a new foundation and a lifting of the centre of consciousness above the mind, the Kingdom of God on earth can only be an ideal, not a fact realised in the general earth-consciousness and earth-life.

RELIGION, MORALITY, IDEALISM AND YOGA

Section Three

RELIGION, MORALITY, IDEALISM AND YOGA

Religion, Morality, Idealism and Yoga

THE spiritual life (*adhyātma-jīvana*), the religious life (*dharma-jīvana*) and the ordinary human life of which morality is a part are three quite different things and one must know which one desires and not confuse the three together. The ordinary life is that of the average human consciousness separated from its own true self and from the Divine and led by the common habits of the mind, life and body which are the laws of the Ignorance. The religious life is a movement of the same ignorant human consciousness, turning or trying to turn away from the earth towards the Divine, but as yet without knowledge and led by the dogmatic tenets and rules of some sect or creed which claims to have found the way out of the bonds of the earth-consciousness into some beatific Beyond. The religious life may be the first approach to the spiritual, but very often it is only a turning about in a round of rites, ceremonies and practices or set ideas and forms without any issue. The spiritual life, on the contrary, proceeds directly by a change of consciousness, a change from the ordinary consciousness, ignorant and separated from its true self and from God, to a greater consciousness in which one finds one's true being and comes first into direct and living contact and then into union with the Divine. For the spiritual seeker this change of consciousness is the one thing he seeks and nothing else matters.

Morality is a part of the ordinary life; it is an attempt to govern the outward conduct by certain mental rules or to form the character by these rules in the image of a certain mental ideal. The spiritual life goes beyond the mind; it enters into the deeper consciousness of the Spirit and acts out of the truth of the Spirit. As for the question about the ethical life and the need to realise God, it depends on what is meant by fulfilment of the objects of life. If an entry into the spiritual consciousness is part of it, then mere morality will not give it to you.

Politics as such has nothing to do with the spiritual life.

If the spiritual man does anything for his country, it is in order to do the will of the Divine and as part of a divinely appointed work and not from any other common human motive. In none of his acts does he proceed from the common mental and vital motives which move ordinary men but acts out of the truth of the Spirit and from an inner command of which he knows the source.

The kind of worship (*pūjā*) spoken of in the letter belongs to the religious life. It can, if rightly done in the deepest religious spirit, prepare the mind and heart to some extent but no more. But if worship is done as a part of meditation or with a true aspiration to the spiritual reality and the spiritual consciousness and with the yearning for contact and union with the Divine, then it can be spiritually effective.

If you have a sincere aspiration to the spiritual change in your heart and soul, then you will find the way and the Guide. A mere mental seeking and questioning are not enough to open the doors of the Spirit.

Obviously to seek the Divine *only* for what one can get out of Him is not the proper attitude; but if it were absolutely forbidden to seek Him for these things, most people in the world would not turn towards Him at all. I suppose therefore it is allowed so that they may make a beginning — if they have faith, they may get what they ask for and think it a good thing to go on and then one day they may suddenly stumble upon the idea that this is after all not quite the one thing to do and that there are better ways and a better spirit in which one can approach the Divine. If they do not get what they want and still come to the Divine and trust in Him, well, that shows they are getting ready. Let us look at it as a sort of infants' school for the unready. But of course that is not the spiritual life, it is only a sort of elementary religious approach. For the spiritual life to give and not to demand is the rule. The sadhak, however, can ask for the Divine Force to aid him in keeping his health or recovering it if he does that as part of his sadhana so that his body may be

able and fit for the spiritual life and a capable instrument for
the Divine Work.

It is correct, religions at best modify only the surface of the
nature. Moreover, they degenerate very soon into a routine of
ceremonial habitual worship and fixed dogmas.

I do not take the same view of the Hindu religion as J. Religion
is always imperfect because it is a mixture of man's spirituality
with his endeavours that come in in trying to sublimate ignorantly
his lower nature. Hindu religion appears to me as a cathedral-
temple, half in ruins, noble in the mass, often fantastic in detail
but always fantastic with a significance — crumbling or badly
outworn in places, but a cathedral-temple in which service is still
done to the Unseen and its real presence can be felt by those who
enter with the right spirit. The outer social structure which it
built for its approach is another matter.

I regard the spiritual history of mankind and especially of India
as a constant development of a divine purpose, not a book that
is closed, the lines of which have to be constantly repeated.
Even the Upanishads and the Gita were not final though everything may be there in seed. In this development the recent
spiritual history of India is a very important stage and the names
I mentioned had a special prominence in my thought at the time
— they seemed to me to indicate the lines from which the future
spiritual development had most directly to proceed, not staying
but passing on. I may say that it is far from my purpose to propagate any religion, new or old, for humanity in the future. A
way to be opened that is still blocked, not a religion to be
founded, is my conception of the matter.

If it is meant by the statement[1] that the form of religion is something permanent and unchangeable, then that cannot be accepted. But if religion here means one's way of communion with the Divine, then it is true that that is something belonging to the inner being and cannot be changed like a house or a cloak for the sake of some personal, social or worldly convenience. If a change is to be made, it can only be for an inner spiritual reason, because of some development from within. No one can be bound to any form of religion or any particular creed or system, but if he changes the one he has accepted for another, for external reasons, that means he has inwardly no religion at all and both his old and his new religion are only an empty formula. At bottom that is, I suppose, what the statement drives at. Preference for a different approach to the Truth or the desire of inner spiritual self-expression are not the motives of the recommendation of change to which objection is made here; — the object proposed is an enhancement of social status and consideration which is no more a spiritual motive than conversion for the sake of money or marriage. If a man has no religion in himself, he can change his credal profession for any motive; if he has, he cannot; he can only change it in response to an inner spiritual need. If a man has a bhakti for the Divine in the form of Krishna, he can't very well say, "I will scrap Krishna for Christ, so that I may become socially respectable."

Vairagya is certainly one way of progressing towards the goal — the traditional way and a drastic if painful one. To lose the desire for human vital enjoyments, to lose the passion for literary or other success, praise, fame, to lose even the insistence on spiritual success, the inner *bhoga* of yoga, have always been recognised as steps towards the goal — provided one keeps the one insistence on the Divine. I prefer myself the calmer way of equality, the way pointed out by Krishna, rather than the

---

[1] These comments are on the following statement of Mahatma Gandhi on Dr. Ambedkar's view about change of religion:

"But religion is not like a house or a cloak which can be changed at will. It is more an integral part of one's self than of one's body. Religion is the tie that binds one to one's creator, and while the body perishes as it has to, religion persists even after that."

more painful one of Vairagya. But if the compulsion in one's nature or the compulsion of one's inner being forcing its way by that means through the difficulties of the nature is on that line, it must be recognised as a valid line. What has to be got rid of in that case is the note of despair in the vital which responds to the cry you speak of — that it will never gain the Divine because it has not yet got the Divine or that there has been no progress. There has certainly been a progress, this greater push of the psychic, this very detachment itself always growing somewhere in you. The thing is to hold on, not to cut the cord which is pulling you up because it hurts the hands, to keep the one insistence if all the others fall away from you.

It is evident that something in you, continuing the unfinished curve of a past life, is pushing you on this path of Vairagya and the more stormy way of Bhakti, — in spite of our preference for a less painful one and yours also, — something that is determined to be drastic with the outer nature so as to make itself free to fulfil its secret aspiration. But do not listen to these suggestions of the voice that says, "You shall not succeed and it is no use trying." That is a thing that need never be said in the Way of the Spirit, however difficult it may seem at the moment to be. Keep through all the aspiration which you express so beautifully in your poems; for it is certainly there and comes out from the depths, and if it is the cause of suffering, — as great aspirations are, in a world and nature where there is so much to oppose them, — it is also the promise and surety of emergence and victory in the future.

I have objected in the past to Vairagya of the ascetic kind and the tamasic kind. By the tamasic kind I mean that spirit which comes defeated from life, not because it is really disgusted with life, but because it could not cope with it or conquer its prizes; for it comes to yoga as a kind of asylum for the maimed or weak and to the Divine as a consolation prize for the failed boys in the world-class. The Vairagya of one who has tasted the world's gifts or prizes but found them insufficient or finally tasteless and turns away towards a higher and more beautiful ideal or the

Vairagya of one who has done his part in life's battles but seen
that something greater is demanded of the soul, is perfectly helpful and a good gate to the yoga. Also the sattwic Vairagya which
has learnt what life is and turns to what is above and behind
life. By the ascetic Vairagya I mean that which denies life and
world altogether and wants to disappear into the Indefinable
— I object to it for those who come to this yoga because it is
incompatible with my aim which is to bring the Divine into life.
But if one is satisfied with life as it is, then there is no reason to
seek to bring the Divine into life, — so Vairagya in the sense of
dissatisfaction with life as it is is perfectly admissible and even
in a certain sense indispensable for my yoga.

I quite acknowledge the utility of a temporary state of Vairagya
as an antidote to the too strong pull of the vital. But Vairagya
always tends to a turning away from life and the tamasic element
in Vairagya — despair, depression, etc. — dilapidates the fire
of the being and may lead in some cases to falling between two
stools so that one loses earth and misses heaven. I therefore prefer to replace Vairagya by a firm and quiet rejection of what has
to be rejected — sex, vanity, ego-centrism, attachment, etc. —
but that does not include rejection of the activities and powers
that can be made instruments of the sadhana and the divine work,
such as art, music, poetry, etc., though these have to find a new
spiritual or psychic base, a deeper inspiration, a turn towards
the Divine or things divine. Yoga can be done without the rejection of life, without killing or impairing the life-joy or the vital
force.

No, I didn't say that you chose the rajasic or tamasic Vairagya.
I only explained how it came, of itself, as a result of the movement of the vital in place of the sattwic Vairagya which is supposed to precede and cause or accompany or result from a
turning away from the world to seek the Divine. The tamasic
Vairagya comes from the recoil of the vital when it feels that it

has to give up the joy of life and becomes listless and joyless; the rajasic Vairagya comes when the vital begins to lose the joy of life but complains that it is getting nothing in its place. Nobody chooses such movements; they come independently of the mind as habitual reactions of the human nature. To refuse these things by detachment, an increasing quiet aspiration, a pure bhakti, an ardent surrender to the Divine, was what I suggested as the true forwarding movement.

There is the sattwic Vairagya — but many people have the rajasic or tamasic kind. The rajasic is carried by a revolt against the conditions of one's own life, the tamasic arises from dissatisfaction, disappointment, a feeling of inability to succeed or face life, a crushing under the grips and pains of life. These bring a sense of the vanity of existence, a desire to seek something less miserable, more sure and happy or else to seek a liberation from existence here, but they do not bring immediately a luminous aspiration or pure aspiration with peace and joy for the spiritual attainment.

The passage through sattwa is the ordinary idea of yoga, it is the preparation and purification by the *yama-niyama* of Patanjali or by other means in other yogas, e.g., saintliness in the bhakti schools, the eightfold path in Buddhism, etc., etc. In our yoga the evolution through sattwa is replaced by the cultivation of equanimity, *samatā*, and by the psychic transformation.

Obviously, the rajasic movements are likely to create more trouble in sadhana than the sattwic ones. The greatest difficulty of the sattwic man is the snare of virtue and self-righteousness, the ties of philanthropy, mental idealisations, family affections, etc., but except the first, these are, though difficult, still not so difficult to surpass or else transform. Sometimes, however, these things are as sticky as the rajasic difficulties.

Sannyasa does not take away attachment — it amounts only to running away from the object of attachment which may help but cannot by itself alone be the radical cure.

This is a feeling (the unimportance of things in Time) that the ascetic discipline sometimes uses in order to get rid of attachment to the world — but it is not good for any positive or dynamic spiritual purpose.

The principle of life which I seek to establish is spiritual. Morality is a question of man's mind and vital, it belongs to a lower plane of consciousness. A spiritual life therefore cannot be founded on a moral basis, it must be founded on a spiritual basis. This does not mean that the spiritual man must be immoral — as if there were no other law of conduct than the moral. The law of action of the spiritual consciousness is higher, not lower than the moral — it is founded on union with the Divine and living in the Divine Consciousness and its action is founded on obedience to the Divine Will.

The beliefs you speak of with regard to right and wrong, beauty and ugliness etc. are necessary for the human being and for the guidance of his life. He cannot do without the distinctions they involve. But in a higher consciousness when he enters into the Light or is touched by it, these distinctions disappear, for he is then approaching the eternal and infinite good and right which he reaches perfectly when he is able to enter into the Truth-Consciousness or supermind. The belief in the guidance of God is also justified by spiritual experience and is very necessary for the sadhana; this also rises to its highest and completest truth when one enters into the Light.

What you say about prayer is correct. That is the highest kind of prayer, but the other kind also (i.e., the more personal) is permissible and even desirable. All prayer rightly offered brings us closer to the Divine and establishes a right relation with Him.

The obstacles you speak of are the ordinary obstacles in the sadhana, brought up by parts of the being, especially through vital disturbance and physical inertia, movements which have to be gradually worked out of the consciousness.

I suppose each man makes or tries to make his own organisation of life out of the mass of possibilities the forces present to him. Self (physical self) and family are the building most make — to earn, to create a family and maintain it, work for or get some position in the means of life one chooses, in business, the profession, etc., etc. Country or humanity are usually added to that by a minority. A few take up some ideal and follow it as the mainstay of their life. It is only the very religious who try to make God the centre of their life — that too rather imperfectly, except for a few. None of these things are secure or certain, even the last being certain only if it is followed with an absoluteness which only a few are willing to give. The life of the Ignorance is a play of forces through which man seeks his way and all depends on his growth through experience to the point at which he can grow out of it into something else. That something else is in fact a new consciousness — whether a new consciousness beyond the earthly life or a new consciousness within it.

Family, society, country are a larger ego — they are not the Divine. One can work for them and say that one is working for the Divine only if one is conscious of the Divine Adesh to act for that purpose or of the Divine Force working within one.

Otherwise it is only an idea of the mind identifying country etc. with the Divine.

Everything depends upon the aim you put before you. If, for the realisation of one's spiritual aim, it is necessary to give up the ordinary life of the Ignorance (*samsāra*), it must be done; the claim of the ordinary life cannot stand against that of the spirit.

If a yoga of works alone is chosen as the path, then one may remain in the *samsāra*, but it will be freely, as a field of action and not from any sense of obligation; for the yogin must be free inwardly from all ties and attachments. On the other hand, there is no necessity to live the family life — one can leave it and take any kind of works as a field of action.

In the yoga practised here the aim is to rise to a higher consciousness and to live out of the higher consciousness alone, not with the ordinary motives. This means a change of life as well as a change of consciousness. But all are not so circumstanced that they can cut loose from the ordinary life; they accept it therefore as a field of experience and self-training in the earlier stages of the sadhana. But they must take care to look at it as a field of experience only and to get free from the ordinary desires, attachments and ideas which usually go with it; otherwise, it becomes a drag and hindrance on their sadhana. When one is not compelled by circumstances there is no necessity to continue the ordinary life.

One becomes tamasic by leaving the ordinary actions and life, only if the vital is so accustomed to draw its motives of energy from the ordinary consciousness and its desires and activities that if it loses them, it loses all joy and charm and energy of existence. But if one has a spiritual aim and an inner life and the vital part accepts them, then it draws its energies from within and there is no danger of one's being tamasic.

It is not absolutely necessary to abandon the ordinary life in order to seek after the Light or to practise yoga. This is usually done by those who want to make a clean cut, to live a purely religious or exclusively inner and spiritual life, to renounce the world entirely and to depart from the cosmic existence by cessation of the human birth and passing away into some higher state or into the transcendental Reality. Otherwise, it is only necessary when the pressure of the inner urge becomes so great that the pursuit of the ordinary life is no longer compatible with the pursuit of the dominant spiritual objective. Till then what is necessary is a power to practise an inner isolation, to be able to retire within oneself and concentrate at any time on the necessary spiritual purpose. There must also be a power to deal with the ordinary outer life from a new inner attitude and one can then make the happenings of that life itself a means for the inner change of nature and the growth in spiritual experience.

As for your friend, it is not possible to say that she can come here; for that depends on many things which are not clearly present here. First, one must enter this Path or it must be seen that one is called to it; afterwards there is the question whether one is meant for the Ashram life here. The question about the family duties can be answered in this way — the family duties exist so long as one is in the ordinary consciousness of the *gṛhastha*; if the call to a spiritual life comes, whether one keeps to them or not depends partly upon the way of yoga one follows, partly on one's own spiritual necessity. There are many who pursue inwardly the spiritual life and keep the family duties, not as social duties but as a field for the practice of Karmayoga, others abandon everything to follow the spiritual call or line and they are justified if that is necessary for the yoga they practise or if that is the imperative demand of the soul within them.

I don't remember the context; but I suppose he means that when one has to escape from the lower Dharma, one has often to renounce it so as to arrive at a larger one, e.g., social duties, paying

debts, looking after family, help to serve your country, etc., etc.
The man who turns to the spiritual life, has to leave all that
behind him often and he is reproached by lots of people for his
Adharma. But if he does not do this Adharma, he is bound for
ever to the lower life — for there is always some duty there to be
done — and cannot take up the spiritual Dharma or can do it
only when he is old and his faculties impaired.

You may get his photograph — it may help to see what kind of
nature he has. But there is no need to go out of the way to *persuade* him; from his letter he does not seem altogether ready for
the spiritual life. His idea of life seems to be rather moral and
philanthropic than spiritual at present; and behind it is the attachment to the family life. If the impulse to seek the Divine of
which he speaks is more than a mental turn suggested by a vague
emotion, if it has really anything psychic in it, it will come out at
its own time; there is no need to stimulate, and a premature stimulation may push him towards something for which he is not
yet fit.

The true object of the yoga is not philanthropy, but to find the
Divine, to enter into the divine consciousness and find one's true
being (which is not the ego) in the Divine.

The "Ripus" cannot be conquered by *damana*: even if it succeeds to some extent, it only keeps them down, but does not destroy them; often compression only increases their force. It is only
by purification through the divine consciousness entering into
the egoistic nature and changing it that this thing can be done.

If the sadhak gives himself from deep within and is absolutely persevering in the Way, then only can he succeed.

The idea of usefulness to humanity is the old confusion due to
second-hand ideas imported from the West. Obviously, to be

"useful" to humanity there is no need of yoga; everyone who leads the human life is useful to humanity in one way or another.

Yoga is directed towards God, not towards man. If a divine supramental consciousness and power can be brought down and established in the material world, that obviously would mean an immense change for the earth including humanity and its life. But the effect on humanity would only be one result of the change; it cannot be the object of the sadhana. The object of the sadhana can only be to live in the divine consciousness and to manifest it in life.

As to the extract about Vivekananda,[1] the point I make there does not seem to me humanitarian. You will see that I emphasise there the last sentences of the page quoted from Vivekananda, not the words about God the poor and sinner and criminal. The point is about the Divine in the world, the All, *sarva-bhūtāni* of the Gita. That is not merely humanity, still less, only the poor or the wicked; surely, even the rich or the good are the part of the All and those also who are neither good nor bad nor rich nor poor. Nor is there any question (I mean in my own remarks) of philanthropic service; so neither *daridrer sevā* is the point. I had formerly not the humanitarian but the humanity view — and something of it may have stuck to my expressions in the *Arya*. But I had already altered my viewpoint from the "Our yoga for the sake of humanity" to "Our yoga for the sake of the Divine". The Divine includes not only the supracosmic but the cosmic and the individual — not only Nirvana or the Beyond but Life and the All. It is that I stress everywhere.

[1] "I have lost all wish for my salvation, may I be born again and again and suffer thousands of miseries so that I may worship the only God that exists, the only God I believe in, the sum-total of all souls, — and above all, my God the wicked, my God the miserable, my God the poor of all races, of all species is the special object of my worship. He who is the high and low, the saint and the sinner, the god and the worm, Him worship, the visible, the knowable, the real, the omnipresent; break all other idols. In whom there is neither past life nor future birth, nor death nor going nor coming, in whom we always have been and always will be one, Him worship; break all other idols." (From a letter of Swami Vivekananda; quoted by Sri Aurobindo in *The Synthesis of Yoga*, Centenary Edition, 1972, pp. 257-58.)

I do not remember what I said about Vivekananda. If I said he
was a great Vedantist, it is quite true. It does not follow that all
he said or did must be accepted as the highest truth or the best.
His ideal of *sevā* was a need of his nature and must have helped
him — it does not follow that it must be accepted as a universal
spiritual necessity or ideal. Whether in declaring it he was the
mouthpiece of Ramakrishna or not, I cannot pronounce. It
seems certain that Ramakrishna expected him to be a great power
for changing the world-mind in a spiritual direction and it may be
assumed that the mission came to the disciple from the Master.
The details of his action are another matter. As for proceeding
like a blind man, that is a feeling that easily comes when a Power
greater than one's mind is pushing one to a large action; for the
mind does not realise intellectually all that it is being pushed to
do and may have its moments of doubt or wonderment about it
— and yet it is obliged to go on. Vedantic (Adwaita) realisation
is the realisation of the silent static or absolute Brahman — one
may have that and yet not have the same indubitable clearness as
to the significance of one's action — for over one's action for the
Adwaitin lies the shadow of Maya.

Today a Kanchanjungha of correspondence has fallen on my
head, so I could not write about Humanity and its progress.
Were not the later views of Lowes Dickinson grayed over by the
sickly cast of a disappointed idealism? I have not myself an exaggerated respect for Humanity and what it is — but to say that
there has been no progress at all is as much an exaggerated
pessimism as the rapturous hallelujahs of the nineteenth
century to a progressive Humanity were an exaggerated
optimism. I shall manage to read through the chapter
you sent me, though how I manage to find time for these
things is a standing miracle and a signal proof of a Divine
Providence.

Yes, the progress you are making is of the genuine kind, —
the signs are recognisable. And after all, the best way to make
Humanity progress is to move on oneself, — that may sound

either individualistic or egoistic, but it isn't: it is only common sense. As the Gita says:

"Whatever the best do is taken as the model by the rest." [1]

There are always unregenerate parts tugging people backwards and who is not divided? But it is best to put one's trust in the soul, the spark of the Divine within and foster that till it rises into a sufficient flame.

It is no use entertaining these feelings. One has to see what the world is without becoming bitter; for the bitterness comes from one's own ego and its disappointed expectations. If one wants the victory of the Divine, one must achieve it in oneself first.

To concentrate most on one's own spiritual growth and experience is the first necessity of the sadhak — to be eager to help others draws away from the inner work. To grow in the spirit is the greatest help one can give to others, for then something flows out naturally to those around that helps them.

All this insistence upon action is absurd if one has not the light by which to act. "Yoga must include life and not exclude it" does not mean that we are bound to accept life as it is with all its stumbling ignorance and misery and the obscure confusion of human will and reason and impulse and instinct which it expresses. The advocates of action think that by human intellect and energy making an always new rush, everything can be put right; the present state of the world after a development of the intellect and a stupendous output of energy for which there is no historical parallel is a signal proof of the emptiness of the illusion under which they labour. Yoga takes the stand that it is only by a change of consciousness that the true basis of life can be discovered; from within outward is indeed the rule. But

---

[1] *Yadyadācarati śreṣṭhastattadevetaro janaḥ.* *Gita*, Ch. III, 21.

within does not mean some quarter inch behind the surface. One must go deep and find the soul, the self, the Divine Reality within us and only then can life become a true expression of what we can be instead of a blind and always repeated confused blur of the inadequate and imperfect thing we were. The choice is between remaining in the old jumble and groping about in the hope of stumbling on some discovery or standing back and seeking the Light within till we discover and can build the Godhead within and without us.

I had never a very great confidence in X's yoga-turn getting the better of his activism, he has two strong ties that prevent it, — ambition and need to act and lead in the vital, and in the mind a mental idealism; these two things are the great fosterers of illusion. The spiritual path needs a certain amount of realism — one has to see the real value of the things that are, which is very little except as steps in evolution. Then one can either follow the spiritual static path of rest and release or the spiritual dynamic path of a greater truth to be brought down into life.

As for your question — Tagore, of course, belonged to an age which had faith in its ideas and whose very denials were creative affirmations. That makes an immense difference. Your strictures on his later development may or may not be correct, but this mixture even was the note of the day and it expressed a tangible hope of a fusion into something new and true — therefore it could create. Now all that idealism has been smashed to pieces by the immense adverse event and everybody is busy exposing its weaknesses — but nobody knows what to put in its place. A mixture of scepticism and slogans, "Heil-Hitler" and the Fascist salute and the Five-Year-Plan and the beating of everybody into one amorphous shape, a disabused denial of all ideals on one side and on the other a blind "shut-my-eyes and shut-everybody's-eyes" plunge into the bog in the hope of finding some firm foundation there, will not carry us very far. And what else is there?

Until new spiritual values are discovered, no great enduring creation is possible.

It is queer these intellectuals go on talking of creation while all they stand for is collapsing into the *Néant* without their being able to raise a finger to save it. What are they going to create, and from what material? Besides what use is it all if a Hitler with his cudgel or a Mussolini with his castor oil can come at any moment and wash it out or beat it into dust?

Yes, but human reason is a very convenient and accommodating instrument and works only in the circle set for it by interest, partiality and prejudice. The politicians reason wrongly or insincerely and have power to enforce the results of their reasoning so as to make a mess of the world's affairs: the intellectuals reason and show what their minds show them, which is far from being always the truth, for it is generally decided by intellectual preference and the mind's inborn education-inculcated angle of vision; but even when they see it, they have no power to enforce it. So between blind power and seeing impotence the world moves, achieving destiny through a mental muddle.

You write as if what is going on in Europe were a war between the powers of the Light and the powers of Darkness — but that is no more so than during the Great War. It is a fight between two kinds of Ignorance. Our aim is to bring down a higher Truth, but that Truth must be able to live by its own strength and not depend upon the victory of one or other of the forces of the Ignorance. That is the reason why we are not to mix in political or social controversies and struggles; it would simply keep down our endeavour to a lower level and prevent the Truth from descending which is none of these things but has a quite

different law and basis. You speak of Brahmatej being over-
powered by Kshatratej, but where is that happening? None of
the warring parties incarnate either.

REASON, SCIENCE AND YOGA

Reason, Science and Yoga

EUROPEAN metaphysical thought — even in those thinkers who try to prove or explain the existence and nature of God or of the Absolute — does not in its method and result go beyond the intellect. But the intellect is incapable of knowing the supreme Truth; it can only range about seeking for Truth, and catching fragmentary representations of it, not the thing itself, and trying to piece them together. Mind cannot arrive at Truth; it can only make some constructed figure that tries to represent it or a combination of figures. At the end of European thought, therefore, there must always be Agnosticism, declared or implicit. Intellect, if it goes sincerely to its own end, has to return and give this report: "I cannot know; there is, or at least it seems to me that there may be or even must be Something beyond, some ultimate Reality, but about its truth I can only speculate; it is either unknowable or cannot be known by me." Or, if it has received some light on the way from what is beyond it, it can say too: "There is perhaps a consciousness beyond Mind, for I seem to catch glimpses of it and even to get intimations from it. If that is in touch with the Beyond or if it is itself the consciousness of the Beyond and you can find some way to reach it, then this Something can be known but not otherwise."

Any seeking of the supreme Truth through intellect alone must end either in Agnosticism of this kind or else in some intellectual system or mind-constructed formula. There have been hundreds of these systems and formulas and there can be hundreds more, but none can be definitive. Each may have its value for the mind, and different systems with their contrary conclusions can have an equal appeal to intelligences of equal power and competence. All this labour of speculation has its utility in training the human mind and helping to keep before it the idea of Something beyond and Ultimate towards which it must turn. But the intellectual Reason can only point vaguely or feel gropingly towards it or try to indicate partial and even conflicting aspects of its manifestation here; it cannot enter into and know it. As long as we remain in the domain of the intellect only, an impartial pondering over all that has been thought and sought after, a constant throwing up of ideas, of all the possible ideas, and the formation of this or that philosophical belief, opinion or conclusion is all that can be done. This kind of disinterested search after Truth would be the only possible attitude for any wide and plastic intelligence. But any conclusion so arrived at would be only speculative; it could have no spiritual value; it would not give the decisive experience or the spiritual certitude for which the soul is seeking. If the intellect is our highest possible instrument and there is no other means of arriving at supraphysical Truth, then a wise and large Agnosticism must be our ultimate attitude. Things in the manifestation may be known to some degree, but the Supreme and all that is beyond the Mind must remain forever unknowable.

It is only if there is a greater consciousness beyond Mind and that consciousness is accessible to us that we can know and enter into the ultimate Reality. Intellectual speculation, logical reasoning as to whether there is or is not such a greater consciousness cannot carry us very far. What we need is a way to get the experience of it, to reach it, enter into it, live in it. If we can get that, intellectual speculation and reasoning must fall necessarily into a very secondary place and even lose their reason for existence. Philosophy, intellectual expression of the Truth may remain, but mainly as a means of expressing this greater discovery and as much of its contents as can at all be expressed in mental terms to those who still live in the mental intelligence.

This, you will see, answers your point about the Western thinkers, Bradley and others, who have arrived through intellectual thinking at the idea of an "Other beyond Thought" or have even, like Bradley, tried to express their conclusions about it in terms that recall some of the expressions in the *Arya*. The idea in itself is not new; it is as old as the Vedas. It was repeated in other forms in Buddhism, Christian Gnosticism, Sufism. Originally, it was not discovered by intellectual speculation, but by the mystics following an inner spiritual discipline. When, somewhere between the seventh and fifth centuries B.C., men began both in the East and West to intellectualise knowledge, this Truth survived in the East; in the West where the intellect began to be accepted as the sole or highest instrument for the discovery of Truth, it began to fade. But still it has there too tried constantly to return; the Neo-Platonists brought it back, and now, it appears, the Neo-Hegelians and others (e.g., the Russian Ouspensky and one or two German thinkers, I believe) seem to be reaching after it. But still there is a difference.

In the East, especially in India, the metaphysical thinkers have tried, as in the West, to determine the nature of the highest Truth by the intellect. But, in the first place, they have not given mental thinking the supreme rank as an instrument in the discovery of Truth, but only a secondary status. The first rank has always been given to spiritual intuition and illumination and spiritual experience; an intellectual conclusion that contradicts this supreme authority is held invalid. Secondly, each philosophy has armed itself with a practical way of reaching to the supreme state of consciousness, so that even when one begins with Thought, the aim is to arrive at a consciousness beyond mental thinking. Each philosophical founder (as also those who continued his work or school) has been a metaphysical thinker doubled with a yogi. Those who were only philosophic intellectuals were respected for their learning but never took rank as truth-discoverers. And the philosophies that lacked a sufficiently powerful means of spiritual experience died out and became things of the past because they were not dynamic for spiritual discovery and realisation.

In the West it was just the opposite that came to pass. Thought, intellect, the logical reason came to be regarded more and more as the highest means and even the highest end; in philosophy, Thought is the be-all and the end-all. It is by intellectual thinking and speculation that the truth is to be discovered; even spiritual experience has been summoned to pass the tests of the intellect, if it is to be held valid — just the reverse of the Indian position. Even those who see that the mental Thought must be overpassed and admit a supramental "Other", do not seem to escape from the feeling that it must be through mental

Thought, sublimating and transmuting itself, that this other Truth must be reached and made to take the place of the mental limitation and ignorance. And again Western thought has ceased to be dynamic; it has sought after a theory of things, not after realisation. It was still dynamic amongst the ancient Greeks, but for moral and aesthetic rather than spiritual ends. Later on, it became yet more purely intellectual and academic; it became intellectual speculation only without any practical ways and means for the attainment of the Truth by spiritual experiment, spiritual discovery, a spiritual transformation. If there were not this difference, there would be no reason for seekers like yourself to turn to the East for guidance; for in the purely intellectual field, the Western thinkers are as competent as any Eastern sage. It is the spiritual way, the road that leads beyond the intellectual levels, the passage from the outer being to the inmost Self, which has been lost by the over-intellectuality of the mind of Europe.

In the extracts you have sent me from Bradley and Joachim, it is still the intellect thinking about what is beyond itself and coming to an intellectual, a reasoned speculative conclusion about it. It is not dynamic for the change which it attempts to describe. If these writers were expressing in mental terms some realisation, even mental, some intuitive experience of this "Other than Thought", then one ready for it might feel it through the veil of the language they use and himself draw near to the same experience. Or if, having reached the intellectual conclusion, they had passed on to the spiritual realisation, finding the way or following one already found, then in pursuing their thought, one might be preparing oneself for the same transition. But there is nothing of the kind in all this strenuous thinking. It remains in the domain of the intellect and in that domain it is no doubt admirable; but it does not become dynamic for spiritual experience.

It is not by "thinking out" the entire reality, but by a change of consciousness that one can pass from the ignorance to the Knowledge — the Knowledge by which we become what we know. To pass from the external to a direct and intimate inner consciousness; to widen consciousness out of the limits of the ego and the body; to heighten it by an inner will and aspiration and opening to the Light till it passes in its ascent beyond Mind; to bring down a descent of the supramental Divine through self-giving and surrender with a consequent transformation of mind, life and body — this is the *integral* way to the Truth.[1] It is this that we call the Truth here and aim at in our yoga.

Yoga is not a thing of ideas but of inner spiritual experience. Merely to be attracted to any set of religious or spiritual ideas does not bring with it any realisation. Yoga means a change of consciousness; a mere mental activity will not bring a change of consciousness, it can only bring a change of mind. And if your mind is sufficiently mobile, it will go on changing from one thing to another till the end without arriving at any sure way or any spiritual harbour. The mind can think and doubt and question and accept and withdraw its acceptance, make formations and unmake them, pass decisions and revoke them, judging always on the surface and by surface indications and therefore never coming to any deep and firm experience of Truth, but by itself it can do no more. There are only three ways by which it can make itself a channel or instrument of Truth. Either it must fall silent in the Self and give room for a wider and greater consciousness; or it must make itself passive to an inner Light and allow that Light to use it as a means of expression; or else, it must itself change from the questioning intellectual superficial mind it now is to an intuitive intelligence, a mind of vision fit for the direct perception of the divine Truth.

If you want to do anything in the path of yoga, you must fix once for all what way you mean to follow. It is no use setting your face towards the future and then always looking back towards the past; in this way you will arrive nowhere. If you are tied to your past, return to it and follow the way you then choose; but if you choose this way instead, you must give your-

---

[1] I have said that the idea of the supermind was already in existence from ancient times. There was in India and elsewhere the attempt to reach it by rising to it; but what was missed was the way to make it integral for the life and to bring it down for transformation of the whole nature, even of the physical nature.

self to it single-mindedly and not look back at every moment.

*
**

As to doubts and argumentative answers to them, I have long given up the practice as I found it perfectly useless. Yoga is not a field for intellectual argument or dissertation. It is not by the exercise of the logical or the debating mind that one can arrive at a true understanding of yoga or follow it. A doubting spirit, "honest doubt" and the claim that the intellect shall be satisfied and be made the judge on every point is all very well in the field of mental action outside. But yoga is not a mental field, the consciousness which has to be established is not a mental, logical or debating consciousness — it is even laid down by yoga that unless and until the mind is stilled, including the intellectual or logical mind, and opens itself in quietude or silence to a higher and deeper consciousness, vision and knowledge, sadhana cannot reach its goal. For the same reason an unquestioning openness to the Guru is demanded in the Indian spiritual tradition; as for blame, criticism and attack on the Guru, it was considered reprehensible and the surest possible obstacle to sadhana.

If the spirit of doubt could be overcome by meeting it with arguments, there might be something in the demand for its removal by satisfaction through logic. But the spirit of doubt doubts for its own sake, for the sake of doubt; it simply uses the mind as its instrument for its particular dharma, and this not the least when that mind thinks it is seeking sincerely for a solution of its honest and irrepressible doubts. Mental positions always differ, moreover, and it is well-known that people can argue for ever without one convincing the other. To go on perpetually answering persistent and always recurring doubts such as for long have filled this Ashram and obstructed the sadhana, is merely to frustrate the aim of the yoga and go against its central principle with no spiritual or other gain whatever. If anybody gets over his fundamental doubts, it is by the growth of the psychic in him or by an enlargement of his consciousness, not otherwise. Questions which arise from the spirit of enquiry, not aggressive or self-assertive, but as a part of a hunger for knowledge can be

answered, but the "spirit of doubt" is insatiable and un-
appeasable.

Out of the thousand mental questions and answers there are
only one or two here and there that are really of any dynamic
assistance — while a single inner response or a little growth of
consciousness will do what those thousand questions and answers
could not do. The yoga does not proceed by *upadeśa* but by inner
influence. To state your condition, experiences, etc. and open to
the help is far more important than question-asking.

*
**

The whole world knows, spiritual thinker and materialist alike,
that the world for the created or naturally evolved being in the
ignorance or the inconscience of Nature is neither a bed of
roses nor a path of joyous Light. It is a difficult journey, a battle
and struggle, an often painful and chequered growth, a life
besieged by obscurity, falsehood and suffering. It has its mental,
vital, physical joys and pleasures, but these bring only a transient taste — which yet the vital self is unwilling to forego — and
they end in distaste, fatigue or disillusionment. What then?
To say the Divine does not exist is easy, but it leads nowhere
— it leaves you where you are with no prospect or issue —
neither Russell nor any materialist can tell you where you are
going or even where you ought to go. The Divine does not manifest himself so as to be recognised in the external world-circum-
stances — admittedly so. These are not the works of an irres-
ponsible autocrat somewhere — they are the circumstances of
a working out of Forces according to a certain nature of being,
one might say a certain proposition or problem of being into
which we have all really consented to enter and co-operate. The
work is painful, dubious, its vicissitudes impossible to forecast?
There are either of two possibilities then, to get out of it into Nirvana by the Buddhist or the illusionist way or to get inside oneself
and find the Divine there since he is not discoverable on the surface. For those who have made the attempt, and there were not

a few but hundreds and thousands, have testified through the ages that he is there and that is why there exists the yoga. It takes long? The Divine is concealed behind a thick veil of his Maya and does not answer at once or at any early stage to our call? Or he gives only a glimpse uncertain and passing and then withdraws and waits for us to be ready? But if the Divine has any value, is it not worth some trouble and time and labour to follow after him and must we insist on having him without any training or sacrifice or suffering or trouble? It is surely irrational to make a demand of such a nature. It is positive that we have to get inside, behind the veil to find him; it is only then that we can see him outside and the intellect be not so much convinced as forced to admit his presence by experience — just as when a man sees what he has denied and can no longer deny it. But for that the means must be accepted and the persistence in the will and patience in the labour.

But why on earth does your despairing friend want everybody to agree with him and follow his own preferred line of conduct or belief? That is the never-realised dream of the politician, or realised only by the violent compression of the human mind and life, which is the latest feat of the man of action. The "incarnate" Gods — Gurus and spiritual men of whom he so bitterly complains — are more modest in their hopes and are satisfied with a handful or, if you like, an Ashramful of disciples, and even these they don't ask for, but they come, they come. So are they not — these denounced "incarnates" — nearer to reason and wisdom than the political leaders? — unless of course one of them makes the mistake of founding a universal religion, but that is not our case. Moreover, he upbraids you for losing your reason in blind faith. But what is his own view of things except a reasoned faith? You believe according to your faith, which is quite natural, he believes according to his opinion, which is natural also, but no better, so far as the likelihood of getting at the true truth of things is in question. His opinion is according to his reason. So are the opinions of his political opponents accord-

ing to their reason, yet they affirm the very opposite idea to his.
How is reasoning to show which is right? The opposite parties
can argue till they are blue in the face — they won't be anywhere nearer a decision. In the end he prevails who has the
greater force or whom the trend of things favours. But who can
look at the world as it is and say that the trend of things is always
(or ever) according to right reason — whatever this thing called
right reason may be? As a matter of fact there is no universal
infallible reason which can decide and be the umpire between
conflicting opinions; there is only my reason, your reason, X's
reason, Y's reason, multiplied up to the discordant innumerable.
Each reasons according to his view of things, his opinion, that is,
his mental constitution and mental preference. So what is the
use of running down faith which after all gives something to hold
on to amidst the contradictions of an enigmatic universe? If
one can get at a knowledge that knows, it is another matter;
but so long as we have only an ignorance that argues, — well,
there is a place still left for faith, — even faith may be a glint from
the knowledge that knows, however far off, and meanwhile
there is not the slightest doubt that it helps to get things done.
There's a bit of reasoning for you!—just like all other reasoning
too, convincing to the convinced, but not to the unconvincible,
that is, to those who don't accept the ground upon which the
reasoning dances. Logic, after all, is only a measured dance of
the mind, nothing else.

Your dream was certainly not moonshine: it was an inner experience and can be given its full value. As for the other questions,
they are full of complications and I do not feel armed to cut the
Gordian knot with a sentence. Certainly, you are right to follow
directly the truth for yourself and need not accept X's or anybody else's proposition or solution. Man needs both faith and
reason so long as he has not reached a surer insight and greater
knowledge. Without faith he cannot certainly walk on any road,
and without reason he might very well be walking, even with the
staff of faith to support him, in the darkness. X himself founds
his faith, if not on Reason yet on reasons; and the rationalist,

the rationaliser or the reasoner must have some faith even if it be faith only in Reason itself as sufficient and authoritative, just as the believer has faith in his faith as sufficient and authoritative. Yet both are capable of error, as they must be since both are instruments of the human mind whose nature is to err, and they share that mind's limitations. Each must walk by the light he has even though there are dark spots in which he stumbles.

All that is, however, another matter than the question about the present human civilisation. It is not this which has to be saved; it is the world that has to be saved and that will surely be done, though it may not be so easily or so soon as some wish or imagine, or in the way that they imagine. The present must surely change, but whether by a destruction or a new construction on the basis of a greater Truth, is the issue. The Mother has left the question hanging and I can only do the same. After all, the wise man, unless he is a prophet or a Director of the Madras Astrological Bureau, must often be content to take the Asquithian position. Neither optimism nor pessimism is the truth: they are only modes of the mind or modes of the temperament.

Let us then, without either excessive optimism or excessive pessimism, "wait and see".

The faith in spiritual things that is asked of the sadhak is not an ignorant but a luminous faith, a faith in light and not in darkness. It is called blind by the sceptical intellect because it refuses to be guided by outer appearances or seeming facts, — for it looks for the truth behind, — and because it does not walk on the crutches of proof and evidence. It is an intuition, an intuition not only waiting for experience to justify it, but leading towards experience. If I believe in self-healing, I shall after a time find out the way to heal myself. If I have a faith in transformation, I can end by laying my hand on and unravelling the process of transformation. But if I begin with doubt and go on with more doubt, how far am I likely to go on the journey?

As for the faith-doubt question, you ardently give to the word faith a sense and a scope I do not attach to it. I will have to write not one but several letters to clear up the position. It seems to me that you mean by faith a mental belief which is in fact put before the mind and senses in the doubtful form of an unsupported asseveration. I mean by it a dynamic intuitive conviction in the inner being of the truth of supersensible things which cannot be proved by any physical evidence but which are a subject of experience. My point is that this faith is a most desirable preliminary (if not absolutely indispensable — for there can be cases of experiences not preceded by faith) to the desired experience. If I insist so much on faith — but even less on positive faith than on the throwing away of *a priori* doubt and denial — it is because I find that this doubt and denial have become an instrument in the hands of the obstructive forces....

Why I call the materialist's denial an *a priori* denial is because he refuses even to consider or examine what he denies but *starts* by denying it like Leonard Woolf with his "quack, quack" on the ground that it contradicts his own theories, so it can't be true. On the other hand, the belief in the Divine and the Grace and yoga and the Guru etc. is not *a priori*, because it rests on a great mass of human experience which has been accumulating through the centuries and the millenniums as well as the personal intuitive perception. Therefore it is an intuitive perception which has been confirmed by the experience of hundreds and thousands of those who have tested it before me.

I have started writing about doubt, but even in doing so I am afflicted by the "doubt" whether any amount of writing or of anything else can ever persuade the eternal doubt in man which is the penalty of his native ignorance. In the first place, to write adequately would mean anything from 60 to 600 pages, but not even 6000 convincing pages would convince doubt. For doubt exists for its own sake; its very function is to doubt always and, even when convinced, to go on doubting still; it is only to persuade its entertainer to give it board and lodging

that it pretends to be an honest truth-seeker. This is a lesson
I have learnt from the experience both of my own mind and of
the minds of others; the only way to get rid of doubt is to take
discrimination as one's detector of truth and falsehood and
under its guard to open the door freely and courageously to
experience.

All the same I have started writing, but I will begin not
with doubt but with the demand for the Divine as a concrete
certitude, quite as concrete as any physical phenomenon caught
by the senses. Now, certainly, the Divine must be such a certitude not only as concrete but more concrete than anything
sensed by ear or eye or touch in the world of Matter; but it is
a certitude not of mental thought but of essential experience.
When the Peace of God descends on you, when the Divine
Presence is there within you, when the Ananda rushes on you
like a sea, when you are driven like a leaf before the wind by the
breath of the Divine Force, when Love flowers out from you on
all creation, when Divine Knowledge floods you with a Light
which illumines and transforms in a moment all that was before
dark, sorrowful and obscure, when all that is becomes part of
the One Reality, when the Reality is all around you, you feel
at once by the spiritual contact, by the inner vision, by the
illumined and seeing thought, by the vital sensation and even
by the very physical sense, everywhere you see, hear, touch only
the Divine. Then you can much less doubt it or deny it than
you can deny or doubt daylight or air or the sun in heaven — for
of these physical things you cannot be sure but they are what
your senses represent them to be; but in the concrete experiences
of the Divine, doubt is impossible.

As to permanence, you cannot expect permanence of the
initial spiritual experiences from the beginning — only a few
have that and even for them the high intensity is not always
there; for most, the experience comes and then draws back
behind the veil waiting for the human part to be prepared and
made ready to bear and hold fast its increase and then its permanence. But to doubt it on that account would be irrational
in the extreme. One does not doubt the existence of air because
a strong wind is not always blowing or of sunlight because

night intervenes between dawn and dusk. The difficulty lies in the normal human consciousness to which spiritual experience comes as something abnormal and is in fact supernormal. This weak limited normality finds it difficult at first even to get any touch of that greater and intenser supernormal experience; or it gets it diluted into its own duller stuff of mental or vital experience, and when the spiritual does come in its own overwhelming power, very often it cannot bear or, if it bears, cannot hold and keep it. Still, once a decisive breach has been made in the walls built by the mind against the Infinite, the breach widens, sometimes slowly, sometimes swiftly, until there is no wall any longer, and there is the permanence.

But the decisive experiences cannot be brought, the permanence of a new state of consciousness in which they will be normal cannot be secured if the mind is always interposing its own reservations, prejudgments, ignorant formulas or if it insists on arriving at the divine certitude as it would at the quite relative truth of a mental conclusion, by reasoning, doubt, enquiry and all the other paraphernalia of Ignorance feeling and fumbling around after Knowledge; these greater things can only be brought by the progressive opening of a consciousness quieted and turned steadily towards spiritual experience. If you ask why the Divine has so disposed it on these highly inconvenient bases, it is a futile question, — for this is nothing else than a psychological necessity imposed by the very nature of things. It is so because these experiences of the Divine are not mental constructions, not vital movements; they are essential things, not things merely thought but realities, not mentally felt but felt in our very underlying substance and essence. No doubt, the mind is always there and can intervene; it can and does have its own type of mentalising about the Divine, thoughts, beliefs, emotions, mental reflections of spiritual Truth, even a kind of mental realisation which repeats as well as it can some kind of figure of the higher Truth, and all this is not without value but it is not concrete, intimate and indubitable. Mind by itself is incapable of ultimate certitude; whatever it believes, it can doubt; whatever it can affirm, it can deny; whatever it gets hold of, it can and does let go. That, if you like, is its freedom, noble right, privilege; it may be all you can say in its praise, but by these methods of mind you cannot hope (outside the reach of physical phenomena and hardly even there) to arrive at anything you can call an ultimate certitude. It is for this compelling reason that mentalising or enquiring about the Divine cannot by its own right bring the Divine. If the consciousness is always busy with small mental movements, — especially accompanied, as they usually are, by a host of vital movements, desires, prepossessions and all else that vitiates human thinking, — even apart from the native insufficiency of reason, what room can there be for a new order of knowledge, for fundamental experiences or for those deep and tremendous upsurgings or descents of the Spirit? It is indeed possible for the mind in the midst of its activities to be suddenly taken by surprise, overwhelmed, swept aside, while all is flooded with a sudden inrush of spiritual experience. But if afterwards it begins questioning, doubting, theorising, surmising what these might be and whether it is true or not, what else can the spiritual power do but retire and wait for the bubbles of the mind to cease?

I would ask one simple question of those who would make the intellectual mind the standard and judge of spiritual experience. Is the Divine something less than mind or is it something greater? Is mental consciousness with its groping enquiry, endless argument, unquenchable doubt, stiff and unplastic logic something superior or even equal to the Divine Consciousness or is it something inferior in its action and status? If it is greater, then there is no reason to seek after the Divine. If it is equal, then spiritual experience is quite superfluous. But if it is inferior, how can it challenge, judge, make the Divine stand as an accused or a witness before its tribunal, summon it to appear as a candidate for admission before a Board of Examiners or pin it like an insect under its examining microscope? Can the vital animal hold up as infallible the standard of its vital instincts, associations and impulses, and judge, interpret and fathom by it the mind of man? It cannot, because man's mind is a greater power working in a wider, more complex way which the animal vital consciousness cannot follow. Is it so difficult to see, similarly, that the Divine Consciousness must be something infinitely wider, more complex than the human mind, filled with greater powers and lights, moving in a way which mere mind cannot judge, interpret or fathom by the standard of its fallible reason and limited half-knowledge? The simple fact is there that Spirit and Mind are not the same thing and that it is the spiritual consciousness into which the yogin has to enter (in all this I am not in the least speaking of the supermind), if he wants to be in permanent contact or union with the Divine. It is not then a freak of the Divine or a tyranny to insist on the mind recognising its limitations, quieting itself, giving up its demands, and opening and surrendering to a greater Light than it can find on its own obscurer level.

This doesn't mean that mind has no place at all in the spiritual life; but it means that it cannot be even the main instrument, much less the authority, to whose judgment all must submit itself, including the Divine. Mind must learn from the greater consciousness it is approaching and not impose its own standards on it; it has to receive illumination, open to a higher Truth, admit a greater power that doesn't work according to mental canons, surrender itself and allow its half-light half-darkness to be flooded from above till where it was blind it can see, where it was deaf it can hear, where it was insensible it can feel, and where it was baffled, uncertain, questioning, disappointed it can have joy, fulfilment, certitude and peace.

This is the position on which yoga stands, a position based upon constant experience since men began to seek after the Divine. If it is not true, then there is no truth in yoga and no necessity for yoga. If it is true, then it is on that basis, from the standpoint of the necessity of this greater consciousness that we can see whether doubt is of any utility for the spiritual life. To believe anything and everything is certainly not demanded of the spiritual seeker; such a promiscuous and imbecile credulity would be not only unintellectual, but in the last degree unspiritual. At every moment of the spiritual life until one has got fully into the higher light, one has to be on one's guard and be able to distinguish spiritual truth from pseudo-spiritual imitations of it or substitutes for it set up by the mind and the vital desire. The power to distinguish between truths of the Divine and the lies of the Asura is a cardinal necessity for yoga. The question is whether that can best be done by the negative and destructive method of doubt, which often kills falsehood but rejects truth too with the same impartial blow, or a more positive, helpful and luminously searching power can be found, which is not compelled by its inherent ignorance to meet truth and falsehood alike with the stiletto of doubt and the bludgeon of denial. An indiscriminateness of mental belief is not the teaching of spirituality or of yoga; the faith of which it speaks is not a crude mental belief but the fidelity of the soul to the guiding light within it, a fidelity which has to remain till the light leads it into knowledge.

I do not ask "undiscriminating faith" from anyone, all I ask is fundamental faith, safeguarded by a patient and quiet discrimination — because it is these that are proper to the consciousness of a spiritual seeker and it is these that I have myself used and found that they removed all necessity for the quite gratuitous dilemma of "either you must doubt everything supraphysical or be entirely credulous", which is the stock-in-trade of the materialist argument. Your doubt, I see, constantly returns to the charge with a repetition of this formula in spite of my denial — which supports my assertion that Doubt cannot be convinced, because by its very nature it does not want to be convinced; it keeps repeating the old ground always.

The abnormal abounds in this physical world, the supernormal is there also. In these matters, apart from any question of faith, any truly rational man with a free mind (not tied up like the rationalists or so-called free-thinkers at every point with the triple cords of *a priori* irrational disbelief) must not cry out at once, "Humbug! Falsehood!" but suspend judgment until he has the necessary experience and knowledge.

To deny in ignorance is no better than to affirm in ignorance.

Whatever the motive immediately pushing the mind or the vital, if there is a true seeking for the Divine in the being, it must lead eventually to the realisation of the Divine. The soul within has always the inherent (*ahaitukī*) yearning for the Divine; the *hetu* or special motive is simply an impulsion used by it to get the mind and the vital to follow the inner urge. If the mind and the vital can feel and accept the soul's sheer love for the Divine for his own sake, then the sadhana gets its full power and many difficulties disappear; but even if they do not, they will get what they seek after in the Divine and through it they will come to realise something, even to pass beyond the limit of the original desire.... I may say that the idea of a joyless God is an absurdity, which only the ignorance of the mind could engender! The Radha love is not based upon any such thing, but means simply that whatever comes on the way to the Divine, pain or joy, *milana* or *viraha*, and however long the sufferings may last, the Radha love is unshaken and keeps its faith and certitude pointing fixedly like a star to the supreme object of Love.

What is this Ananda, after all? The mind can see in it nothing but a pleasant psychological condition, — but if it were only that, it could not be the rapture which the bhaktas and the mystics find in it. When the Ananda comes into you, it is the Divine who comes into you, just as when the Peace flows into you, it is the Divine who is invading you, or when you are flooded with Light, it is the flood of the Divine himself that is around you. Of course, the Divine is something much more, many other things besides, and in them all a Presence, a Being, a Divine Person; for the Divine is Krishna, is Shiva, is the Supreme Mother. But through the Ananda you can perceive the Anandamaya Krishna, for the Ananda is the subtle body and being of Krishna; through the Peace you can perceive the Shantimaya Shiva; in the Light, in the delivering Knowledge, the Love, the fulfilling and uplifting Power you can meet the presence of the Divine Mother. It is this percep-

tion that makes the experiences of the bhaktas and mystics so
rapturous and enables them to pass more easily through the
nights of anguish and separation; when there is this soul-
perception, it gives to even a little or brief Ananda a force or
value it could not otherwise have, and the Ananda itself gathers
by it a growing power to stay, to return, to increase.

I cannot very well answer the strictures of Russell, for the
conception of the Divine as an external omnipotent Power who
has "created" the world and governs it like an absolute and
arbitrary monarch — the Christian or Semitic conception — has
never been mine; it contradicts too much my seeing and experience during thirty years of sadhana. It is against this conception that the atheistic objection is aimed, — for atheism in
Europe has been a shallow and rather childish reaction against
a shallow and childish exoteric religionism and its popular
inadequate and crudely dogmatic notions. But when I speak
of the Divine Will, I mean something different, — something
that has descended here into an evolutionary world of Ignorance, standing at the back of things, pressing on the Darkness
with its Light, leading things presently towards the best possible
in the conditions of a world of Ignorance and leading it eventually towards a descent of a greater power of the Divine, which
will be not an omnipotence held back and conditioned by the
law of the world as it is, but in full action and therefore bringing
the reign of light, peace, harmony, joy, love, beauty and Ananda,
for these are the Divine Nature. The Divine Grace is there ready
to act at every moment, but it manifests as one grows out of the
Law of Ignorance into the Law of Light, and it is meant, not as
an arbitrary caprice, however miraculous often its intervention,
but as a help in that growth and a Light that leads and eventually delivers. If we take the facts of the world as they are and
the facts of spiritual experience as a whole, neither of which
can be denied or neglected, then I do not see what other Divine
there can be. This Divine may lead us often through darkness,
because the darkness is there in us and around us, but it is to
the Light he is leading and not to anything else.

*
**

The point about the intellect's misrepresentation of the "Formless" (the result of a merely negative expression of something that is inexpressibly intimate and positive) is very well made and hits the truth in the centre. No one who has had the Ananda of the Brahman can do anything but smile at the charge of coldness; there is an absoluteness of immutable ecstasy in it, a concentrated intensity of silent and inalienable rapture that is impossible even to suggest to anyone who has not had the experience. The eternal Reality is neither cold nor dry nor empty; you might as well talk of the midsummer sunlight as cold or the ocean as dry or perfect fullness as empty. Even when you enter into it by elimination of form and everything else, it surges up as a miraculous fullness — that is truly the Purnam; when it is entered affirmatively as well as by negation, there can obviously be no question of emptiness or dryness! All is there and more than one could ever dream of as the all. That is why one has to object to the intellect thrusting itself in as the *sab-jāntā* (all-knowing) judge: if it kept to its own limits, there would be no objection to it. But it makes constructions of words and ideas which have no application to the Truth, babbles foolish things in its ignorance and makes its constructions a wall which refuses to let in the Truth that surpasses its own capacities and scope.

If one is blind, it is quite natural — for the human intelligence is after all rather an imbecile thing at its best — to deny daylight: if one's highest natural vision is that of glimmering mists, it is equally natural to believe that all high vision is but a mist or a glimmer. But Light exists for all that — and Spiritual Truth is more than a mist and a glimmer.

In reference to what Prof. Sorley has written on *The Riddle of this World*, the book, of course, was not meant as a full or direct statement of my thought and, as it was written to sadhaks mostly, many things were taken for granted there. Most of the major ideas — e.g. overmind — were left without elucidation. To make the ideas implied clear to the intellect, they must be put with precision in an intellectual form — so far as that is possible with supra-intellectual things. What is written in the book can be clear to those who have gone far enough in experience, but for most it can only be suggestive.

I do not think, however, that the statement of supra-intellectual things necessarily involves a making of distinctions in the terms of the intellect. For, fundamentally, it is not an expression of ideas arrived at by speculative thinking. One has to arrive at spiritual knowledge through experience and a consciousness of things which arises directly out of that experience or else underlies or is involved in it. This kind of knowledge, then, is fundamentally a consciousness and not a thought or formulated idea. For instance, my first major experience — radical and overwhelming, though not, as it turned out, final and exhaustive — came after and by the exclusion and silencing of all thought — there was, first, what might be called a spiritually substantial or concrete consciousness of stillness and silence, then the awareness of some sole and supreme Reality in whose presence things existed only as forms, but forms not at all substantial or real or concrete; but this was all apparent to a spiritual perception and essential and impersonal sense and there was not the least concept or idea of reality or unreality or any other notion, for all concept or idea was hushed or rather entirely absent in the absolute stillness. These things were known directly through the pure consciousness and not through the mind, so there was no need of concepts or words or names. At the same time this fundamental character of spiritual experience is not absolutely limitative; it can do without thought, but it can do with thought also. Of course, the first idea of the mind would be that the resort to thought brings one back at once to the domain of the intellect — and at first and for a long time it may be so; but it is not my experience that this is unavoidable. It happens so when one tries to make an intellectual statement of what one has experienced; but there is another kind of thought that springs out as if it were a body or form of the experience or of the consciousness involved in it — or of a part of that consciousness — and this does not seem to me to be intellectual in its character. It has another light, another power in it, a sense within the sense. It is very clearly so with those thoughts that come without the need of words to embody them, thoughts that are of the nature of a direct seeing in the consciousness, even a kind of intimate sense or contact formulating itself into a precise expression of its awareness (I hope this is not too mystic or unintelligible); but it might be said that directly the thoughts turn into words they belong to the kingdom of intellect — for words are a coinage of the intellect. But is it so really or inevitably? It has always seemed to me that words came originally from somewhere else than the thinking mind, although the thinking mind secured hold of them, turned them to its use and coined them freely for its purposes. But even otherwise, is it not possible to use words for the expression of something that is not intellectual? Housman contends that poetry is perfectly poetical only when it is non-intellectual, when it is non-sense. That is too paradoxical, but I suppose what he means is that if it is put to the strict test of the intellect, it appears extravagant because it conveys something that expresses and is real to some other kind of seeing than that which intellectual thought brings to us. Is it not possible that words may spring from, that language may be used to express — at least up to a certain point and in a certain way — the supra-intellectual consciousness which is the essential power of spiritual experience? This, however, is by the way — when one tries to explain spiritual experience to the intellect itself, then it is a different matter.

The interpenetration of the planes is indeed for me a capital and fundamental part of spiritual experience without which yoga as I practise it and its aim could not exist. For that aim is to manifest, reach or embody a higher consciousness upon earth and not to get away from earth into a higher world or some supreme Absolute. The old yogas (not quite all of them) tended the other way — but that was, I think, because they found the earth as it is a rather impossible place for any spiritual being and the resistance to change too obstinate to be borne; earth-nature looked to them in Vivekananda's simile like the dog's tail which, every time you straighten it, goes back to its original curl. But the fundamental proposition in this matter was proclaimed very definitely in the Upanishads which went so far as to say that Earth is the foundation and all the worlds are on the earth and to imagine a clean-cut or irreconcilable difference between them is ignorance: here and not elsewhere, not by going to some other world, the divine realisation must come. This statement was used to justify a purely individual realisation, but it can equally be the basis of a wider endeavour.

About polytheism, I certainly accept the truth of the many forms and personalities of the One which since the Vedic times has been the spiritual essence of Indian polytheism — a secondary aspect in the seeking for the One and only Divine. But the passage referred to by Professor Sorley[1] is concerned with something else — the little godlings and Titans spoken of there are supraphysical beings of other planes. It is not meant to be suggested that they are real Godheads and entitled to worship — on the contrary, it is indicated that to accept their influence is to move towards error and confusion or a deviation from the true spiritual way. No doubt, they have some power to create, they are makers of forms in their own way and in their limited domain, but so are men too creators of outward and of inward things in their own domain and limits — and, even, man's creative powers can have repercussions on the supraphysical levels.

I agree that asceticism can be overdone. It has its place as one means — not the only one — of self-mastery; but asceticism that cuts away life is an exaggeration, though one that had many remarkable results which perhaps could hardly have come otherwise. The play of forces in this world is enigmatic, escaping from any rigid rule of the reason, and even an exaggeration like that is often employed to bring about something needed for the full development of human achievement and knowledge and experience. But it was an exaggeration all the same and not, as it claimed to be, the indispensable path to the true goal.

[1] "Or there is the opposite danger that he may become the instrument of some apparently brilliant but ignorant formation; for these intermediate planes are full of little Gods or strong Daityas..."

I find nothing to object to in Prof. Sorley's comment on the still, bright and clear mind, for it adequately indicates the process by which the mind makes itself ready for the reflection of the higher Truth in its undisturbed surface or substance. One thing perhaps needs to be kept in view — this pure stillness of the mind is always the required condition, the desideratum, but to bring it about there are more ways than one. It is not, for instance, only by an effort of the mind itself to get clear of all intrusive emotion or passion or of its own characteristic vibrations or of the obscuring fumes of a physical inertia which brings about the sleep or torpor of the mind instead of its wakeful silence that the thing can be done — for this is only the ordinary process of the yogic path of knowledge. It can happen also by a descent from above of a great spiritual stillness imposing silence on the mind and heart and the life stimuli and the physical reflexes. A sudden descent of this kind or a series of descents accumulative in force and efficacy is a well-known phenomenon of spiritual experience. Or again one may start a process of one kind or another for the purpose which would normally mean a long labour and be seized, even at the outset, by a rapid intervention or manifestation of the Silence with an effect out of all proportion to the means used at the beginning. One commences with a method, but the work is taken up by a Grace from above, from That to which one aspires or an irruption of the infinitudes of the Spirit. It was in this last way that I myself came by the mind's absolute silence, unimaginable to me before I had its actual experience.

There is another point of some importance, — the exact nature of this brightness, clearness, stillness, — of what it is constituted, whether it is merely a psychological condition or something more. Professor Sorley says these words are after all metaphors and he wants to express and succeeds in expressing the same thing in a more abstract language. But I was not conscious of using metaphors when I wrote the phrase, though I am aware that the words could to others have that appearance. I think even that they would seem to one who had half the same experience not only a more vivid but a more accurate description of this inner state than any more abstract language could give. It is true that metaphors, symbols, images are constant auxiliaries summoned by the mystic for the expression of his experiences: that is inevitable because he has to express, in a language made or at least developed and manipulated by the mind, the phenomena of a consciousness other than the mental and at once more complex and more subtly concrete. It is this subtle concrete, supersensuously sensible reality of the pheno-mena of that consciousness to which the mystic arrives, that justi-fies the use of metaphor and image as a more living and accurate transcription than the abstract terms which intellectual reflection employs for its own characteristic process. If the images used are misleading or not descriptively accurate, it is because the writer has a force of expression inadequate to the intensity of his experience. The scientist speaks of light-waves or of sound-waves and in doing so he uses a metaphor, but one which corres-ponds to the physical fact and is perfectly applicable — for there is no reason why there should not be a wave, a constant flowing movement of light or of sound as well as of water. But when I speak of the mind's brightness, clearness, stillness, I have no idea of calling metaphor to my aid. It was meant to be a descrip-tion as precise and positive as if I were describing in the same way an expanse of air or a sheet of water. For the mystic's experience of mind — especially when it falls still — is not that of an abstract condition or a falling off or of some unseizable element of the consciousness, it is an experience of an extended subtle substance in which there can be and are waves, currents, vibra-tions not material but still as definite, perceptible, controllable by an inner sense as any movement of material energy or subs-tance by the physical senses. The stillness of the mind means first the falling to rest of the habitual thought movements, thought formations, thought currents which agitate the mind-substance, and that for many is a sufficient mental silence. But even in this repose of all thought movements or movements of feelings, when one looks more closely at it, one sees that this mind-substance is in a constant state of very subtle vibration, not at first easily observable, but afterwards quite evident — and that state of constant vibration may be as harmful to the exact reflection or reception of the descending Truth as any more formed thought movement — for it is the source of a mentalisation which can diminish or distort the authenticity of the higher Truth or break it up into mental refractions. When I speak of a still mind, I mean one in which these disturbances are no longer there. As they fall quiet one can feel the increasing stillness and a resultant clearness as palpable as one can perceive the stillness and clearness of a physical atmosphere. What I describe as the brightness — there is another element — is resolved into a phenomenon of Light common in mystic experience. That Light is not a metaphor — as when Goethe called for more light in his last moments — it presents itself as a very positive illumination actually seen and felt by the inner sense. The brightness of the still and clear mind is also a positive reflection of this Light before the Light itself manifests — and this reflection of the Light is a very necessary condition for a growing capacity of penetrability by the Truth one has to receive and harbour. I have emphasised this part of the subject at a little length because it helps to bring out the difference between the abstract mental and the concrete mystic perception of supraphysical things which is the source of much misunderstanding between the spiritual seeker and the intellectual thinker. Even when they speak the same language it is a different order of perceptions to which the language refers the products of two different grades of consciousness and even in their agreement there is often a certain gulf of difference.

That brings us straight to the question raised by Professor Sorley, what is the relation of mystic or spiritual experience and is it true, as it is contended, that the mystic must, whether as to the validity of his experience itself or the validity of his expression of it, accept the intellect as the judge. It is very plain that in the experience itself the intellect cannot claim to put its limits or its law on an endeavour whose very aim, principle and matter is to go beyond the domain of the ordinary earth-ruled and sense-ruled mental intelligence. It is as if I were asked to climb a mountain with a rope around my feet attaching me to the terrestrial level or to fly only on condition that I keep my feet on the earth while I do it. It may be the safest thing to walk on earth and be on firm ground always and to ascend on wings or otherwise may be to risk a collapse and all sorts of accidents of error, illusion, extravagance, hallucination or what not — the usual charges of the positive earth-walking intellect against mystic experience; but I have to take the risk if I want to do it at all. The reasoning intellect bases itself on man's normal experience and on the workings of a surface external perception and conception of things which is at its ease only when working on a mental basis formed by terrestrial experience and its accumulated data. The mystic goes beyond into a region where this mental basis falls away, where these data are exceeded, where there is another law and canon of perception and knowledge. His entire business is to break through these borders into another consciousness which looks at things in a different way and though this new consciousness may include the data of the ordinary external intelligence it cannot be limited by them or bind itself to see from the intellectual standpoint or in accordance with its way of conceiving, reasoning, established interpretation of experience. A mystic entering the domain of the occult or of the spirit with the intellect as his only or his supreme light or guide would risk seeing nothing or else arriving only at a mental realisation already laid down for him by the speculations of the intellectual thinker.

There is, no doubt, a strain of spiritual thought in India which compromises with the modern intellectual demand and admits Reason as a supreme judge, but they speak of a Reason which in its turn is prepared to compromise and accept the data of spiritual experience as valid *per se*. That, in a sense, is just what the Indian philosophers have always done; for they have tried to establish generalisations drawn from spiritual experience by the light of metaphysical reasoning, but on the basis of that experience and with the evidence of the spiritual seekers as a supreme proof ranking higher than intellectual speculation or experience. In that way the freedom of spiritual and mystic experience is preserved, the reasoning intellect comes in only on the second line as a judge of the generalised statements drawn from the experience. This is, I presume, something akin to

Prof. Sorley's position — he concedes that the experience itself is of the domain of the Ineffable, but as soon as I begin to interpret it, to state it, I fall back into the domain of the thinking mind, I use its terms and ways of thought and expression and must accept the intellect as judge. If I do not, I knock away the ladder by which I have climbed — through mind to Beyond-Mind — and I am left in the air. It is not quite clear whether the truth of my experience itself is supposed to be invalidated by this unsustained position in the air, but it remains at any rate something aloof and incommunicable without support or any consequences for thought or life. There are three propositions, I suppose, which I can take as laid down or admitted here and joined together. First, the spiritual experience is itself of the Beyond-Mind, ineffable and, I presume, unthinkable. Next, in the expression, the interpretation of the experience, you are obliged to fall back into the domain of the consciousness you have left and must abide by its judgments, accept the terms and the canons of its law, submit to its verdict; you have abandoned the freedom of the Ineffable and are no longer your master. Last, spiritual truth may be true in itself, to its own self-experience, but any statement of it is liable to error and here the intellect is the sole judge.

I do not think I am prepared to accept any of these affirmations completely as they are. It is true that spiritual and mystic experience carries one first into domains of Other-Mind (and also Other-Life) and then into the Beyond-Mind; it is true also that the ultimate Truth is described as unthinkable, ineffable, unknowable — speech cannot reach there nor mind arrive to it; I may observe that it is so to human mind, but not to itself — for to itself it is described as self-conscient, in some direct supramental way knowable, known, eternally self-aware. And here the question is not of the ultimate realisation of the ultimate Ineffable which, according to many, can only be reached in a supreme trance, *samādhi*, withdrawn from all outer mental or other awareness, but of an experience in a luminous silence of the mind which looks up into the boundlessness of the last illimitable silence into which it is to pass and disappear, but before that unspeakable experience of the Ultimate or disappearance into it, there is possible a descent of at least some Power or Presence of the Reality into the substance of mind along with a modification of mind-substance, an illumination of it, and of this experience an expression of some kind, a rendering into thought ought to be possible. Or let us suppose the Ineffable and Unknowable may have aspects, presentations of it that are not utterly unthinkable and ineffable.

If it were not so, all account of spiritual truth and experience would be impossible. At most one could speculate about it, but that would be an activity very much in the air, even in a void, without support or data, a mere manipulation of all the possible ideas of what might be the Supreme and Ultimate. Apart from that there could be only a certain unaccountable transition by one way or another from consciousness to an incommunicable Supraconscience. That is indeed what much mystical seeking actually reached both in Europe and India. The Christian mystics spoke of a total darkness, a darkness complete and untouched by any mental lights, through which one must pass into that luminous Ineffable. The Indian Sannyasis sought to shed mind altogether and pass into a thought-free trance from which if one returns, no communication or expression could be brought back of what was there except a remembrance of inexpressible existence and bliss. But still there were previous experiences of the supreme mystery, formulations of the Highest or the occult universal Existence which were held to be spiritual truth and on the basis of which the seers and mystics did not hesitate to formulate their experience and the thinkers to build on it numberless philosophies and books of exegesis. The only question that remains is what creates the possibility of this communication and expression, this transmission of the facts of a different order of consciousness to the mind and what determines the validity of the expression or, even, of the original experience. If no valid account were possible there could be no question of the judgment of the intellect — only the grotesque contradiction of sitting down to speak of the Ineffable, think of the Unthinkable, comprehend the Incommunicable and Unknowable.

*
**

I have read Leonard Woolf's article, but I do not propose to deal with it in my comments on Professor Sorley's letter — for apart from the ignorant denunciation and cheap satire in which it deals, there is nothing much in its statement of the case against spiritual thought or experience; its reasoning is superficial and springs from an entire misunderstanding of the case for the mystic. There are four main arguments he sets against it and none of them has any value.

Argument number one. Mysticism and mystics have always risen in times of decadence, of the ebb of life and their loud quacking is a symptom of the decadence. This argument is absolutely untrue. In the East the great spiritual movements have arisen in the full flood of a people's life and culture or on a rising tide and they have themselves given a powerful impulse of expression and richness to its thought and Art and life; in Greece the mystics and the mysteries were there at the prehistoric beginning and in the middle (Pythagoras was one of the greatest of mystics) and not only in the ebb and decline; the mystic cults flourished in Rome when its culture was at high tide; many great spiritual personalities of Italy, France, Spain sprang up in a life that was rich, vivid and not in the least touched with decadence. This hasty and stupid generalisation has no truth in it and therefore no value.

Argument number two. A spiritual experience cannot be taken as a truth (it is a chimera) unless it is proved just as the presence of a chair in the next room can be proved by showing it to the eye. Of course, a spiritual experience cannot be proved in that way, for it does not belong to the order of physical facts and is not physically visible or touchable. The writer's proposition would amount to this that only what is or can easily be evident to everybody without any need of training, development, equipment or personal discovery is to be taken as true. This is a position which, if accepted, would confine knowledge or truth within very narrow limits and get rid of a great deal of human culture. A spiritual peace — the peace that passeth all understanding — is a common experience of the mystics all over the world, it is a fact but a spiritual fact, a fact of the invisible, and when one enters it or it enters into one, one knows that it is a truth of existence and is there all the time behind life and visible things. But how am I to prove these invisible facts to Mr. Leonard Woolf? He will turn away saying that this is the usual decadent quack-quack and pass contemptuously on — perhaps to write another cleverly shallow article on some subject of which he has no personal knowledge or experience.

Argument number three. The generalisations based on spiritual experience are irrational as well as unproven. Irrational in what way? Are they merely foolish and inconceivable or do they belong to a suprarational order of experience to which the ordinary intellectual canons do not apply because these are founded on phenomena as they appear to the external mind and sense and not to an inner realisation which surpasses these phenomena? That is the contention of the mystics and it cannot be dismissed by merely saying that as these generalisations do not agree with the ordinary experience, therefore they are nonsense and false. I do not undertake to defend all that Joad or Radhakrishnan may have written — such as the statement that the "universe is good" — but I cannot admit about many of these statements condemned by the writer that they are irrational at all. "Integrating the personality" may have no meaning to him, it has a very clear meaning to me, for it is a truth of experience — and, if modern psychology is to be believed, it is not irrational, since there is in our being not only a conscious but an unconscious or subconscious or concealed subliminal part and it is not impossible to become aware of both and make some kind of integration. To transcend both also may have a rational meaning if we admit that as there is a subconscious so there may be a superconscious part of our being; to reconcile disparate parts of our nature or our experience is also not such a ridiculous or meaningless phrase. It is not absurd to say that the doctrine of Karma reconciles determinism and free-willism, since it supposes that our own past action and therefore our past will determine to a great extent the present results, but not so as to exclude a present will modifying them and creating a fresh determinism of our existence yet to be. The phrase about the value of the world is quite intelligible when we see that it refers to a progressive value, not determined by the good or bad experience of the moment, a value of existence developing through time and taken as a whole. As for the statement about God, it has no meaning if it is taken in connection with the superficial idea of the Divine current in popular religion, but it is a perfectly logical result of the premises that there is an Infinite and Eternal which is manifesting in itself Time and things that are phenomenally finite. One may accept or reject this complex idea of the Divine which is founded on co-ordination of the data of long spiritual experience passed through by thousands of seekers in all times, but I fail to see why it should be considered unreasonable. If it is because that means "to have it not only in both ways but in every way", I do not see why that should be so reprehensible and inadmissible. There can be after all a synthetic and global view and consciousness of things which is not bound by the oppositions and divisions of a mere analytical and selective or dissecting intelligence.

Argument number four. The plea of intuition is only a cover for the inability to explain or establish by the use of reason — Joad and Radhakrishnan reason, but take refuge in intuition where their reasoning fails. Can the issue be settled in so easy and trenchant a way? The fact is that the mystic depends on an inner knowledge, an inner experience; but if he. philosophises, he must try to explain to the reason, though not necessary always by the reason alone, what he has seen to be the Truth. He cannot but say, "I am explaining a truth which is beyond outer phenomena and the intelligence which depends on phenomena; it really depends on a certain kind of direct experience and the intuitive knowledge which arises from that experience, it cannot be adequately communicated by symbols appropriate to the world of outer phenomena, yet I am obliged to do as well as I can with these to help me towards some statement which will be intellectually acceptable to you." There is no wickedness or deceitful cunning therefore in using metaphors and symbols with a cautionary "as it were", as in the simile of the focus, which is surely not intended as an argument but as a suggestive image. I may observe in passing that the writer himself takes refuge in metaphor frequently, beginning with the quack-quack and Joad might well reply that he does so in order to damn the opposite

side, while avoiding the necessity of a sound philosophical reply
to the philosophy he dislikes and repudiates. An intensity of belief is not the measure of truth, but neither is an intensity of
unbelief the right measure.

As to the real nature of intuition and its relation to the intellectual mind, that is quite another and very large and complex
question which I cannot deal with here. I have confined myself
to pointing out that this article is quite inadequate and superficial criticism. A case can be made against spiritual experience
and spiritual philosophy and its positions, but to deserve a serious
reply it must be put forward by a better advocate and it must
touch the real centre of the problem, which lies here. As there is
a category of facts to which our senses are our best available but
very imperfect guides, as there is a category of truths which we
seek by the keen but still imperfect light of our reason, so according to the mystic, there is a category of more subtle truths
which surpass the reach both of the senses and the reason but
can be ascertained by an inner direct knowledge and direct experience. These truths are supersensuous, but not the less real for
that: they have immense results upon the consciousness changing
its substance and movement, bringing especially deep peace and
abiding joy, a great light of vision and knowledge, a possibility
of the overcoming of the lower animal nature, vistas of a spiritual
self-development which without them do not exist. A new outlook on things arises which brings with it, if fully pursued into its
consequences, a great liberation, inner harmony, unification
— many other possibilities besides. These things have been
experienced, it is true, by a small minority of the human race,
but still there has been a host of independent witnesses to them
in all times, climes and conditions and numbered among them
are some of the greatest intelligences of the past, some of the
world's most remarkable figures. Must these possibilities be
immediately condemned as chimeras because they are not only
beyond the average man in the street but also not easily seizable
even by many cultivated intellects or because their method is
more difficult than that of the ordinary sense or reason? If there
is any truth in them, is not this possibility opened by them worth
pursuing as disclosing a highest range of self-discovery and world

discovery by the human soul? At its best, taken as true, it must be that — at its lowest taken as only a possibility, as all things attained by man have been only a possibility in their earlier stages, it is a great and may well be a most fruitful adventure.

II

I do not think anything can be said that would convince one who starts from exactly the opposite viewpoint to the spiritual, the way of looking at things of a Victorian agnostic. His points of doubt about the value — other than subjective and purely individual — of yoga experience are that it does not aim at scientific truth and cannot be said to achieve ultimate truth because the experiences are coloured by the individuality of the seer. One might ask whether Science itself has arrived at any ultimate truth; on the contrary, ultimate truth even on the physical plane seems to recede as Science advances. Science started on the assumption that the ultimate truth must be physical and objective — and the objective Ultimate (or even less than that) would explain all subjective phenomena. Yoga proceeds on the opposite view that the ultimate Truth is spiritual and subjective and it is in that ultimate Light that we must view objective phenomena. It is the two opposite poles and the gulf is as wide as it can be.

Yoga, however, is scientific to this extent that it proceeds by subjective experiment and bases all its findings on experience; mental intuitions are admitted only as a first step and are not considered as realisation — they must be confirmed by being translated into and justified by experience. As to the value of the experience itself, it is doubted by the physical mind because it is subjective, not objective. But has the distinction much value? Is not all knowledge and experience subjective at bottom? Objective external physical things are seen very much in the same way by human beings because of the construction of the mind and senses; with another construction of mind and sense quite another account of the physical world would be given — Science itself has made that very clear. But your friend's point is that the

yoga experience is individual, coloured by the individuality of
the seer. It may be true to a certain extent of the precise form
or transcription given to the experience in certain domains; but
even here the difference is superficial. It is a fact that yogic experience runs everywhere on the same lines. Certainly, there are,
not one line, but many; for, admittedly, we are dealing with a
many-sided Infinite to which there are and must be many ways
of approach; but yet the broad lines are the same everywhere
and the intuitions, experiences, phenomena are the same in ages
and countries far apart from each other and systems practised
quite independently from each other. The experiences of the
mediaeval European *bhakta* or mystic are precisely the same in
substance, however differing in names, forms, religious colouring,
etc., as those of the mediaeval Indian *bhakta* or mystic — yet
these people were not corresponding with one another or aware
of each other's experiences and results as are modern scientists
from New York to Yokohama. That would seem to show that
there is something there identical, universal and presumably true
— however the colour of the translation may differ because of
the difference of mental language.

As for ultimate Truth, I suppose both the Victorian agnostic
and, let us say, the Indian Vedantin may agree that it is veiled but
there. Both speak of it as the Unknowable; the only difference
is that the Vedantin says it is unknowable by the mind and inexpressible by speech, but still attainable by something deeper or
higher than the mental perception, while even mind can reflect
and speech express the thousand aspects it presents to the mind's
outward and inward experience. The Victorian agnostic would,
I suppose, cancel this qualification; he would pronounce for the
doubtful existence and, if existent, for the absolute unknowable-
ness of this Unknowable.

You ask me whether you have to give up your predilection for
testing before accepting and to accept everything in yoga *a priori*
— and by testing you mean testing by the ordinary reason. The
only answer I can give to that is that the experiences of yoga
belong to an inner domain and go according to a law of their

own, have their own method of perception, criteria and all the rest of it which are neither those of the domain of the physical senses nor of the domain of rational or scientific enquiry. Just as scientific enquiry passes beyond that of the physical senses and enters the domain of the infinite and infinitesimal about which the senses can say nothing and test nothing — for one cannot see and touch an electron or know by the evidence of the sense-mind whether it exists or not or decide by that evidence whether the earth really turns round the sun and not rather the sun round the earth as our senses and all our physical experience daily tell us — so the spiritual search passes beyond the domain of scientific or rational enquiry and it is impossible by the aid of the ordinary positive reason to test the data of spiritual experience and decide whether those things exist or not or what is their law and nature. As in Science, so here you have to accumulate experience on experience, following faithfully the methods laid down by the Guru or by the systems of the past, you have to develop an intuitive discrimination which compares the experiences, see what they mean, how far and in what field each is valid, what is the place of each in the whole, how it can be reconciled or related with others that at first might seem to contradict it, etc., etc., until you can move with a secure knowledge in the vast field of spiritual phenomena. That is the only way to test spiritual experience. I have myself tried the other method and I have found it absolutely incapable and inapplicable. On the other hand, if you are not prepared to go through all that yourself, — as few can do except those of extraordinary spiritual stature — you have to accept the leading of a Master, as in Science you accept a teacher instead of going through the whole field of Science and its experimentation all by yourself — at least until you have accumulated sufficient experience and knowledge. If that is accepting things *a priori*, well, you have to accept *a priori*. For I am unable to see by what valid tests you propose to make the ordinary reason the judge of what is beyond it.

You quote the sayings of V or X. I would like to know before assigning a value to these utterances what they actually did for the testing of their spiritual perceptions and experiences. How did V test the value of his spiritual experiences — some of them not easily credible to the ordinary positive mind any more than the miracles attributed to some famous yogis? I know nothing about X, but what were his tests and how did he apply them? What are his methods? his criteria? It seems to me that no ordinary mind will accept the apparition of Buddha out of a wall or the half hour's talk with Hayagriva as valid facts by any kind of testing. It would either have to accept them *a priori* or on the sole evidence of V, which comes to the same thing, or to reject them *a priori* as hallucinations or mere mental images accompanied in one case by an auditive hallucination. I fail to see how it could "test" them. Or how was I to test by the ordinary mind my experience of Nirvana? To what conclusion could I come about it by the aid of the ordinary positive reason? How could I test its validity? I am at a loss to imagine. I did the only thing I could — to accept it as a strong and valid truth of experience, let it have its full play and produce its full experimental consequences until I had sufficient yogic knowledge to put it in its place. Finally, how without inner knowledge or experience can you or anyone else test the inner knowledge and experience of others?

I have often said that discrimination is not only perfectly admissible but indispensable in spiritual experience. But it must be a discrimination founded on knowledge, not a reasoning founded on ignorance. Otherwise you tie up your mind and hamper experience by preconceived ideas which are as much *a priori* as any acceptance of a spiritual truth or experience can be. Your idea that surrender can only come by love is a point in instance. It is perfectly true in yogic experience that surrender by true love, which means psychic and spiritual love, is the most powerful, simple and effective of all, but one cannot, putting that forward as a dictum arrived at by the ordinary reason, shut up the whole of possible experience of surrender into that formula or announce on its strength that one must wait till one loves perfectly before one can surrender. Yogic experience shows that surrender can also be made by the mind and will, a clear and sincere mind seeing the necessity of surrender and a clear and sincere will enforcing it on the recalcitrant members. Also, experience shows that not only can surrender come by love, but love also can come by surrender or grow with it from an imperfect to a perfect love. One starts by an intense idea and will to know or reach the Divine and surrenders more and more one's ordinary personal ideas, desires, attachments, urges to action or habits of action so that the Divine may take up everything. Surrender means that, to give up our little mind and its mental ideas and preferences into a divine Light and a greater Knowledge, our petty personal troubled blind stumbling will into a great, calm, tranquil, luminous Will and Force, our little, restless, tormented feelings into a wide intense divine Love and Ananda, our small suffering personality into the one Person of which it is an obscure outcome. If one insists on one's own ideas and reasonings, the greater Light and Knowledge cannot come or else is marred and obstructed in the coming at every step by a lower interference; if one insists on one's desires and fancies, that great luminous Will and Force cannot act in its own true power — for you ask it to be the servant of your desires; if one refuses to give up one's petty ways of feeling, eternal Love and supreme Ananda cannot descend or are mixed and spilt from the effervescing crude emotional vessel. No amount of ordinary reasoning can get rid of the necessity of surmounting the lower in order that the higher may be there.

And if some find that retirement is the best way of giving oneself to the Higher, to the Divine by avoiding as much as possible occasions for the bubbling up of the lower, why not? The aim they have come for is that, and why blame or look with distrust and suspicion on the means they find best or daub it with disparaging adjectives to discredit it — grim, inhuman and the rest? It is your vital that shrinks from it and your vital mind that supplies these epithets which express only your shrinking and not what the retirement really is. For it is the vital or its social part that shrinks from solitude; the thinking mind does not but rather courts it. The poet seeks solitude with himself or with Nature to listen to his inspiration; the thinker plunges into solitude to meditate on things and commune with a deeper knowledge; the scientist shuts himself up in his laboratory to pore by experiment into the secrets of Nature; these retirements are not grim and inhuman. Neither is the retirement of the sadhak into the exclusive concentration of which he feels the need; it is a means to the end — to the end on which his whole heart is set. As for the yogin or Bhakta who has already begun to have the fundamental experience, he is not in a grim and inhuman solitude. The Divine and all the world are there in the being of the one, the supreme Beloved or his Ananda is there in the heart of the other.

I say this as against your depreciation of retirement founded on ignorance of what it really is; but I do not, as I have often said, recommend a total seclusion, for I hold that to be a dangerous expedient which may lead to morbidity and much error. Nor do I impose retirement on anyone as a method or approve of it unless the person himself seeks it, feels its necessity, has the joy of it and the personal proof that it helps to the spiritual experience. It is not to be imposed on anyone as a principle, for that is the mental way of doing things, the way of the ordinary mind — it is as a need that it has to be accepted, when it is felt as a need, not as a general law or rule.

What you describe in your letter as the response of the Divine would not be called that in the language of yogic experience — this feeling of great peace, light, ease, trust, difficulties lessening, certitude would rather be called a response of your own nature to the Divine. There is a Peace or Light which is the response of the Divine, but that is a wide Peace, a great Light which is felt as a presence other than one's personal self, not part of one's personal nature, but something that comes from above, though in the end it possesses the nature — or there is the Presence itself which carries with it indeed the absolute liberation, happiness, certitude. But the first responses of the Divine are not often like that — they come rather as a touch, a pressure one must be in a condition to recognise and to accept, or it is a voice of assurance, sometimes a very "still small voice", a momentary Image or Presence, a whisper of Guidance sometimes, there are many forms it may take. Then it withdraws and the preparation of the nature goes on till it is possible for the touch to come again and again, to last longer, to change into something more pressing and near and intimate. The Divine in the beginning does not impose himself — he asks for recognition, for acceptance. That is one reason why the mind must fall silent, not put tests, not make claims — there must be room for the true intuition which recognises at once the true touch and accepts it.

Then for the tumultuous activity of the mind which prevents your concentration. But that or else a more tiresome, obstinate, grinding, mechanical activity is always the difficulty when one tries to concentrate and it takes a long time to get the better of it. That or the habit of sleep which prevents either the waking concentration or the conscious samadhi or the absorbed and all-excluding trance which are the three forms that yogic concentration takes. But it is surely ignorance of yoga, its process and its difficulties that makes you feel desperate and pronounce yourself unfit for ever because of this quite ordinary obstacle. The insistence of the ordinary mind and its wrong reasonings, sentiments and judgments, the random activity of the thinking mind in concentration or its mechanical activity, the slowness of response to the veiled or the initial touch are the ordinary obstacles the mind imposes, just as pride, ambition, vanity, sex, greed, grasping of things for one's own ego are the difficulties and obstacles offered by the vital. As the vital difficulties can be fought down and conquered, so can the mental. Only one has to see that these are inevitable obstacles and neither cling to them nor be terrified or overwhelmed because they are there. One has to persevere till one can stand back from the mind as from the vital and feel the deeper and larger mental and vital Purushas within one which are capable of silence, capable of a straight receptivity of the true Word and Force as of the true silence. If the nature takes the way of fighting down the difficulties first, then the first half of the way is long and tedious and the complaint of the want of the response of the Divine arises. But really the Divine is there all the time, working behind the veil as well as waiting for the recognition of his response and for the response to the response to be possible.

One feels here a stream from the direct sources of Truth that one does not meet so often as one could desire. Here is a mind that can not only think but see — and not merely see the surfaces of things with which most intellectual thought goes on wrestling without end or definite issue and as if there were nothing else, but look into the core. The Tantriks have a phrase *paśyantī vāk* to describe one level of the Vak-Shakti, the seeing Word; here is *paśyantī buddhi*, a seeing intelligence. It might be because the seer within has passed beyond thought into experience, but there are many who have a considerable wealth of experience without its clarifying their eye of thought to this extent; the soul feels, but the mind goes on with mixed and imperfect transcriptions, blurs and confusions in the idea. There must have been the gift of right vision lying ready in this nature.

It is an achievement to have got rid so rapidly and decisively of the shimmering mists and fogs which modern intellectualism takes for Light of Truth. The modern mind has so long and persistently wandered — and we with it — in the Valley of the False Glimmer that it is not easy for anyone to disperse its mists with the sunlight of clear vision so soon and entirely as has here been done. All that is said here about modern humanism and humanitarianism, the vain efforts of the sentimental idealist and the ineffective intellectual, about synthetic eclecticism and other kindred things is admirably clear-minded, it hits the target. It is not by these means that humanity can get that radical change of its ways of life which is yet becoming imperative, but only by reaching the bed-rock of Reality behind, — not through mere ideas and mental formations, but by a change of the consciousness, an inner and spiritual conversion. But that is a truth for which it would be difficult to get a hearing in the present noise of all kinds of many-voiced clamour and confusion and catastrophe.

A distinction, the distinction very keenly made here, between the plane of phenomenal process, of externalised Prakriti, and the plane of Divine Reality ranks among the first words of the inner wisdom. The turn given to it in these pages is not merely an ingenious explanation; it expresses very soundly one of the clear certainties you meet when you step across the border and look at the outer world from the standing-ground of the inner spiritual experience. The more you go inward or upward, the more the view of things changes and the outer knowledge Science organises takes its real and very limited place. Science, like most mental and external knowledge, gives you only truth of process.

I would add that it cannot give you even the whole truth of process; for you seize some of the ponderables, but miss the all-important imponderables; you get, hardly even the how, but the conditions under which things happen in Nature. After all the triumphs and marvels of Science the explaining principle, the rationale, the significance of the whole is left as dark, as mysterious and even more mysterious than ever. The scheme it has built up of the evolution not only of this rich and vast and variegated material world, but of life and consciousness and mind and their workings out of a brute mass of electrons, identical and varied only in arrangement and number, is an irrational magic more baffling than any the most mystic imagination could conceive. Science in the end lands us in a paradox effectuated, an organised and rigidly determined accident, an impossibility that has somehow happened, — it has shown us a new, a material Maya, *aghaṭana-ghaṭana-paṭīyasī*, very clever at bringing about the impossible, a miracle that cannot logically be and yet somehow is there actual, irresistibly organised, but still irrational and inexplicable. And this is evidently because Science has missed something essential; it has seen and scrutinised what has happened and in a way how it has happened, but it has shut its eyes to something that made this impossible possible, something it is there to express. There is no fundamental significance in things if you miss the Divine Reality; for you remain embedded in a huge surface crust of manageable and utilisable appearance. It is the magic of the Magician you are trying to analyse, but only when you enter into the consciousness of the Magician himself can you begin to experience the true origination, significance and circles of the Lila. I say "begin" because the Divine Reality is not so simple that at the first touch you can know all of it or put it into a single formula; it is the Infinite and opens before you an infinite knowledge to which all Science put together is a bagatelle. But still you do touch the essential, the eternal behind things and in the light of That all begins to be profoundly luminous, intimately intelligible.

I have once before told you what I think of the ineffective peckings of certain well-intentioned scientific minds on the surface or apparent surface of the spiritual Reality behind things and

I need not elaborate it. More important is the prognostic of a greater danger coming in the new attack by the adversary, the sceptics, against the validity of spiritual and supraphysical experience, their new strategy of destruction by admitting and explaining it in their own sense. There may well be a strong ground for the apprehension; but I doubt whether, if these things are once admitted to scrutiny, the mind of humanity will long remain satisfied with explanations so ineptly superficial and external, explanations that explain nothing. If the defenders of religion take up an unsound position, easily capturable, when they affirm only the subjective validity of spiritual experience, the opponents also seem to me to be giving away, without knowing it, the gates of the materialistic stronghold by their consent at all to admit and examine spiritual and supraphysical experience. Their entrenchment in the physical field, their refusal to admit or even examine supraphysical things was their tower of strong safety; once it is abandoned, the human mind pressing towards something less negative, more helpfully positive will pass to it over the dead bodies of their theories and the broken debris of their annulling explanations and ingenious psychological labels. Another danger may then arise, — not of a final denial of the Truth, but the repetition in old or new forms of a past mistake, on one side some revival of blind fanatical obscurantist sectarian religionism, on the other a stumbling into the pits and quagmires of the vitalistic occult and the pseudo-spiritual — mistakes that made the whole real strength of the materialistic attack on the past and its credos. But these are phantasms that meet us always on the border line or in the intervening country between the material darkness and the perfect Splendour. In spite of all, the victory of the supreme Light even in the darkened earth-consciousness stands as the one ultimate certitude.

Art, poetry, music are not yoga, not in themselves things spiritual any more than philosophy is a thing spiritual or Science. There lurks here another curious incapacity of the modern intellect — its inability to distinguish between mind and spirit, its readiness to mistake mental, moral and aesthetic idealisms for spirituality and their inferior degrees for spiritual values. It is mere truth that the mental intuitions of the metaphysician or the poet for the most part fall far short of a concrete spiritual experience; they are distant flashes, shadowy reflections, not rays from the centre of Light. It is not less true that, looked at from the peaks, there is not much difference between the high mental eminences and the lower climbings of this external existence. All the energies of the Lila are equal in the sight from above, all are disguises of the Divine. But one has to add that all can be turned into a first means towards the realisation of the Divine. A philosophic statement about the Atman is a mental formula, not knowledge, not experience; yet sometimes the Divine takes it as a channel of touch; strangely, a barrier in the mind breaks down, something is seen, a profound change operated in some inner part, there enters into the ground of the nature something calm, equal, ineffable. One stands upon a mountain ridge and glimpses or mentally feels a wideness, a pervasiveness, a nameless Vast in Nature; then suddenly there comes the touch, a revelation, a flooding, the mental loses itself in the spiritual, one bears the first invasion of the Infinite. Or you stand before a temple of Kali beside a sacred river and see what? — a sculpture, a gracious piece of architecture, but in a moment mysteriously, unexpectedly there is instead a Presence, a Power, a Face that looks into yours, an inner sight in you has regarded the World-Mother. Similar touches can come through art, music, poetry to their creator or to one who feels the shock of the word, the hidden significance of a form, a message in the sound that carries more perhaps than was consciously meant by the composer. All things in the Lila can turn into windows that open on the hidden Reality. Still so long as one is satisfied with looking through windows, the gain is only initial; one day one will have to take up the pilgrim's staff and start out to journey there where the Reality is for ever manifest and present. Still less can it be spiritually satisfying to remain with shadowy reflections, a search imposes itself for the Light which they strive to figure. But since this Reality and this Light are in ourselves no less than in some high region above the mortal plane, we can in the seeking for it use many of the figures and activities of life; as one offers a flower, a prayer, an act to the Divine, one can offer too a created form of beauty, a song, a poem, an image, a strain of music, and gain through it a contact, a response or an experience. And when that divine consciousness has been entered or when it grows within, then too its expression in life through these things is not excluded from yoga; these creative activities can still have their place, though not intrinsically a greater place than any other that can be put to divine use and service. Art, poetry, music, as they are in their ordinary functioning, create mental and vital, not spiritual values; but they can be turned to a higher end, and then, like all things that are capable of linking our consciousness to the Divine, they are transmuted and become spiritual and can be admitted as part of a life of yoga. All takes new values not from itself, but from the consciousness that uses it; for there is only one thing essential, needful, indispensable, to grow conscious of the Divine Reality and live in it and live it always.

The difficulty is that you are a non-scientist trying to impose your ideas on the most difficult because most material field of science — physics. It is only if you were a scientist yourself basing your ideas on universally acknowledged scientific facts or else your own discoveries — though even then with much difficulty — that you could get a hearing or your opinion have any weight. Otherwise you open yourself to the accusation of pronouncing in a field where you have no authority, just as the scientist himself does when he pronounces on the strength of his discoveries that there is no God. When the scientist says that "scientifically speaking, God is a hypothesis which is no longer necessary" he is talking arrant nonsense — for the existence of God is not and cannot be and never was a scientific hypothesis or problem at all, it is and always has been a spiritual or a metaphysical problem. You cannot speak scientifically about it at all either pro or con. The metaphysician or the spiritual seeker has a right to point out that it is nonsense; but if you lay down the law to the scientist in the field of science, you run the risk of having the same objection turned against you.

As to the unity of all knowledge, that is a thing *in posse*, not yet *in esse*. The mechanical method of knowledge leads to certain results, the higher method leads to certain others, and they at many points fundamentally disagree. How is the difference to be bridged — for each seems valid in its own field; it is a problem to be solved, but you cannot solve it in the way you propose. Least of all in the field of physics. In psychology one can say that the mechanical or physiological approach takes hold of the thing by the blind end and is the least fruitful of all — for psychology is not primarily a thing of mechanism and measure, it opens to a vast field beyond the physical instrumentalities of the body-consciousness. In biology one can get a glimpse of something beyond mechanism, because there is from the beginning a stir of consciousness progressing and organising itself more and more for self-expression. But in physics you are in the very domain of the mechanical law where process is everything and the driving consciousness has chosen to conceal itself with the greatest thoroughness — so that, "scientifically speaking", it does not exist there. One can discover it there only by occultism and yoga, but the methods of occult science and of yoga are not measurable or followable by the means of physical science — so the gulf remains still in existence. It may be bridged one day, but the physicist is not likely to be the bridge-builder, so it is no use asking him to try what is beyond his province.

The desire [of the occultists and the spiritists] to satisfy the physical scientists is absurd and illogical. The physical scientists have their own field with its own instruments and standards. To apply the same tests to phenomena of a different kind is as foolish as to apply physical tests to spiritual truth. One can't dissect God or see the soul under a microscope. So also the subjection of disembodied spirits or even of psycho-physical phenomena to tests and standards valid only for material phenomena is a most false and unsatisfactory method. Moreover, the physical scientist is for the most part resolved not to admit what cannot be neatly packed and labelled and docketed in his own system and its formulas. Dr. Jules Romains, himself a scientist as well as a great writer, makes experiments to prove that man can see and read with the eyes blindfolded, the scientists refuse even to admit or record the results. Khuda Baksh comes along and proves it patently, indubitably, under all legitimate tests, the scientists are quite unwilling to cede and record the fact even though his results are undeniable. He walks on fire unhurt and disproves all hitherto suggested explanations, — they simply cast about for another and still more silly explanation! What is the use of trying to convince people who are determined not to believe?

The scientific mind refuses to leave anything unclassed. Has it not classified the Divine also?

The minds of these people [the scientists] are too much accustomed to deal with physical things and things measurable by instruments and figures to be much good for any other provinces. Einstein's views outside his domain are crude and childish, a sort of unsubstantial commonplace idealism without grasp on realities. As a man can be a great scholar and yet simple and foolish, so a man can be a great scientist but his mind and ideas negligible in other things.

Psychologists of course having to deal with mental movements more easily recognise that there can be no real equation between them and physiological processes and at the most mind and body react on each other as is inevitable since they are lodging together. But even a great physical scientist like Huxley recognised that mind was something quite different from matter and could not possibly be explained in the terms of matter. Only since then physical Science became very arrogant and presumptuous and tried to subject everything to itself and its processes. Now in theory it has begun to recognise its limitations in a general way, but the old mentality is still too habitual in most scientists to shake off yet.

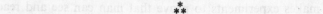

[1] The article reads as if it had been written by a professor rather than a philosopher. What you speak of is, I suppose, a survival of the nineteenth-century scientific contempt for metaphysics; all thinking must be based on scientific *facts* and the generalisations of science, often so faulty and ephemeral, must be made the basis for any sound metaphysical thinking. That is to make philosophy the handmaid of science, metaphysics the camp-follower of physics and to deny her her sovereign rights in her own city. It ignores the fact that the philosopher has his own domain and his own instruments; he may use scientific discoveries as material just as he may use any other facts of existence, but whatever generalisations science offers he must judge by his own standards — whether they are valid for transference to the metaphysical plane and, if so, how far. Still in the heyday of physical science before it discovered its own limitations and the shakiness of its scheme of things floating precariously in a huge infinity or boundless Finite of the Unknown, there was perhaps some excuse for such an attitude. But spiritualism glorified under the name of psychical research? That is not a science; it is a mass of obscure and ambiguous documents from which you can draw only a few meagre and doubtful genera-

---

[1] This is in reply to the points raised by a disciple in the following letter to Sri Aurobindo:

"On p. 511 of *The Listener* of March 28, 1934 there are a couple of surprising assumptions — first, that metaphysics is one among the experimental sciences and has a darkened *séance* room for its laboratory — and secondly, that *survival* need not be distinguished from *immortality*. In the interests of clearness, most philosophical thinkers have made this distinction; it is odd that it should be ignored when such a polemic is being launched against them.... Of course, if one has a turn for practical experimenting in *science*, it is no doubt admirable to employ it in psychical investigation — but (unless it is assumed that all cultured human beings, or all philosophers at least, should possess and cultivate this gift) why are the majority of philosophers to be blamed for finding the results up-to-date obscure and meagre and for following their bent in confining themselves to *metaphysical* studies proper?"

(Regarding a dream about a long-distance telephone conversation with an acquaintance.) "In actual life I think a telephone can be far less satisfactory than an exchange of letters. Is there not something very symbolic about the emergence of telephony and cinematography just at an epoch when human behaviour and relationship is breaking down? Owing to falsehood and callousness and self-centred indifference to others, each person is to every other more and more a meaningless shadow and a deceptive voice. In *The Manchester Guardian's* musical critic's remarks on an Elgar Memorial Concert there are some good points about 'the reaction working against nobility and tenderness in art'. I fail to see any further need for human beings either as creators or enjoyers of such 'art' as can still fall within the canons of fashion; perhaps, however, in an Asuric civilisation, men are anyhow superfluous and only 'incarnated Asuras' are required?"

lisations. Moreover, so far as it belongs to the occult, it touches only the inferior regions of the occult — what we would call the lowest vital worlds — where there is as much falsehood and fake and confused error as upon the earth and even more. What is a philosopher to do with all that obscure and troubled matter? I do not catch the point of many of his remarks. Why should a prediction of a future event alter our conception — at least any philosophic conception — of Time? It can alter one's ideas of the relation of events to each other or of the working out of forces or of the possibilities of consciousness, but Time remains the same as before.

The dream is, of course, the rendering of an attempt at communication on the subtle plane. As for the telephone and cinema, there is something of what you say, but it seems to me that these and other modern things could have taken on a different character if they had been accepted and used in a different spirit. Mankind was not ready for these discoveries, in the spiritual sense, nor even, if the present confusions are a sign, intellectually ready. The aesthetic downfall is perhaps due to other causes, a disappointed idealism in its recoil generating its opposite, a dry and cynical intellectualism which refuses to be duped by the ideal, romantic or the emotional or anything that is higher than the reason walking by the light of the senses. The Asuras of the past were after all often rather big beings; the trouble about the present ones is that they are not really Asuras, but beings of the lower vital world, violent, brutal and ignoble, but above all narrow-minded, ignorant and obscure. But this kind of cynical narrow intellectualism that is rampant now, does not last — it prepares its own end by increasing dryness — men begin to feel the need of new springs of life.

I do not think the two questions you put are of much importance from the viewpoint of spiritual sadhana.

1. The question about science and spirituality would have been of some moment some twenty years ago and it filled the minds of men in the earlier years of the twentieth century, but it

is now out of date. Science itself has come to the conclusion that it cannot, as it once hoped, determine what is the truth of the things or their real nature, or what is behind physical phenomena; it can only deal with the process of physical things and how they come about or on what lines men can deal with and make use of them. In other words, the field of physical science has been now definitely marked off and limited and questions about God or the ultimate Reality or other metaphysical or spiritual problems are outside it. This is at least the case all over continental Europe and it is only in England and America that there is still some attempt to reason about these things on the basis of physical science.

The so-called sciences which deal with the mind and men (psychology, etc.) are so much dependent on physical science that they cannot go beyond narrow limits. If science is to turn her face towards the Divine, it must be a new science not yet developed which deals directly with the forces of the life-world and of Mind and so arrives at what is beyond Mind; but present-day science cannot do that.

2. From the spiritual point of view such temporary phenomena as the turn of the educated Hindus towards materialism are of little importance. There have always been periods when the mind of nations, continents or cultures turned towards materialism and away from all spiritual belief. Such periods came in Europe in the nineteenth century, but they are usually of short duration. Western Europe has already lost its faith in materialism and is seeking for something else, either turning back to old religions or groping for something new. Russia and Asia are now going through the same materialistic wave. These waves come because of a certain necessity in human development — to destroy the bondage of old forms and leave a field for new truth and new forms of truth and action in life as well as for what is behind life.

I think X bases his ideas on the attempt of Jeans, Eddington and other English scientists to thrust metaphysical conclusions into scientific facts; it is necessary that he should appreciate fully

the objections of more austerely scientific minds to such a mixture. Moreover, spiritual seeking has its own accumulated knowledge which does not depend in the least on the theories or
discoveries of science in the purely physical sphere. X's attempt
like that of Jeans and others is a reaction against the illegitimate
attempts of some scientific minds in the nineteenth century and
of many others who took advantage of the march of scientific
discovery to discredit or abolish as far as possible the religious
spirit and to discredit also metaphysics as a cloudy verbiage,
exalting science as the only clue to the truth of the universe.
But I think that attitude is now dead or moribund; the scientists
recognise, as you point out, the limits of their sphere. I may
observe that the conflict between religion and science never arose
in India (until the days of European education) because religion
did not interfere with scientific discovery and scientists did not
question religious or spiritual truth because the two things were
kept on separate but not opposing lines.

The defect in what X writes about Science seems to be that he is
insisting vehemently on the idea that Science is still materialistic
or at least that scientists, Jeans and Eddington excepted, are still
fundamentally materialists. This is not the fact. Most continental scientists have now renounced the idea that Science can
explain the fundamentals of existence. They hold that Science is
only concerned with process and not with fundamentals. They
declare that it is not the business of Science nor is it within its
means to decide anything about the great questions which concern philosophy and religion. This is the enormous change which
the latest developments of Science have brought about. Science
itself nowadays is neither materialistic nor idealistic. The rock
on which materialism was built and which in the 19th century
seemed unshakable has now been shattered. Materialism has
now become a philosophical speculation just like any other
theory; it cannot claim to found itself on a sort of infallible
Biblical authority, based on the facts and conclusions of Science.
This change can be felt by one like myself who grew up in the

heyday of absolute rule of scientific materialism in the 19th century. The way which had been almost entirely barred, except by rebellion, now lies wide open to spiritual truths, spiritual ideas, spiritual experiences. That is the real revolution. Mentalism is only a half-way house, but mentalism and vitalism are now perfectly possible as hypotheses based on the facts of existence, scientific facts as well as any others. The facts of Science do not compel anyone to take any particular philosophical direction. They are now neutral and can even be used on one side or another though most scientists do not consider such a use as admissible. Nobody here ever said that the new discoveries of Physics supported the ideas of religion or churches; they merely contended that Science had lost its old materialistic dogmatism and moved away by a revolutionary change from its old moorings.

It is this change which I expected and prophesied in my poems in the first *Ahana* volume, "A Vision of Science" and "In the Moonlight".

*
**

I am afraid I have lost all interest in these speculations; things are getting too serious for me to waste time on these inconclusive intellectualities. I do not at all mind your driving your point triumphantly home and replacing a dogmatism from materialistic science on its throne of half a century ago from which it could victoriously ban all thought surpassing its own narrow bounds as mere wordy metaphysics and mysticism and moonshine. Obviously, if material energies alone can exist in the material world, there can be no possibility of a life divine on the earth. A mere metaphysical "sleight of mind", as one might call it, could not justify it against the objections of scientific negation and concrete common sense. I had thought that even many scientific minds on the Continent had come to admit that science could no longer claim to decide what was the real reality of things, that it had no means of deciding it and could only discover and describe the how and process of the operations of material Force in the physical front of things. That left the field open to higher thought and speculation, spiritual experience and even to mysticism, occultism and all those greater things which almost everyone had come to disbelieve as impossible nonsense. That was the condition of things when I was in England. If that is to return or if Russia and her dialectical materialism are to lead the world, well, fate must be obeyed and life divine must remain content to wait perhaps for another millennium. But I do not like the idea of one of our periodicals being the arena for a wrestle of that kind. That is all. I am writing under the impression of your earlier article on this subject, as I have not gone carefully through the later ones; I dare say these later ones may be entirely convincing and I would find after reading them that my own position was wrong and that only an obstinate mystic could still believe in such a conquest of Matter by the Spirit as I had dared to think possible. But I am just such an obstinate mystic; so, if I allowed your exposition of the matter to be published in one of our own periodicals, I would be under the obligation of returning to the subject in which I have lost interest and therefore the inclination to write, so as to re-establish my position and would have to combat the claim of materialistic Science to pronounce anything on these matters on which it has no means of enquiry nor any possibility of arriving at a valid decision. Perhaps I would have practically to rewrite *The Life Divine* as an answer to the victorious "negation of the materialist"! This is the only explanation which I can give, apart from sheer want of time to tackle the subject, for my long and disappointing silence.

I know it is the Russian explanation of the recent trend to spirituality and mysticism that it is a phenomenon of capitalist society in its decadence. But to read an economic cause, conscious or unconscious, into all phenomena of man's history is part of the Bolshevik gospel born of the fallacy of Karl Marx. Man's nature is not so simple and one-chorded as all that — it has many lines and each line produces a need of his life. The spiritual or mystic line is one of them and man tries to satisfy it in various ways, by superstitions of all kinds, by ignorant religionism, by spiritism, demonism and what not, in his more enlightened parts by spiritual philosophy, the higher occultism and the rest, at his highest by the union with the All, the Eternal or the Divine. The tendency towards the search for spirituality began in Europe with a recoil from the nineteenth century's scientific materialism, a dissatisfaction with the pretended all-sufficiency of the reason and the intellect and a feeling out for something deeper. That was a pre-war phenomenon, and began when there was no menace of Communism and the capitalistic world was at its height of insolent success and triumph, and it came rather as a revolt against the materialistic bourgeois life and its ideals, not as an attempt to serve or sanctify it. It has been at once served and opposed by the post-war disillusionment — opposed because the post-war world has fallen back either on cynicism and the life of the senses or on movements like Fascism and Communism; served because with the deeper minds the dissatisfaction with the ideals of the past or the present, with all mental or vital or material solutions of the problem of life has increased and only the spiritual path is left. It is true that the European mind having little light on these things dallies with vital will-o'-the wisps like spiritism or theosophy or falls back upon the old religionism; but the deeper minds of which I speak either pass by them or pass through them in search of a greater Light. I have had contact with many and the above tendencies are very clear. They come from all countries and it was only a minority who hailed from England or America. Russia is different — unlike the others it has lingered in mediaeval religionism and not passed through any period of revolt — so when the revolt came it was naturally anti-religious and atheistic. It is only when this phase is exhausted that Russian mysticism can receive and take not a narrow religious but the spiritual direction. It is true that mysticism *à revers*, turned upside down, has made Bolshevism and its endeavour a creed rather than a political theme and a search for the paradisal secret millennium on earth rather than the building of a purely social structure. But for the most part Russia is trying to do on the communistic basis all that nineteenth-century idealism hoped to get at — and failed — in the midst of or against an industrial competitive environment. Whether it will really succeed any better is for the future to decide — for at present it only keeps what it has got by a tension and violent control which is not over.

The Isha Upanishad passage[1] is of course a much larger statement of the nature of universal existence than the Einstein theory which is confined to the physical universe. You can deduce too a much larger law of relativity from the statement in the verse. What it means from this point of view — for it contains much more in it — is that the absolute Reality exists, but it is immovable and always the same, the universal movement is a motion of consciousness in this Reality of which only the Transcendent itself can seize the truth, which is self-evident to It, while the apprehension of it by the Gods (the mind, senses, etc.) must necessarily be imperfect and relative, since they can try to follow but none can really overtake (apprehend or seize) that Truth, each being limited by its own viewpoint[2], lesser instrumentality or capacity of consciousness, etc. This is the familiar attitude of the Indian or at least the Vedantic mind which held that our knowledge, perception and experience of things in the world and of the world itself must be *vyāvahārika*, relative, practical or pragmatic only, — so declared Shankara, — it is in fact an illusory knowledge, the real Truth of things lying beyond our mental and sensory consciousness. Einstein's relativity is a scientific, not a metaphysical statement. The form and field of it are different — but, I suppose, if one goes back from it and beyond it to its essential significance, the real reason for its being so, one can connect it with the Vedantic conclusion. But to justify that to the intellect, you would have to go through a whole process to show how the connection comes — it does not self-evidently follow.

As for Jeans, many would say that his conclusions are not at all legitimate. Einstein's law is a scientific generalisation based upon certain relations proper to the domain of physics and, if

---

[1] "One unmoving that is swifter than Mind, That the Gods reach not, for It progresses ever in front. That, standing, passes beyond others as they run." *Isha Upanishad*, Verse 4. Sri Aurobindo's translation. See Sri Aurobindo, *Eight Upanishads* (1965 Edition), p. 5.

[2] The Gods besides are in and subject to Space and Time, part of the motion in Space and Time, not superior to it.

valid, valid there in the limits of that domain, or, if you like, in the general domain of scientific observation and measurement of physical processes and motions; but how can you transform that at once into a metaphysical generalisation? It is a jump over a considerable gulf — or a forceful transformation of one thing into another, of a limited physical result into an unlimited all-embracing formula. I don't quite know what Einstein's law really amounts to, but does it amount to more than this that our scientific measurements of time and other things are, in the conditions under which they have to be made, relative because subject to the unavoidable drawback of these conditions? What metaphysically follows from that — if anything at all does follow — it is for the metaphysicians, not the scientists to determine. The Vedantic position was that the Mind itself (as well as the senses) is a limited power making its own representations, constructions, formations and imposing them on the Reality. That is a much bigger and more intricate affair shooting down into the very roots of our existence. I think myself there are many positions taken by modern Science which tend to be helpful to that view — though in the nature of things they cannot be sufficient to prove it.

I state the objections only; I myself see certain fundamental truths underlying all the domains and the one Reality everywhere. But there is also a great difference in the instruments used and the ways of research followed by the seekers in these different ways (the physical, the occult and the spiritual) and for the intellect at least the bridge between them has still to be built. One can point out analogies, but it can be maintained very well that Science cannot be used for yielding or buttressing results of spiritual knowledge. The other side can be maintained also and it is best that both should be stated — so this is not meant to discourage your thesis.

How does Sir James Jeans or any other scientist know that it was by a "mere accident" that life came into existence or that there is no life anywhere else in the universe or that life elsewhere must either be exactly the same as life here under the same conditions or not existent at all? These are mere mental speculations without any conclusiveness in them. Life can be an accident only if the whole world also is an accident — a thing created by Chance and governed by Chance. It is not worthwhile to waste time on this kind of speculation, for it is only the bubble of a moment.

The material universe is only the façade of an immense building which has other structures behind it, and it is only if one knows the whole that one can have some knowledge of the truth of the material universe. There are vital, mental and spiritual ranges behind which give the material its significance. If the earth is the only field of the spiritual evolution in Matter — (assuming that) — then it must be as part of the total design. The idea that all the rest must be a waste is a human idea which would not trouble the vast Cosmic Spirit whose consciousness and life are everywhere, in the stone and dust as much as in the human intelligence. But this is a speculative question which is quite alien to our practical purpose. For us it is the development of the spiritual consciousness in the human body that matters.

In this development there are stages — the whole truth cannot be known till all are passed and the final stage is there. The stage in which you are is one in which the self is beginning to be realised, the self free from all embodiment and not depending on embodiment for its perpetual existence. It is therefore natural that you should feel the embodiment to be something quite subordinate and like the earth-life of Jeans almost accidental. It is because of this stage that the Mayavadins, taking it for final, thought the world to be an illusion. But this is only a stage of the journey. Beyond this Self which is static, separate, formless, there is a greater Consciousness in which the Silence and the Cosmic Activity are united but in another knowledge than the walled-in ignorance of the embodied human being. This Self is only one aspect of the Divine Reality. It is when one gets to that greater Consciousness that cosmic existence and form and life and mind no longer appear to be an accident but find their significance. Even there there are two stages, the overmental and the supramental, and it is not till one gets to the last that the full truth of existence can become entirely real to the consciousness. Observe what you experience and know that it has its value and is indispensable as a stage, but do not take the experience of a stage for the final knowledge.

I have not read him [Bergson] sufficiently to pronounce. So far as I know, he seems to have some perception of the dynamic creative intuition involved in Life, but none of the truly supra-rational intuition above. If so, his Intuition which he takes to be the sole secret of things is only a secondary manifestation of something transcendent which is itself only the "rays of the Sun".

No, it [Bergson's "élan vital"] is not the supramental. But Bergson's "intuition" seems to be a Life Intuition which is of course the supramental fragmented and modified to act as a Knowledge in "Life-in-Matter". I can't say definitively yet, but that is the impression it gave me.

He [Bergson] sees Consciousness (Chit) not in its essential truth but as a creative Force=a sort of transcendent Life-Energy descending into Matter and acting there.

[Élan Vital:] Not Sachchidananda but Chit-shakti in the disguise of Pranashakti. Bergson is, I believe, a vitalist (as opposed to a materialist on one side and an idealist on the other) with a strong perception of Time (in Upanishadic times they speculated whether Time was not the Brahman and some schools held that idea). So for him Brahman=Consciousness-Force=Time-Force=Life-Force. But the last two he sees vividly while the first which is the real thing behind creation he sees very dimly.

Instinct and intuition as described by him [Bergson] are vital, but it is possible to develop a corresponding mental intuition, and that is probably what he suggests — and which depends not on thought but a sort of mental direct contact with things. This is not exactly mysticism, though it is a first step towards it.

I suppose Bergson must already know what the "mystics" say about the matter and has put his own interpretation or value upon it. So he would not at all be impressed by your suggestion. He would say, "I know all about that already."

These extraordinary occurrences which go outside the ordinary course of physical Nature, happen frequently in India and are not unknown elsewhere; they are akin to what is called poltergeist phenomena in Europe. Scientists do not speak or think about such supernormal happenings except to pooh-pooh them or to prove that they are simply the tricks of children simulating supernatural manifestations.

Scientific laws only give a schematic account of material process of Nature — as a valid scheme they can be used for reproducing or extending at will a material process, but obviously they cannot give an account of the thing itself. Water, for instance, is not merely so much oxygen and hydrogen put together — the combination is simply a process or device for enabling the materialisation of a new thing called water; what that new thing really is, is quite another matter. In fact, there are different planes of substance, gross, subtle and more subtle going back to what is called causal (Karana) substance. What is more gross can be reduced to the subtle state and the subtle brought into the gross state; that accounts for dematerialisation and rematerialisation. These are occult processes and are vulgarly regarded as magic. Ordinarily the magician knows nothing of the why and wherefore of what he is doing, he has simply learned the formula or process or else controls elemental beings of the subtler states (planes or worlds) who do the thing for him. The Tibetans indulge widely in occult processes; if you see the books of Madame David Neel who has lived in Tibet you will get an idea of their expertness in these things. But also the Tibetan Lamas know something of the laws of occult (mental and vital) energy and how it can be made to act on physical things. That is something which goes beyond mere magic. The direct power of mind-force or life-force upon Matter can be extended to an almost illimitable degree. It must be remembered that Energy is fundamentally one in all the planes, only taking more and more dense forms, so there is nothing *a priori* impossible in mind-energy or life-energy acting directly on material energy and substance; if they do, they can make a material object do things or rather can do things with a material object which would be to that object in its ordinary poise or "law" unhabitual and therefore apparently impossible.

I do not see how cosmic rays can explain the origination of Matter; it is like Sir Oliver Lodge's explanation of life on earth that it comes from another planet; it only pushes the problem one step farther back — for how do the cosmic rays come into existence? But it is a fact that Agni is the basis of forms as the Sankhya pointed out long ago, i.e. the fiery principle in the three powers radiant, electric and gaseous (the Vedic trinity of Agni) is the agent in producing liquid and solid forms of what is called Matter.

Obviously, a layman cannot do these things, unless he has a native "psychic" (that is, occult) faculty and even then he will have to learn the law of the thing before he can use it at will. It is always possible to use spiritual force or mind-power or will-power or a certain kind of vital energy to produce effects in men, things and happenings; but knowledge and much practice is needed before this possibility ceases to be occasional and haphazard and can be used quite consciously, at will or to perfection. Even then, to have "a control over the whole material world" is too big a proposition, a local and partial control is more possible or, more widely, certain kinds of control over Matter.

**

All the world, according to Science, is nothing but a play of Energy — a material Energy it used to be called, but it is now doubted whether Matter, scientifically speaking, exists except as a phenomenon of Energy. All the world, according to Vedanta, is a play of a power of a spiritual entity, the power of an original consciousness, whether it be Maya or Shakti, and the result an illusion or real. In the world so far as man is concerned we are aware only of mind-energy, life-energy, energy in Matter; but it is supposed that there is a spiritual energy or force also behind them from which they originate. All things, in either case, are the results of a Shakti, energy or force. There is no action without a Force or Energy doing the action and bringing about its consequence. Further, anything that has no Force in it is either something dead or something unreal or something inert and without consequence. If there is no such thing as spiritual consciousness, there can be no reality of yoga, and if there is no yoga-force, spiritual force, yoga shakti, then also there can be no effectivity in yoga. A yoga-consciousness or spiritual consciousness which has no power or force in it, may not be dead or unreal, but it is evidently something inert and without effect or consequence. Equally, a man who sets out to be a yogi or Guru and has no spiritual consciousness or no power in his spiritual consciousness — a yoga-force or spiritual force — is making a false claim and is either a charlatan or a self-deluded imbecile; still more is he so if having no spiritual force he claims to have made a path others can follow. If yoga is a reality, if spirituality is anything better than a delusion, there must be such a thing as yoga-force or spiritual force.

It is evident that if spiritual force exists, it must be able to produce spiritual results — therefore there is no irrationality in the claim of those sadhaks who say that they feel the force of the Guru or the force of the Divine working in them and leading towards spiritual fulfilment and experience. Whether it is so or not in a particular case is a personal question, but the statement cannot be denounced as *per se* incredible and manifestly false, because such things cannot be. Further, if it be true that spiritual force is the original one and the others are derivative from it, then there is no irrationality in supposing that spiritual force can produce mental results, vital results, physical results. It may act through mental, vital or physical energies and through the means which these energies use, or it may act directly on mind, life or Matter as the field of its own special and immediate action. Either way is *prima facie* possible. In a case of cure of illness, someone is ill for two days, weak, suffering from pains and fever; he takes no medicine, but finally asks for cure from his Guru; the next morning he rises well, strong and energetic. He has at least some justification for thinking that a force has been used on him and put into him and that it was a spiritual power that acted. But in another case, medicines may be used, while at the same time the invisible force may be called for to aid the material means, for it is a known fact that medicines may or may not succeed — there is no certitude. Here for the reason of an outside observer (one who is neither the user of the force nor the doctor nor the patient) it remains uncertain whether the patient was cured by the medicines only or by the spiritual force with the medicines as an instrument. Either is possible, and it cannot be said that because medicines were used, therefore the working of a spiritual force is *per se* incredible and demonstrably false. On the other hand, it is possible for the doctor to have felt a force working in him and guiding him or he may see the patient improving with a rapidity which, according to medical science, is incredible. The patient may feel the force working in himself bringing health, energy, rapid cure. The user of the force may watch the results, see the symptoms he works on diminishing, those he did not work upon increasing till he does work on them and then immediately diminishing, the doctor working according to his unspoken suggestions, etc., etc., until the cure is done. (On the other hand, he may see forces working against the cure and conclude that the spiritual force has to be contented with a withdrawal or an imperfect success.) In all that the doctor, the patient or the user of force is justified in believing that the cure is at least partly or even fundamentally due to the spiritual force. Their experience is valid of course for themselves only, not for the outside rationalising observer. But the latter is not logically entitled to say that their experience is incredible and must be false.

Another point. It does not follow that a spiritual force must either succeed in all cases or, if it does not, that proves its non-existence. Of no force can that be said. The force of fire is to burn, but there are things it does not burn; under certain circumstances it does not burn even the feet of the man who walks barefoot on red-hot coals. That does not prove that fire cannot burn or that there is no such thing as force of fire, Agni Shakti.

I have no time to write more; it is not necessary either. My object was not to show that spiritual force must be believed in, but that the belief in it is not necessarily a delusion and that this belief can be rational as well as possible.

The invisible Force producing tangible results both inward and outward is the whole meaning of the yogic consciousness. Your question about yoga bringing merely a feeling of Power without any result was really very strange. Who would be satisfied with such a meaningless hallucination and call it Power? If we had not had thousands of experiences showing that the Power within could alter the mind, develop its powers, add new ones, bring in new ranges of knowledge, master the vital movements, change the character, influence men and things, control the conditions and functionings of the body, work as a concrete dynamic Force on other forces, modify events, etc., etc., we would not speak of it as we do. Moreover, it is not only in its results but in its movements that the Force is tangible and concrete. When I speak of feeling Force or Power, I do not mean simply having a vague sense of it, but feeling it concretely and consequently being able to direct it, manipulate it, watch its movement, be conscious of its mass and intensity and in the same way of that of other, perhaps opposing forces; all these things are possible and usual by the development of yoga.

It is not, unless it is supramental Force, a Power that acts without conditions and limits. The conditions and limits under which yoga or sadhana has to be worked out are not arbitrary or capricious; they arise from the nature of things. These including the will, receptivity, assent, self-opening and surrender of the sadhak have to be respected by the yoga-force, unless it receives a sanction from the Supreme to override everything and get something done, but that sanction is sparingly given. It is only if the supramental Power came fully down, not merely sent its influences through the overmind, that things could be very radically directed towards that object — for then the sanction would not be rare. For the Law of the Truth would be at work, not constantly balanced by the law of the Ignorance.

Still the yoga-force is always tangible and concrete in the way I have described and has tangible results. But it is invisible — not like a blow given or the rush of a motor car knocking somebody down which the physical senses can at once perceive. How is the mere physical mind to know that it is there and working? By its results? But how can it know that the results were that of the yogic force and not of something else? One of two things it must be. Either it must allow the consciousness to go inside, to become aware of inner things, to believe in the experience of the invisible and the supraphysical, and then by experience, by the opening of new capacities, it becomes conscious of these forces and can see, follow and use their workings, just as the Scientist uses the unseen forces of Nature. Or one must have faith and watch and open oneself and then it will begin to see how things happen, it will notice that when the Force was called in, there began after a time to be a result, then repetitions, more repetitions, more clear and tangible results, increasing frequency, increasing consistency of results, a feeling and awareness of the Force at work — until the experience becomes daily, regular, normal, complete. These are the two main methods, one internal, working from in outward, the other external, working from outside and calling the inner force out till it penetrates and is visible in the exterior consciousness. But neither can be done if one insists always on the extrovert attitude, the external concrete only and refuses to join to it the internal concrete — or if the physical mind at every step raises a dance of doubts which refuses to allow the nascent experience to develop. Even the Scientist carrying on a new experiment would never succeed if he allowed his mind to behave in that way.

*
**

Concrete? What do you mean by concrete? Spiritual force has
its own concreteness; it can take a form (like a stream, for instance) of which one is aware and can send it quite concretely on
whatever object one chooses.

This is a statement of fact about the power inherent in spiritual consciousness. But there is also such a thing as a willed use
of any subtle force — it may be spiritual, mental or vital — to secure a particular result at some point in the world. Just as there
are waves of unseen physical forces (cosmic waves etc.) or currents of electricity, so there are mind-waves, thought-currents,
waves of emotion, — for example, anger, sorrow, etc., — which
go out and affect others without their knowing whence they come
or that they come at all, they only feel the result. One who has
the occult or inner senses awake can feel them coming and invading him. Influences good or bad can propagate themselves in
that way; that can happen without intention and naturally, but
also a deliberate use can be made of them. There can also be a
purposeful generation of force, spiritual or other. There can
be too the use of the effective will or idea acting directly without
the aid of any outward action, speech or other instrumentation
which is not concrete in that sense, but is all the same effective.
These things are not imaginations or delusions or humbug, but
true phenomena.

The fact that you don't feel a force does not prove that it is not
there. The steam-engine does not feel a force moving it, but the
force is there. A man is not a steam-engine? He is very little
better, for he is conscious only of some bubbling on the surface
which he calls 'himself' and is absolutely unconscious of all the
subconscient, subliminal, superconscient forces moving him.
(This is a fact which is being more and more established by modern psychology, though it has got hold only of the lower force
and not the higher, — so you must not turn up your rational nose
at it.) He twitters intellectually, foolishly about the surface
results and attributes them all to his 'noble self', ignoring the fact
that his noble self is hidden far away from his own view behind
the veil of his dimly sparkling intellect and the reeking fog of his

vital feelings, emotions, impulses, sensations and impressions. So your argument is utterly absurd and futile. Our aim is to bring the secret forces out and unwalled into the open, so that instead of getting some shadows or lightnings of themselves out through the veil or being wholly obstructed, they may pour down and flow in rivers. But to expect that all at once is a presumptuous demand which shows an impatient ignorance and inexperience. If they begin to trickle at first, that is enough to justify the faith in a future downpour. You admit that you once or twice felt a force coming down; it proves that the force was and is there and at work and it is only your sweating Herculean labour that prevents you feeling it. Also, it is the trickle that gives the assurance of the possibility of the downpour. One has only to go on and by one's patience deserve the downpour or else, without deserving, slide on until one gets it. In yoga the experience itself is a promise and foretaste but gets shut off till the nature is ready for the fulfilment. This is a phenomenon familiar to every yogi when he looks back on his past experience. Such were the brief visitations of Ananda you had sometimes before. It does not matter if you have not a leech-like tenacity — leeches are not the only type of yogis. If you can stick anyhow or get stuck, that is sufficient.

These things should not be spoken of but kept under a cover.... Even in ordinary non-spiritual things the action of invisible or subjective forces is open to doubt and discussion in which there could be no material certitude, while the spiritual force is invisible in itself and also invisible in its action. So it is idle to try to prove that such and such a result was the effect of spiritual force. Each must form his own idea about that, for if it is accepted, it cannot be as a result of proof and argument, but only as a result of experience, of faith or of that insight in the deeper heart or the deeper intelligence which looks behind appearances and sees what is behind them. The spiritual consciousness does not claim in that way, it can state the truth about itself but not fight for a personal acceptance. A general and impersonal truth about spiritual force is another matter, but I doubt whether the time has come for it or whether it could be understood by mere reasoning intelligence.

If I write about these questions from the yogic point of view, even though on a logical basis, there is bound to be much that is in conflict with the current opinions, e.g., about miracles, the limits of judgment by sense-data, etc. I have avoided as much as possible writing about these subjects because I would have to propound things that cannot be understood except by reference to other data than those of the physical senses or of reason founded on these alone. I might have to speak of laws and forces not recognised by reason or physical science. In my public writings and my writings to sadhaks I have not dealt with these because they go out of the range of ordinary knowledge and the understanding founded on it. These things are known to some, but they do not usually speak about them, while the public view of much of those as are known is either credulous or incredulous, but in both cases without experience or knowledge.

*
**

As for what you write about your experience and your ideas, it looks as if it were simply the old thoughts and movements rising, as they often do, to interfere with the straight course of the sadhana. Mental realisations and ideas of this kind are at best only half-truths and not always even that; once one has taken up a sadhana that goes beyond the mind, it is a mistake to give them too much importance. They can easily become by misapplication a fruitful ground for error.

If you examine the ideas that have come to you, you will see that they are quite inadequate. For example:

1. Matter is *jaḍa* only in appearance. As even modern Science admits, Matter is only energy in action, and, as we know in India, energy is force of consciousness in action.

2. Prakriti in the material world seems to be *jaḍa*, but this

too is only an appearance. Prakriti is in reality the conscious power of the Spirit.

3. A bringing down of the Spirit into Matter cannot lead to a *laya* in *jaḍa prakṛti*. A descent of the Spirit could only mean a descent of light, consciousness and power, not a growth of unconsciousness and inertia which is what is meant by the *jaḍa-laya*.

4. The Spirit is there already in Matter as everywhere else; it is only a surface apparent unconsciousness or involved consciousness which veils its presence. What we have to do is to awake Matter to the spiritual consciousness concealed in it.

5. What we aim at bringing down into the material world is the supramental consciousness, light and energy, because it is this alone that can truly transform it.

If there is at any time a growth of unconsciousness and inertia, it is because of the resistance of the ordinary nature to the spiritual change. But this is usually raised up in order to be dealt with and eliminated. If it is allowed to remain concealed and not raised up, the difficulty will never be grappled with and no real transformation will take place.

If there were no creative power in the material energy, there would be no material universe. Matter is not unconscious or without dynamism — only it is an involved force and consciousness that work in it. It is what the psychologists call the inconscient from which all comes — but it is not really inconscient.

[1] There is no need to put "the" before "quality" — in English that would alter the sense. Matter is not regarded in this passage as a quality of being perceived by sense; I don't think that would have any meaning. It is regarded as a result of a certain power

---

[1] This explanation is apropos of the following passage in *The Yoga and Its Objects* (1968 Edition), p. 13:

"Matter itself, you will one day realise, is not material, it is not substance but form of consciousness, *guṇa*, the result of quality of being perceived by sense-knowledge."

and action of consciousness which presents forms of itself to
sense perception and it is this quality of sense-perceivedness, so
to speak, that gives them the appearance of Matter, i.e. of a certain kind of substantiality inherent in themselves — but in fact
they are not self-existent substantial objects but forms of consciousness. The point is that there is no such thing as the self-
existent Matter posited by nineteenth century Science.

You are reasoning on the analogy of your own very cabined and
limited sense-consciousness and its rather clumsy relations with
the happenings in material space. What is space after all but an
extension of conscious being in which Consciousness-Force
builds its own surroundings? In the subtle physical plane there
are, not one, but many layers of consciousness and each moves
in its own being, that is to say, in its own space. I have said that
each subtle plane is a conglomeration or series of worlds. Each
space may at any point meet, penetrate or coincide with another; accordingly at one point of meeting or coincidence there
might be several subtle objects occupying what we might rather
arbitrarily call the same space, and yet they may not be in any
actual relation with each other. If there is a relation created, it
is the multiple consciousness of the seer in which the meeting-
place becomes apparent that creates it.

On the other hand, there may be a relation between objects
in different regions of space correlated to each other as in the
case of the gross physical object and its subtle counterpart.
There you can more easily reason of relations between one space
and another.

Time and Space are not limited, they are infinite — they are the
terms of an extension of consciousness in which things take place
or are arranged in a certain relation, succession, order. There
are again different orders of Time and Space; that too depends
on the consciousness. The Eternal is extended in Time and Space,
but he is also beyond all Time and Space. Timelessness and Time

are two terms of the eternal existence. The Spaceless Eternal is not one indivisible infinity of Space, there is in it no near or far, no here or there — the Timeless Eternal is not measurable by years or hours or aeons, the experience of it has been described as the eternal moment. But for the mind this state cannot be described except by negatives, — one has to go beyond and to realise it.

The objection[1] is founded on human three dimensional ideas of space and division in space, which are again founded upon the limited nature of the human senses. To some beings space is one dimensional, to others two dimensional, to others three dimensional — but there are other dimensions also. It is well recognised in metaphysics that the Infinite can be in a point and not only in extension of space — just as there is an eternity of extension in Time but also an Eternity which is independent of Time so that it can be felt in the moment — one has not to think of millions and millions of years in order to realise it. So too the rigid distinction of One against Many, a One that cannot be many or of an All that is made up by addition and not self-existent are crude mental notions of the outer finite mind that cannot be applied to the Infinite. If the All were of this material and unspiritual character, tied down to a primary arithmetic and geometry, the realisation of the universe in oneself, of the all in each and each in all, of the universe in the Bindu would be impossible. Your Xs are evidently innocent of the elements of metaphysical thinking or they would not make such objections.

It is only by feeling all things as one spiritual substance that one can arrive at unity — unity is in the spiritual consciousness. The material point is only one point among millions of millions — so that is not the base of unity. But once you get the unity in consciousness, you can feel through that the unity of mind

---

[1] "How can the Divine, who is the all-pervading and all-containing Infinite, incarnate in the small space of a human body?"

substance, mind force, etc., the unity of life substance (mobile) and life force, the unity of material substance and energies. Being — Consciousness of being — energy of consciousness — form of consciousness, all things are really that.

It is quite true that the word "superstition" has been habitually used as a convenient club to beat down any belief that does not agree with the ideas of the materialistic reason, that is to say, the physical mind dealing with the apparent law of physical process and seeing no farther. It has also been used to dismiss ideas and beliefs not in agreement with one's own idea of what is the rational norm of supraphysical truths as well. For many ages man cherished beliefs that implied a force behind which acted on principles unknown to the physical mind and beyond the witness of the outward reason and the senses. Science came in with a method of knowledge which extended the evidence of this outer field of consciousness, and thought that by this method all existence would become explicable. It swept away at once without examination all the ancient beliefs as so many "superstitions" — true, half-true or false, all went into the dust-bin in one impartial sweep, because they did not rely on the method of physical Science and lay outside its data or were or seemed incompatible with its standpoint. Even in the field of supraphysical experience only so much was admitted as could give a mentally rational explanation of itself according to a certain range of ideas — all the rest, everything that seemed to demand an occult, mystic or below-the-surface origin to explain it, was put aside as so much superstition. Popular beliefs that were the fruit sometimes of imagination but sometimes also of a traditional empirical knowledge or of a right instinct shared naturally the same fate. That all this was a hasty and illegitimate operation, itself based on the "superstition" of the all-sufficiency of the new method which really applies only to a limited field, is now becoming more and more evident. I agree with you that the word superstition is one which should be used either not at all or with great caution. It is evidently an anachronism to apply it to beliefs not accepted by the form of religion one happens oneself to follow or favour.

The growing reversal of opinion with regard to many things that were then condemned but are now coming into favour once more is very striking. In addition to the instances you quote a hundred others might be added. One does not quite know why a belief in graphology should be condemned as irrational or superstitious; it seems to me quite rational to believe that a man's handwriting is the result of or consistent with his temperament and nature and, if so, it may very well prove on examination to be an index of character. It is now a known fact that each man is an individual by himself with his own peculiar formation different from others and made by minute variations in the general human plan, — this is true of small physical characteristics, it is evidently equally true of psychological characteristics; it is not unreasonable to suppose a correlation between the two. On that basis cheiromancy may very well have a truth in it, for it is a known fact that the lines in an individual hand are different from the lines in others and that this, as well as differences of physiognomy, may carry in it psychological indications is not impossible. The difficulty for minds trained under rationalistic influences becomes greater when these lines or the data of astrology are interpreted as signs of destiny, because modern rationalism resolutely refused to admit that the future was determined or could be determinable. But this looks more and more like one of the "superstitions" of the modern mind, a belief curiously contradictory of the fundamental notions of Science. For Science has believed, at least until yesterday, that everything is determined in Nature and it attempts to find the laws of that determination and to predict future physical happenings on that basis. If so, it is reasonable to suppose that there are unseen connections determining human events in the world and that future events may therefore be predictable. Whether it can be done on the lines of astrology or cheiromancy is a matter of enquiry and one does not get any farther by dismissing the possibility with a summary denial. The case for astrology is fairly strong; a case seems to exist for cheiromancy also.

On the other hand, it is not safe to go too hastily in the other direction. There is the opposite tendency to believe everything in these fields and not keep one's eyes open to the element of limitation or error in these difficult branches of knowledge — it was the excess of belief that helped to discredit them, because their errors were patent. It does not seem to me established that the stars determine the future — though that is possible, but it does look as if they indicate it — or rather, some certitudes and potentialities of the future. Even the astrologers admit that there is another element of determination in man himself which limits the field of astrological prediction and may even alter many of its ascertained results. There is a very tangled and difficult complex of forces making up any determination of things in the world and when we have disentangled one thread of the skein and follow it we may get many striking results, but we cannot rely on it as the one wholly reliable clue. The mind's methods are too rigid and conveniently simple to unravel the true or whole truth whether of the Reality or of its separate phenomena.

I would accept your statement about the possibility of knowing much about a man from observations of a small part of his being, physical or psychological, but I think it is to go too far to say that one can reconstruct a whole man from one minute particle of a hair. I should say from my knowledge of the complexity and multiplicity of elements in the human being that such a procedure would be hazardous and would leave a large part of the Unknown overshadowing the excessive certitude of this inferential structure

I suppose we cannot go so far as to deny that there is such a thing as superstition — a fixed belief without any ground in something that is quite unsound and does not hang together. The human mind readily claps on such beliefs to things which can be or are in themselves true, and this is a mixture which very badly confuses the search for knowledge. But precisely because of this mixture, because somewhere behind the superstition or not far off from it there is very usually some real truth, one ought to be cautious in using the word or sweeping away with it as a convenient broom the true, the partly true and the unfounded together and claiming that the bare ground left is the only truth of the matter.

When I wrote that sentence about "a fixed blind belief", I was not thinking really of religious beliefs, but of common popular ideas and beliefs. Your feeling about the matter, in any case, is quite sound. One can and ought to believe and follow one's own path without condemning or looking down on others for having beliefs different from those one thinks or sees to be the best or the largest in truth. The spiritual field is many-sided and full of complexities and there is room for an immense variety of experiences. Besides, all mental egoism — and spiritual egoism — has to be surmounted and this sense of superiority should therefore not be cherished.

P.S. A sincere, whole-hearted and one-pointed following of this yoga should lead to a level where these rigid mental divisions do not exist, for they are mental walls put round one part of Truth and Knowledge so as to cut it off from the rest, but this view from above the mind is comprehensive and everything falls into its place in the whole.

PLANES AND PARTS OF THE BEING

Planes and Parts of the Being

MEN do not know themselves and have not learned to distinguish the different parts of their being; for these are usually lumped together by them as mind, because it is through a mentalised perception and understanding that they know or feel them; therefore they do not understand their own states and actions, or, if at all, then only on the surface. It is part of the foundation of yoga to become conscious of the great complexity of our nature, see the different forces that move it and get over it a control of directing knowledge. We are composed of many parts each of which contributes something to the total movement of our consciousness, our thought, will, sensation, feeling, action, but we do not see the origination or the course of these impulsions; we are aware only of their confused and pell-mell results on the surface upon which we can at best impose nothing better than a precarious shifting order.

The remedy can only come from the parts of the being that are already turned towards the Light. To call in the light of the Divine Consciousness from above, to bring the psychic being to the front and kindle a flame of aspiration which will awaken spiritually the outer mind and set on fire the vital being, is the way out.

Each part of the being has its own nature or even different natures contained in the same part.

Consciousness is not, to my experience, a phenomenon dependent on the reactions of personality to the forces of Nature and amounting to no more than a seeing or interpretation of these reactions. If that were so, then when the personality becomes silent and immobile and gives no reactions, as there would be no seeing or interpretative action, there would therefore be no consciousness. That contradicts some of the fundamental experiences of yoga, e.g., a silent and immobile consciousness infinitely spread out, not dependent on the personality but impersonal and universal, not seeing and interpreting contacts but motionlessly self-aware, not dependent on the reactions, but persistent in itself even when no reactions take place. The subjective personality itself is only a formation of consciousness which is a power inherent, not in the activity of the temporary manifested personality, but in the being, the Self or Purusha.

Consciousness is a reality inherent in existence. It is there even when it is not active on the surface, but silent and immobile; it is there even when it is invisible on the surface, not reacting on outward things or sensible to them, but withdrawn and either active or inactive within; it is there even when it seems to us to be quite absent and the being to our view unconscious and inanimate.

Consciousness is not only power of awareness of self and things, it is or has also a dynamic and creative energy. It can determine its own reactions or abstain from reactions; it can not only answer to forces, but create or put out from itself forces. Consciousness is Chit but also Chit Shakti.

Consciousness is usually identified with mind, but mental consciousness is only the human range which no more exhausts all the possible ranges of consciousness than human sight exhausts all the gradations of colour or human hearing all the gradations of sound — for there is much above or below that is to man invisible and inaudible. So there are ranges of consciousness above and below the human range, with which the normal human has no contact and they seem to it unconscious, — supramental or overmental and submental ranges.

When Yajnavalkya says there is no consciousness in the Brahman state, he is speaking of consciousness as the human being knows it. The Brahman state is that of a supreme existence supremely aware of itself, *svayamprakāśa*, — it is Sachchidananda, Existence-Consciousness-Bliss. Even if it be spoken of as beyond That, *parātparam*, it does not mean that it is a state of Non-existence or Non-consciousness, but beyond even the highest spiritual substratum (the "foundation above" in the luminous paradox of the Rig Veda) of cosmic existence and consciousness. As it is evident from the description of Chinese Tao and the Buddhist Shunya that that is a Nothingness in which all is, so with the negation of consciousness here. Superconscient and subconscient are only relative terms; as we rise into the superconscient we see that it is a consciousness greater than the highest we yet have and therefore in our normal state inaccessible to us and, if we can go down into the subconscient, we find there a consciousness other than our own at its lowest mental limit and therefore ordinarily inaccessible to us. The Inconscient itself is only an involved state of consciousness which like the Tao or Shunya, though in a different way, contains all things suppressed within it so that under a pressure from above or within all can evolve out of it — "an inert Soul with a somnambulist Force."

The gradations of consciousness are universal states not dependent on the outlook of the subjective personality; rather the outlook of the subjective personality is determined by the grade of consciousness in which it is organised according to its typal nature or its evolutionary stage.

It will be evident that by consciousness is meant something which is essentially the same throughout but variable in status, condition and operation, in which in some grades or conditions the activities we call consciousness can exist either in a suppressed or an unorganised or a differently organised state; while in other states some other activities may manifest which in us are suppressed, unorganised or latent or else are less perfectly manifested, less intensive, extended and powerful than in those higher grades above our highest mental limit.

It all depends upon where the consciousness places itself and concentrates itself. If the consciousness places or concentrates itself within the ego, you are identified with the ego — if in the mind, it is identified with the mind and its activities and so on. If the consciousness puts its stress outside, it is said to live in the external being and becomes oblivious of its inner mind and vital and inmost psychic; if it goes inside, puts its centralising stress there, then it knows itself as the inner being or, still deeper, as the psychic being; if it ascends out of the body to the planes where self is naturally conscious of its wideness and freedom it knows itself as the Self and not the mind, life or body. It is this stress of consciousness that makes all the difference. That is why one has to concentrate the consciousness in heart or mind in order to go within or go above. It is the disposition of the consciousness that determines everything, makes one predominantly mental, vital, physical or psychic, bound or free, separate in the Purusha or involved in the Prakriti.

Consciousness has no need of a clear individual "I" to dispose variously the centralising stress, — wherever the stress is put the "I" attaches itself to that, so that one thinks of oneself as a mental being or physical being or whatever it may be. The consciousness in me can dispose its stress in this way or the other way — it may go down into the physical and work there in the physical nature keeping all the rest behind or above for the time or it may go up into the overhead level and stand above mind, life and body seeing them as instrumental lower forms of itself or not seeing them at all and merged in the free undifferentiated Self or it may throw itself into an active dynamic cosmic consciousness and identify with that or do any number of other things without resorting to the help of this much overrated and meddlesome fly on the wheel which you call the clear individual "I". The real "I" — if you want to use that word — is not "clear individual," that is, a clear-cut limited separative ego, it is as wide as the universe and wider and can contain the universe in itself, but that is not the Ahankar, it is the Atman.

Consciousness is a fundamental thing, the fundamental thing in existence — it is the energy, the motion, the movement of consciousness that creates the universe and all that is in it — not only the macrocosm but the microcosm is nothing but consciousness arranging itself. For instance, when consciousness in its movement or rather a certain stress of movement forgets itself in the action it becomes an apparently "unconscious" energy; when it forgets itself in the form it becomes the electron, the atom, the material object. In reality it is still consciousness that works in the energy and determines the form and the evolution of form. When it wants to liberate itself, slowly, evolutionarily, out of Matter, but still in the form, it emerges as life, as animal, as man and it can go on evolving itself still farther out of its involution and become something more than mere man. If you can grasp that, then it ought not to be difficult to see further that it can subjectively formulate itself as a physical, a vital, a mental, a psychic consciousness — all these are present in man, but as they are all mixed up together in the external consciousness with their real status behind in the inner being, one can only become fully aware of them by releasing the original limiting stress of the consciousness which makes us live in our external being and become awake and centred within in the inner being. As the consciousness in us, by its external concentration or stress, has to put all these things behind — behind a wall or veil, it has to break down the wall or veil and get back in its stress into these inner parts of existence — that is what we call living within; then our external being seems to us something small and superficial, we are or can become aware of the large and rich and inexhaustible kingdom within. So also consciousness in us has drawn a lid or covering or whatever one likes to call it between the lower planes of mind, life, body supported by the psychic and the higher planes which contain the spiritual kingdoms where the self is always free and limitless, and it can break or open the lid or covering and ascend there and become the Self free and wide and luminous or else bring down the influence, reflection, finally even the presence and power of the higher consciousness into the lower nature.

Now that is what consciousness is — it is not composed of parts, it is fundamental to being and itself formulates any parts it chooses to manifest — developing them from above downward by a progressive coming down from spiritual levels towards involution in Matter or formulating them in an upward working in the front by what we call evolution. If it chooses to work in you through the sense of ego, you think that it is the clear-cut indi-

vidual "I" that does everything — if it begins to release itself
from that limited working, you begin to expand your sense of
"I" till it bursts into infinity and no longer exists or you shed it
and flower into spiritual wideness. Of course, this is not what
is spoken of in modern materialistic thought as consciousness,
because that thought is governed by science and sees consciousness only as a phenomenon that emerges out of inconscient
Matter and consists of certain reactions of the system to outward
things. But that is a phenomenon of consciousness, it is not consciousness itself, it is even only a very small part of the possible
phenomenon of consciousness and can give no clue to Consciousness the Reality which is of the very essence of existence.

      That is all at present. You will have to fix yourself in that
— for it is fundamental — before it can be useful to go any
further.

Consciousness is made up of two elements, awareness of self and
things and forces and conscious-power. Awareness is the first
thing necessary, you have to be aware of things in the right consciousness, in the right way, seeing them in their truth; but
awareness by itself is not enough. There must be a Will and a
Force that make the consciousness effective. Somebody may
have the full consciousness of what has to be changed, what has
to go and what has to come in its place, but may be helpless to
make the change. Another may have the will-force, but for want
of a right awareness may be unable to apply it in the right way
at the right place. The advantage of being in the true consciousness is that you have the right awareness and its will being in
harmony with the Mother's will, you can call in the Mother's
Force to make the change. Those who live in the mind and the
vital are not so well able to do this; they are obliged to use mostly
their personal effort and as the awareness and will and force
of the mind and vital are divided and imperfect, the work done
is imperfect and not definitive. It is only in the supermind that
Awareness, Will, Force are always one movement and automatically effective.

II

Sachchidananda is the One with a triple aspect. In the Supreme the three are not three but one — existence is consciousness, consciousness is bliss, and they are thus inseparable, not only inseparable but so much each other that they are not distinct at all. In the superior planes of manifestation they become triune — although inseparable, one can be made more prominent and base or lead the others. In the lower planes below they become separable in appearance, though not in their secret reality, and one can exist phenomenally without the others so that we become aware of what seems to us an inconscient or a painful existence or a consciousness without Ananda. Indeed, without this separation of them in experience pain and ignorance and falsehood and death and what we call inconscience could not have manifested themselves — there could not have been this evolution of a limited and suffering consciousness out of the universal nescience of Matter.

Supermind is between the Sachchidananda and the lower creation. It alone contains the self-determining Truth of the Divine Consciousness and is necessary for a Truth-creation.

One can of course realise Sachchidananda in relation to the mind, life and body also — but then it is something stable, supporting by its presence the lower Prakriti, but not transforming it. The supermind alone can transform the lower nature.

It is the supramental Power that transforms mind, life and body — not the Sachchidananda consciousness which supports impartially everything. But it is by having experience of the Sachchidananda, pure existence-consciousness-bliss, that the ascent to the supramental and the descent of the supramental become (at a much later stage) possible. For first one must get free from the ordinary limitation by the mental, vital and physical formations, and the experience of the Sachchidananda peace, calm, purity and wideness gives this liberation.

The supermind has nothing to do with passing into a blank. It is the Mind overpassing its own limits and following a negative and quietistic way to do it that reaches the big blank. The Mind, being the Ignorance, has to annul itself in order to enter into the supreme Truth — or, at least, so it thinks. But the supermind being the Truth-Consciousness and the Divine Knowledge has no need to annul itself for the purpose.

In the supramental consciousness, there are no problems — the problem is created by the division set up by the Mind. The supramental sees the Truth as a single whole and everything falls into its place in that whole. The supramental is also spiritual, but the old yogas reach Sachchidananda through the spiritualised mind and depart into the eternally static oneness of Sachchidananda or rather pure Sat (Existence), absolute and eternal or else a pure Non-existence, absolute and eternal. Ours having realised Sachchidananda in the spiritualised mind plane proceeds to realise it in the supramental plane.

The supreme supracosmic Sachchidananda is above all. Supermind may be described as its power of self-awareness and world-awareness, the world being known as within itself and not outside. So to live consciously in the supreme Sachchidananda one must pass through the supermind. If one is in the supracosmic apart from the manifestation, there is no place for problems or solutions. If one lives in the transcendence and the cosmic view at the same time, that can only be by the supramental consciousness in the supreme Sachchidananda consciousness — so why should the question arise? Why should there be a difference between the supreme Sachchidananda version of the cosmos and the supermind's version of it? Your difficulty probably comes from thinking of both in terms of the mind.

The supermind is an entirely different consciousness not only from the spiritualised Mind, but from the planes above spiritualised Mind which intervene between it and the supramental plane. Once one passes beyond overmind to supermind, one enters into a consciousness to which the norms of the other planes do not at all apply and in which the same Truth, e.g. Sachchidananda and truth of this universe, is seen in quite a different way and has a different dynamic consequence. This necessarily results from the fact that supermind has an indivisible knowledge, while overmind proceeds by union in division and Mind by division taking division as the first fact, for that is the natural process of its knowledge.

In all planes the essential experience of Sachchidananda, pure Existence, Consciousness, Bliss is the same and Mind is often contented with it as the sole Truth and dismisses all else as part of the grand Illusion, but there is also a dynamic experience of the Divine or of Existence (e.g. as One and Many, Personal and Impersonal, the Infinite and Finite, etc.) which is essential for the integral knowledge. The dynamic experience is not the same in the lower planes as in the higher, in the intermediate spiritual planes and in the supramental. In these the oppositions can only be put together and harmonised, in the supermind they fuse together and are inseparably one; that makes an enormous difference.

The universe is dynamism, movement — the essential experience of Sachchidananda apart from the dynamism and movement is static. The full dynamic truth of Sachchidananda and the universe and its consequence cannot be grasped by any other consciousness than the supermind, because the instrumentation in all other (lower) planes is inferior and there is therefore a disparity between the fullness of the static experience and the incompleteness of the dynamic power, knowledge, result of the inferior light and power of other planes. This is the reason why the consciousness of the other spiritual planes, even if it descends, can make no radical change in the earth-consciousness, it can only modify or enrich it. The radical transformation needs the descent of a supramental power and nature.

One cannot speak of two classes of Sachchidananda, for Sachchidananda is the same always — but the knowledge of Sachchidananda and the universe differs according to the degree of the consciousness which has the experience.

The personal realisation of the Divine may be sometimes with Form, sometimes without Form. Without Form, it is the Presence of the living Divine Person, felt in everything. With Form, it comes with the image of the One to whom worship is offered. The Divine can always manifest himself in a form to the bhakta or seeker. One sees him in the form in which one worships or seeks him or in a form suitable to the Divine Personality who is the object of the adoration. How it manifests depends on many things and it is too various to be reduced to a single rule. Sometimes it is in the heart that the Presence with the form is seen, sometimes in any of the other centres, sometimes above and guiding from there, sometimes it is seen outside and in front as if an embodied Person. Its advantages are an intimate relation and constant guidance or if felt or seen within, a very strong and concrete realisation of the constant Presence. But one must be very sure of the purity of one's adoration and seeking — for the disadvantage of this kind of embodied relation is that Other Forces can imitate the Form or counterfeit the voice and the guidance and this gets more force if it is associated with a constructed image which is not the true thing. Several have been misled in this way because pride, vanity or desire was strong in them and robbed them of the finer psychic perception that is not mental and can at once turn the Mother's light on such misleadings or errors.

1. I mean by the supracosmic Reality the supreme Sachchidananda who is above this and all manifestation, not bound by any, yet from whom all manifestation proceeds and all universe.

2. The supramental and the supracosmic are not the same. If it were so there could be no supramental world and no descent of the supramental principle into the material world — we would be brought back to the idea that the divine Truth and Reality can only exist beyond and the universe — any universe — can only be half-truth or an illusion of ignorance.

3. I mean by the supramental the Truth-Consciousness whether above or in the universe by which the Divine knows not only his own essence and being but his manifestation also. Its

fundamental character is knowledge by identity, by that the Self is known, the Divine Sachchidananda is known, but also the truth of manifestation is known, because this too is That — *sarvam khalvidam brahma, vāsudevaḥ sarvam*, etc. Mind is an instrument of the Ignorance trying to know — supermind is the Knower possessing knowledge, because one with it and the known, therefore seeing all things in the light of His own Truth, the light of their true self which is He. It is a dynamic and not only a static Power, not only a Knowledge, but a Will according to Knowledge — there is a supramental Power or Shakti which can manifest direct its world of Light and Truth in which all is luminously based on the harmony and unity of the One, not disturbed by a veil of Ignorance or any disguise. The supermind therefore does not transcend all possible manifestation, but it is above the triplicity of mind, life and Matter which is our present experience of this manifestation.

4. The overmind is a sort of delegation from the supermind (this is a metaphor only) which supports the present evolutionary universe in which we live here in Matter. If supermind were to start here from the beginning as the direct creative Power, a world of the kind we see now would be impossible; it would have been full of the divine Light from the beginning, there would be no involution in the inconscience of Matter, consequently no gradual striving evolution of consciousness in Matter. A line is therefore drawn between the higher half of the universe of consciousness, *parārdha*, and the lower half, *aparārdha*. The higher half is constituted of Sat, Chit, Ananda, Mahas (the supramental) — the lower half of mind, life, Matter. This line is the intermediary overmind which, though luminous itself, keeps from us the full indivisible supramental Light, depends on it indeed, but in receiving it, divides, distributes, breaks it up into separated aspects, powers, multiplicities of all kinds, each of which it is possible by a further diminution of consciousness, such as we reach in Mind, to regard as the sole or the chief Truth and all the rest as subordinate or contradictory to it. To this action of the overmind may be applied the words of the Upanishad, "The face of the Truth is covered by a golden Lid", or those of the Vedic *ṛtena ṛtam apihitam*. Here there is the working of a sort of

vidyā-avidyāmayī māyā which makes possible the predominance
of *avidyā*. It is by this primitive divisional principle that the
Mind is enabled to regard, for example, the Impersonal as the
Truth, the Personal as only a mask or the personal Divine as the
greatest Truth and impersonality as only an aspect; it is so too
that all the conflicting philosophies and religions arise, each exalting one aspect or potentiality of Truth presented to Mind as the
whole sufficient explanation of things or exalting one of the
Divine's Godheads above all others as the true God than whom
there can be no other or none so high or higher. This divisional
principle pursues man's mental knowledge everywhere and even
when he thinks he has arrived at the final unity, it is only a constructed unity, based on an Aspect. It is so that the scientist seeks
to found the unity of knowledge on some original physical aspect
of things, Energy or Matter, Electricity or Ether, or the Mayavadin thinks he has arrived at the absolute Adwaita by cutting
existence into two, calling the upper side Brahman and the lower
side Maya. It is the reason why mental knowledge can never
arrive at a final solution of anything, for the aspects of Existence
as distributed by overmind are numberless and one can go on
multiplying philosophies and religions for ever.

In the overmind itself there is not this confusion, for the
overmind knows the One as the support, essence, fundamental
power of all things, but in the dynamic play proper to it it lays
emphasis on its divisional power of multiplicity and seeks to give
each power or Aspect its full chance to manifest, relying on the
underlying Oneness to prevent disharmony or conflict. Each
Godhead, as it were, creates his own world, but without conflict
with others; each Aspect, each Idea, each Force of things can
be felt in its full separate energy or splendour and work out its
values, but this does not create a disharmony, because the overmind has the sense of the Infinite and in the true (not spatial)
Infinite many concording infinities are possible. This peculiar
security of overmind is however not transferable to the lesser
planes of consciousness which it supports and governs, because
as one descends in the scale the stress on division and mutiplicity
increases and in the Mind the underlying oneness becomes vague,
abstract, indeterminate and indeterminable and the only apparent

concreteness is that of the phenomenal which is by its nature a form and representation — the self-view of the One has already begun to disappear. Mind acts by representations and constructions, by the separation and weaving together of its constructed data; it can make a synthetic construction and see it as the whole, but when it looks for the reality of things, it takes refuge in abstractions — it has not the concrete vision, experience, contact sought by the mystic and the spiritual seeker. To know Self and Reality directly or truly, it has to be silent and reflect some light of these things or undergo self-exceeding and transformation, and this is only possible either by a higher Light descending into it or by its ascent, the taking up or immergence of it into a higher Light of existence. In Matter, descending below Mind, we arrive at the acme of fragmentation and division; the One, though secretly there, is lost to knowledge and we get the fullness of the Ignorance, even a fundamental Inconscience out of which the universe has to evolve consciousness and knowledge.

5. If we regard Vaikuntha or Goloka each as the world of a Divinity, Vishnu or Krishna, we would be naturally led to seek its place or its origin in the overmind plane. The overmind is the plane of the highest worlds of the Gods. But Vaikuntha and Goloka are human conceptions of states of being that are beyond humanity. Goloka is evidently a world of Love, Beauty and Ananda full of spiritual radiances (the cow is the symbol of spiritual Light) of which the souls there are keepers or possessors, Gopas and Gopis. It is not necessary to assign any single plane to this manifestation — in fact, there can be a reflection or possession of it or of its conditions on any plane of consciousness — the mental, vital or even the subtle physical plane. The explanation of it which you mention is not therefore excluded, it is quite feasible.

6. It is not possible to situate Nirvana as a world or plane, for the Nirvana push is to a withdrawal from world and world-values; it is therefore a state of consciousness or rather of super-consciousness without habitation or level. There is more than one kind of Nirvana (extinction or dissolution) possible. Man being a mental being in a body, *manomaya puruṣa*, makes this attempt at retreat from the cosmos through the spiritualised

mind, he cannot do otherwise and it is this that gives it the appearance of an extinction or dissolution, *laya, nirvāṇa*; for extinction of the mind and all that depends on it including the separative ego in something Beyond is the natural way, almost the indispensable way for such a withdrawal. In a more affirmative yoga seeking transcendence but not withdrawal there would not be this indispensability, for there would be the way already alluded to of self-exceeding or transformation of the mental being. But it is possible also to pass to that through a certain experience of Nirvana, an absolute silence of mind and cessation of activities, constructions, representations, which can be so complete that not only to the silent mind but also to the passive senses the whole world is emptied of its solidity and reality and things appear only as unsubstantial forms without any real habitations or else floating in Something that is a nameless infinite: this infinite or else something still beyond is That which alone is real; an absolute calm, peace, liberation would be the resulting state. Action would continue, but no initiation or participation in it by the silent liberated consciousness; a nameless power would do all until there began the descent from above which would transform the consciousness, making its silence and freedom a basis for a luminous knowledge, action, Ananda. But such a passage would be rare; ordinarily a silence of the mind, a liberation of the consciousness, a renunciation of its belief in the final value or truth of the mind's imperfect representations or constructions would be enough for the higher working to be possible.

7. Now about the cosmic consciousness and Nirvana. Cosmic consciousness is a complex matter. To begin with, there are two sides to it, the experience of the Self free, infinite, silent, inactive, one in all and beyond all, and the direct experience of the cosmic Energy and its forces, workings and formations, this latter experience not being complete till one has the sense of being commensurate with the universe or pervading, exceeding and containing it. Till then there may be direct contacts, communications, interchanges with cosmic forces, beings, movements, but not the full unity of mind with the cosmic Mind, of life with the cosmic Life, of body and physical consciousness with

the cosmic material Energy and its substance. Again, there may be a realisation of the Cosmic Self which is not followed by the realisation of the dynamic universal oneness. Or, on the contrary, there may be some dynamic universalising of consciousness without the experience of the free static Self omnipresent everywhere, — the preoccupation with and pleasure of the greater energies that one would thus experience would stop the way to that liberation. Also the identification or universalisation may be more on one plane or level than on another, predominantly mental or predominantly emotional (through universal sympathy or love) or vital of another kind (experience of the universal life forces) or physical. But in any case, even with the full realisation and experience it should be evident that this cosmic play would be something that one would finally feel as limited, ignorant, imperfect from its very nature. The free soul might regard it untouched and unmoved by its imperfections and vicissitudes, do some appointed work, try to help all or be an instrument of the Divine, but neither the work nor the instrumentation would have anything like the perfection or even the full light, power, bliss of the Divine. This could only be gained by an ascension into higher planes of cosmic existence or their descent into one's consciousness — and, if this were not envisaged or accepted, the push to Nirvana would still remain as a way of escape. The other way would be the ascent after death into these higher planes — the heavens of the religions signify after all nothing but such an urge to a greater, luminous, beatific Divine Existence.

But, one might ask, if the higher planes or if the overmind itself were to manifest their consciousness with all their power, light, freedom and vastness and these things were to descend into an individual consciousness here, would not that make unnecessary both the cosmic negation or the Nirvanic push and the urge towards some Divine Transcendence? But in the result though one might live in a union with the Divine in a luminous wide free consciousness embracing the universe in itself and be a channel of great energies or creations, spiritual or external, yet this world here would remain fundamentally the same — there would be a gulf of difference between the Spirit within and its medium and stuff on which it acted, between the inner consciousness and the world in which it is working. The achievement inner, subjective, individual might be perfect, but the dynamic outcome insufficient, disparate, a mixture, not a perfect harmony of the inner and the outer, a new integral rhythm of existence here that could be called truly divine. Only a consciousness like the supramental, unconditioned and in perfect unity with its source, a Truth-Consciousness empowered to create its own free determinations would be able to establish some perfect harmony and rhythm of the higher hemisphere in this lowest rung of the lower hemisphere. Whether it is to do so or not depends on the significance of the evolutionary existence; it depends on whether that existence is something imperfect in its very nature and doomed to frustration — in which case either a negative way of transcendence by some kind of Nirvana or a positive way of transcendence, perhaps by breaking the shining shield of overmind, *hiraṇmaya pātra*, into what is above it, would be the final end of the soul escaping from this meaningless universe; unless indeed like the Amitabha Buddha one were held by compassion or else the Divine Will within to continue helping and sharing the upward struggle towards the Light of those here still in the darkness of the Ignorance. If, on the contrary, this world is a Lila of spiritual involution and evolution in which one power after another up to the highest is to appear, as Matter, Life and Mind have already appeared out of an apparent indeterminate Inconscience, then another culmination is possible.

The push to Nirvana has two motive forces behind it. One is the sense of the imperfection, sorrow, death, suffering of this world — the original motive force of the Buddha. But for escape from these afflictions Nirvana might not be necessary, if there are higher worlds into which one can ascend where there is no such imperfection, sorrow, death or suffering. But this other possibility of escape is met by the idea that these higher worlds too are transient and part of the Ignorance, that one has to return here always till one overcomes the Ignorance, that the Reality and the cosmic existence are as Truth and Falsehood, opposite, incompatible. This brings in the second motive force, that of the call to transcendence. If the Transcendent is not only supra-cosmic but an aloof Incommunicable, *avyavahāryam*, which one cannot reach except by a negation of all that is here, then some kind of Nirvana, an absolute Nirvana even is inevitable. If, on the other hand, the Divine is transcendent but not incommunicable, the call will still be there and the soul will leave the chequered cosmic play for the beatitude of the transcendent existence, but an absolute Nirvana would not be indispensable; a beatific union with the Divine offers itself as the way before the seeker. This is the reason why the Cosmic Consciousness is not sufficient and the push away from it is so strong, — it is only if the golden lid of the overmind is overpassed and opened and the dynamic contact with the supermind and a descent of its Light and Power here is intended that it can be otherwise.

The Divine is everywhere on all the planes of consciousness seen by us in different ways and aspects of His being. But there is a Supreme which is above all these planes and ways and aspects and from which they come.

The Divine can be and is everywhere, masked or half-manifest or beginning to be manifest, in all the planes of consciousness; in the Supramental it begins to be manifest without disguise or veil in its own *svarūpa.*

I do not think exact correlations can always be traced between one system of spiritual and occult knowledge and another. All deal with the same material, but there are differences of standpoint, differences of view-range, a divergence in the mental idea of what is seen and experienced, disparate pragmatic purposes and therefore a difference in the paths surveyed, cut out or followed; the systems vary, each constructs its own schema and technique.

In the ancient Indian system there is only one triune supernal, Sachchidananda. Or if you speak of the upper hemisphere as the supernal, there are three, Sat plane, Chit plane and Ananda plane. The supermind could be added as a fourth, as it draws upon the other three and belongs to the upper hemisphere. The Indian systems did not distinguish between two quite different powers and levels of consciousness, one which we can call overmind and the other the true supermind or Divine Gnosis. That is the reason why they got confused about Maya (overmind-Force or Vidya-Avidya), and took it for the supreme creative power. In so stopping short at what was still a half-light they lost the secret of transformation — even though the Vaishnava and Tantra yogas groped to find it again and were sometimes on the verge of success. For the rest, this, I think, has been the stumbling-block of all attempts at the discovery of the dynamic divine Truth; I know of none that has not imagined, as soon as it felt the overmind lustres descending, that this was the true illumination, the Gnosis, with the result that they either stopped short there and could get no farther, or else concluded that this too was only Maya or Lila and that the one thing to do was to get beyond it into some immovable and inactive silence of the Supreme.

Perhaps, what may be meant by supernals is rather the three *fundamentals* of the present manifestation. In the Indian system, these are Ishwara, Shakti and Jiva, or else Sachchidananda, Maya and Jiva. But in our system which seeks to go beyond the present manifestation, these could very well be taken for granted and, looked at from the point of view of the planes of consciousness, the three highest — Ananda (with Sat and Chit resting upon it), supermind and overmind might be called the three Supernals. Overmind stands at the top of the lower hemisphere, and you have to pass through and beyond overmind, if you would reach supermind, while still above and beyond supermind are the worlds of Sachchidananda.

You speak of the gulf below the overmind. But is there a gulf — or any other gulf than human unconsciousness? In all the series of the planes or grades of consciousness there is nowhere any real gulf, always there are connecting gradations and one can ascend from step to step. Between the overmind and the human mind there are a number of more and more luminous gradations; but, as these are superconscient to human mind (except one or two of the lowest of which it gets some direct touches), it is apt to

regard them as a superior Inconscience. So one of the Upanishads speaks of the Ishwara consciousness as *suṣupti*, deep Sleep,
because it is only in Samadhi that man usually enters into it, so
long as he does not try to turn his waking consciousness into a
higher state.

There are in fact two systems simultaneously active in the
organisation of the being and its parts: one is concentric, a series
of rings or sheaths with the psychic at the centre; another is verti-
cal, an ascension and descent, like a flight of steps, a series of
superimposed planes with the supermind-overmind as the crucial
nodus of the transition beyond the human into the Divine. For
this transition, if it is to be at the same time a transformation,
there is only one way, one path. First, there must be a conversion
inwards, a going within to find the inmost psychic being and bring
it out to the front, disclosing at the same time the inner mind,
inner vital, inner physical parts of the nature. Next, there must
be an ascension, a series of conversions upwards and a turning
down to convert the lower parts. When one has made the inward
conversion, one psychicises the whole lower nature so as to make
it ready for the divine change. Going upwards, one passes beyond the human mind and at each stage of the ascent, there is a
conversion into a new consciousness and an infusion of this new
consciousness into the whole of the nature. Thus rising beyond
intellect through illuminated higher mind to the intuitive consciousness, we begin to look at everything not from the intellect
range or through intellect as an instrument, but from a greater
intuitive height and through an intuitivised will, feeling, emotion,
sensation and physical contact. So, proceeding from Intuition to
a greater overmind height, there is a new conversion and we
look at and experience everything from the overmind consciousness and through a mind, heart, vital and body surcharged with
the overmind thought, sight, will, feeling, sensation, play of force
and contact. But the last conversion is the supramental, for once
there — once the nature is supramentalised, we are beyond the
Ignorance and conversion of consciousness is no longer needed,
though a farther divine progression, even an infinite development
is still possible.

*
**

There is a world of Ignorance, there are worlds also of Truth. Creation has no beginning and no end. It is only a particular creation that can be said to have a beginning and an end.

You must remember that there are reflections of the Higher worlds in the lower planes which can easily be experienced as supreme for that stage of the evolution. But the supreme Sachchidananda is not a world, it is supracosmic. The Sat (Satyaloka) world is the highest of the scale connected with this universe.

That is the original Tapoloka in which the principle is Chit and its power of Tapas, but there are other worlds of Tapas on the other planes below. There is one in the mental, another in the vital range. It is one of these Tapas worlds from which the being you saw must have come.

There is a vital plane (self-existent) above the material universe which we see; there is a mental plane (self-existent) above the vital and material. These three together, — mental, vital, physical, — are called the triple universe of the lower hemisphere. They have been established in the earth-consciousness by evolution — but they exist in themselves before the evolution, above the earth-consciousness and the material plane to which the earth belongs.

If we regard the gradation of worlds or planes as a whole, we see them as a great connected complex movement; the higher precipitate their influences on the lower, the lower react to the higher and develop or manifest in themselves within their own formula something that corresponds to the superior power and its action. The material world has evolved life in obedience to a pressure from the vital plane, mind in obedience to a pressure from the mental plane. It is now trying to evolve supermind in obedience to a pressure from the supramental plane. In more detail, particular forces, movements, powers, beings of a higher world can throw themselves on the lower to establish appropriate and corresponding forms which will connect them with the material domain and, as it were, reproduce or project their action here. And each thing created here has, supporting it, subtler envelopes or forms of itself which make it subsist and connect it with forces acting from above. Man, for instance, has, besides his gross physical body, subtler sheaths or bodies by which he lives behind the veil in direct connection with supraphysical planes of consciousness and can be influenced by their powers, movements and beings. What takes place in life has always behind it pre-existent movements and forms in the occult vital planes; what takes place in mind presupposes pre-existent movements and forms in the occult mental planes. That is an aspect of things which becomes more and more evident, insistent and important, the more we progress in a dynamic yoga.

But all this must not be taken in too rigid and mechanical a sense. It is an immense plastic movement full of the play of possibilities and must be seized by a flexible and subtle tact or sense in the seeing consciousness. It cannot be reduced to a too rigorous logical or mathematical formula. Two or three points must be pressed in order that this plasticity may not be lost to our view.

First, each plane, in spite of its connection with others above and below it, is yet a world in itself, with its own movements, forces, beings, types, forms existing as if for its and their own sake, under its own laws, for its own manifestation without apparent regard for the other members of the great series. Thus, if we regard the vital or the subtle physical plane, we see great ranges of it, (most of it), existing in themselves, without any relation with the material world and with no movement to affect or influence it, still less to precipitate a corresponding manifestation in the physical formula. At most we can say that the existence of anything in the vital, subtle physical or any other plane creates a possibility for a corresponding movement of manifestation in the physical world. But something more is needed to turn that static or latent possibility into a dynamic potentiality or an actual urge towards a material creation. That something may be a call from the material plane, e.g., some force or someone on the physical existence entering into touch with a supraphysical power or world or part of it and moved to bring it down into the earth-life. Or it may be an impulse in the vital or other plane itself, e.g., a vital being moved to extend his action towards the earth and establish there a kingdom for himself or the play of the forces for which he stands in his own domain. Or it may be a pressure from above; let us say, some supramental or mental power precipitating its formation from above and developing forms and movements on the vital level as a means of transit to its self-creation in the material world. Or it may be all these things acting together, in which case there is the greatest possibility of an effective creation.

Next, as a consequence, it follows that only a limited part of the action of the vital or other higher plane is concerned with the earth-existence. But even this creates a mass of possibilities which is far greater than the earth can at one time manifest or contain in its own less plastic formulas. All these possibilities do not realise themselves; some fail altogether and leave at the most an idea that comes to nothing; some try seriously and are repelled and defeated and, even if in action for a time, come to nothing. Others effectuate a half manifestation, and this is the most usual result, the more so as these vital or other supraphysical forces come into conflict and have not only to overcome the resistance of the physical consciousness and of matter, but their own internecine resistance to each other. A certain number succeed in precipitating their results in a more complete and successful creation, so that if you compare this creation with its original in the higher plane, there is something like a close resemblance or even an apparently exact reproduction or translation from the supraphysical to the physical formula. And yet even there the exactness is only apparent; the very fact of translation into another substance and another rhythm of manifestation makes a difference. It is something new that has manifested and it is that that makes the creation worth while. What for instance would be the utility of a supramental creation on earth if it were just the same thing as a supramental creation on the supramental plane? It is that, in principle, but yet something else, a triumphant new self-discovery of the Divine in conditions that are not elsewhere.

No doubt, the subtle physical is closest to the physical, and most like it. But yet the conditions are different and the thing too different. For instance, the subtle physical has a freedom, plasticity, intensity, power, colour, wide and manifold play (there are thousands of things there that are not here) of which, as yet, we have no possibility on earth. And yet there is something here, a potentiality of the Divine which the other, in spite of its greater liberties, has not, something which makes creation more difficult, but in the last result justifies the labour.

Most things happen in the vital before they happen in the physical, but all that happens in the vital does not realise itself in the physical, or not in the same way. There is always or at least usually a change in the form, time, circumstances due to the different conditions of the physical plane.

These perceptions are correct on the whole. Each plane is true in itself but only in partial truth to the supermind. When these higher truths come into the physical they try to realise themselves there, but can do so only in part and under the conditions of the material plane. It is only the supermind that can overcome this difficulty.

The heavenly worlds are above the body. What the parts of the body correspond to are planes — subtle physical, higher, middle and lower vital, mental. Each plane is in communication with various worlds that belong to it.

It is the external consciousness, the inner consciousness, the superconscient that are meant.[1] The terms waking, dream, sleep are applied because in the ordinary consciousness of man the external only is awake, the inner being is mostly subliminal and acts directly only in a state of sleep when its movements are felt like things of dream and vision; while the superconscient (supermind, overmind, etc.) is beyond even that range and is to the mind like a deep sleep.

But why do you want to connect these things with the soul? These four names[2] are given to four conditions of transcendent and universal Brahman or Self, — they are merely conditions of Being and Consciousness — the Self that supports the waking state or *sthūla* consciousness, the Self that supports the Dream State or subtle consciousness, the Self that supports the Deep Sleep State or Causal consciousness, *kāraṇa,* and the Self in the supracosmic consciousness. The individual of course participates, but these are conditions of the Self, not the Self and soul. The meaning of these expressions is fixed in the Mandukya Upanishad.

These two sets of three names each mean the same things. Visva or Virat=the Spirit of the external universe, Hiranyagarbha or Taijasa (the Luminous)=the Spirit in the inner planes, Prajna or Ishwara=the Superconscient Spirit, Master of all things and the highest Self on which all depends. The Mental cannot be Ishwara.

Virat is the outer manifestation and if we take all that as Brahman without knowing what is behind the manifestation we shall fall into the intellectual error of Pantheism, not realising that the Divine is more than this outer manifestation and cannot be

---

[1] *Vaiśvānara, Taijasa* and *Prājña* in the Mandukya Upanishad.

[2] *Vaiśvānara, Taijasa, Prājña* and *Kūṭastha.*

known by it alone. In the vital we may fall into the error of accepting what is dark and imperfect on the same terms as that which makes for the light and divine perfection. There may be many other consequent errors also.

III

By the supermind is meant the full Truth-Consciousness of the Divine Nature in which there can be no place for the principle of division and ignorance; it is always a full light and knowledge superior to all mental substance or mental movement. Between the supermind and the human mind are a number of ranges, planes or layers of consciousness — one can regard it in various ways — in which the element or substance of mind and consequently its movements also become more and more illumined and powerful and wide. The overmind is the highest of these ranges; it is full of lights and powers; but from the point of view of what is above it, it is the line of the soul's turning away from the complete and indivisible knowledge and its descent towards the Ignorance. For although it draws from the Truth, it is here that begins the separation of aspects of the Truth, the forces and their working out as if they were independent truths and this is a process that ends, as one descends to ordinary Mind, Life and Matter, in a complete division, fragmentation, separation from the indivisible Truth above. There is no longer the essential, total, perfectly harmonising and unifying knowledge, or rather knowledge for ever harmonious because for ever one, which is the character of supermind. In the supermind, mental divisions and oppositions cease, the problems created by our dividing and fragmenting mind disappear and Truth is seen as a luminous whole. In the overmind there is not yet the actual fall into Ignorance, but the first step is taken which will make the fall inevitable.

The supermind is the One Truth deploying and determining the manifestation of its Powers — all these Powers working as a multiple Oneness, in harmony, without opposition or collision, according to the One Will inherent in all. The overmind takes these Truths and Powers and sets each working as a force in itself with its necessary consequences — there can be harmony in their action, but it is rather synthetic and mostly partial than inherent and inevitable and as one descends from the highest overmind, separation, collision and conflict of forces increase, separability dominates, ignorance grows, existence becomes a clash of possibilities, a mixture of conflicting half-truths, an unsolved and apparently unsolvable riddle and puzzle.

If the supermind were not to give us a greater and completer truth than any of the lower planes, it would not be worth while trying to reach it. Each plane has its own truths. Some of them are no longer true on a higher plane; e.g. desire and ego were truths of the mental, vital and physical Ignorance — a man there without ego or desire would be a tamasic automaton. As we rise higher, ego and desire appear no longer as truths, they are falsehoods disfiguring the true person and the true will. The struggle between the Powers of Light and the Powers of Darkness is a truth here — as we ascend above, it becomes less and less of a truth and in the supermind it has no truth at all. Other truths remain but change their character, importance, place in the whole. The difference or contrast between the Personal and Impersonal is a truth of the overmind — there is no separate truth of them in the supermind, they are inseparably one. But one who has not mastered and lived the truths of overmind cannot reach the supramental Truth. The incompetent pride of man's mind makes a sharp distinction and wants to call all else untruth and leap at once to the highest truth whatever it may be — but that is an ambitious and arrogant error. One has to climb the stairs and rest one's feet firmly on each step in order to reach the summit.

I do not understand. The Personal Divine does not mean the

Avatar. What I said was that the scission between the two aspects of the Divine is a creation of the overmind which takes various aspects of the Divine and separates them into separate entities. Thus it divides Sat, Chit and Ananda, so that they become three separate aspects different from each other. In fact in the Reality there is no separateness, the three aspects are so fused into each other, so inseparably one that they are a single undivided reality. It is the same with the Personal and Impersonal, the Saguna and Nirguna, the Silent and the Active Brahman. In the Reality they are not contrasted and incompatible aspects; what we call Personality and what we call Impersonality are inseparably fused together into a single Truth. In fact "fused together" even is a wrong phrase, because there they were never separated so that they have to be fused. All the quarrels about either the Impersonal being the only true truth or the Personal being the only highest truth are mind-created quarrels derivative from this dividing aspect of the overmind. The overmind does not deny any in the aspects as the Mind does, it admits them all as aspects of the One Truth, but by separating them it originates the quarrel in the more ignorant and more limited and divided Mind, because the Mind, cannot see how two opposite things can exist together in one Truth, how the Divine can be *nirguṇo guṇi* ; — having no experience of what is behind the two words it takes each in an absolute sense. The Impersonal is Existence, Consciousness, Bliss, not a Person, but a state. The Person is the Existent, the Conscious, the Blissful; consciousness, existence, bliss taken as separate things are only states of his being. But in fact the two (personal being and eternal state) are inseparable and are one reality.

It is hardly possible to say what the supermind is in the language of Mind, even spiritualised Mind, for it is a different consciousness altogether and acts in a different way. Whatever may be said of it is likely to be not understood or misunderstood. It is only by growing into it that we can know what it is and this also cannot be done until after a long process by which mind heightening and illuminating becomes pure Intuition (not the mixed thing that ordinarily goes by that name) and masses itself into overmind; after that overmind can be lifted into and suffused with supermind till it undergoes a transformation.

In the supermind all is self-known self-luminously, there are no divisions, oppositions or separated aspects as in Mind whose principle is division of Knowledge into parts and setting each part against another. Overmind approaches this at its top and is often mistaken for supermind, but it cannot reach it — except by uplifting and transformation.

*
**

It is (sometimes directly, sometimes indirectly) by the power of the overmind releasing the mind from its close partitions that the cosmic consciousness opens in the seeker and he becomes aware of the cosmic spirit and the play of the cosmic forces.

It is from or at least through the overmind plane that the original pre-arrangement of things in this world is effected; for from it the determining vibrations originally come. But there are corresponding movements on all the planes, the mind, the vital, the physical even and it is possible in a very clear or illumined condition of the lower consciousness to become aware of these movements and understand the plan of things and be either a conscious instrument or even, to a limited extent, a determinant Will or Force. But the stuff of the lower planes always mixes with the overmind forces when they descend and diminishes or even falsifies and perverts their truth and power.

It is even possible for the overmind to transmit to the lower planes of consciousness something of the supramental Light; but, so long as the supermind does not directly manifest, its Light is modified in the overmind itself and still further modified in the application by the needs, the demands, the circumscribing possibilities of the individual nature. The success of this diminished and modified Light, e.g. in purifying the physical, cannot be immediate and absolute as the full and direct supramental action would be; it is still relative, conditioned by the individual nature and the balance of the universal forces, resisted by adverse powers, baulked of its perfect result by the unwillingness of the lower workings to cease, limited either in its scope or in its efficacy by the want of a complete consent in the physical nature.

The overmind has to be reached and brought down before the supermind descent is at all possible — for the overmind is the passage through which one passes from Mind to supermind.

It is from the overmind that all these different arrangements of the creative Truth of things originate. Out of the overmind they come down to the Intuition and are transmitted from it to the Illumined and Higher Mind to be arranged there for our intelligence. But they lose more and more of their power and certitude in the transmission as they come down to the lower levels. What energy of directly perceived Truth they have is lost in the human mind; for to the human intellect they present themselves only as speculative ideas, not as realised Truth, not as direct sight, a dynamic vision coupled with a concrete undeniable experience.

There are different planes of the overmind. One is mental, directly creative of all the formations that manifest below in the mental world — that is the mental overmind. Above is the overmind intuition. Still above are the planes of overmind that are more and more connected with the supermind and have a partly supramental character. Highest in the overmind ranges is the supramental overmind or overmind gnosis. But these are things you cannot understand until you get a higher experience. You cannot do it at present. Only those who have got fully into cosmic consciousness can do it and even they cannot do it at first. One must first go fully through the experience of higher mind and illumined mind and intuition before it can be done.

It is not so simple as that — but it [the overmind] can for convenience be divided into four planes — mental overmind and the three you have written (intuitive overmind, true overmind and supramental overmind), but there are many layers in each and each of these can be regarded as a plane in itself.

That is not impossible — it is perfectly possible on any of the larger planes — infinity is everywhere, once one breaks the individual limits.

There are many stages in the transition from mental overmind to supramentalised overmind and from there to supermind. Do not be in a hurry to say, "This is the last highest overmind."

What you call supramental overmind[1] is still overmind — not a part of the true supermind. One cannot get into the true supermind (except in some kind of trance or Samadhi) unless one has first objectivised the overmind truth in life, speech, action, external knowledge and not only experienced it in meditation and inner experience.

At the time when the last chapters of *The Synthesis of Yoga* were written in the *Arya*, the name "overmind" had not been found, so there is no mention of it. What is described in those chapters is the action of the supermind when it descends into the overmind plane and takes up the overmind workings and transforms them. The highest supermind or Divine gnosis existent in itself, is something that lies beyond still and quite above. It was intended in latter chapters to show how difficult even this was and how many levels there were between the human mind and supermind and how even supermind descending could get mixed with

---

[1] This expression is a misnomer since overmind cannot be supramental: it can at most receive some light and truth from the higher source.

the lower action and turned into something that was less than the true Truth. But these latter chapters were not written.

The distinction [between the overmind and the supermind] has not been made in the *Arya* because at that time what I now call the overmind was supposed to be an inferior plane of the supermind. But that was because I was seeing them from the Mind. The true defect of overmind, the limitation in it which gave rise to a world of ignorance is seen fully only when one looks at it from the physical consciousness, from the result (Ignorance in Matter) to the cause (overmind division of the Truth). In its own plane overmind seems to be only a divided, many-sided play of the Truth, so can easily be taken by the Mind as a supramental province. Mind also when flooded by the overmind lights feels itself living in a surprising revelation of divine Truth. The difficulty comes when we deal with the vital and still more with the physical. Then it becomes imperative to face the difficulty and to make a sharp distinction between overmind and supermind — for it then becomes evident that the overmind Power (in spite of its lights and splendours) is not sufficient to overcome the Ignorance because it is itself under the law of Division out of which came the Ignorance. One has to pass beyond and supramentalise overmind so that mind and all the rest may undergo the final change.

Probably what he calls overmind is the first "above-mind" layers of consciousness. Or it may be experiences from the larger Mind or Vital ranges. To the human mind all these are so big that it is easy to take them for overmind or even supermind. One can get indirect overmind touches if one opens into the cosmic consciousness, still more if one enters freely into that consciousness. Direct overmind experience cannot come unless part of the being at least is seated in the wideness and peace.

Intuition is above illumined Mind which is simply higher Mind raised to a great luminosity and more open to modified forms of intuition and inspiration.

The Intuition is the first plane in which there is a real opening to the full possibility of realisation — it is through it that one goes farther — first to overmind and then to supermind.

Intuition sees the truth of things by a direct inner contact, not like the ordinary mental intelligence by seeking and reaching out for indirect contacts through the senses etc. But the limitation of the Intuition as compared with the supermind is that it sees things by flashes, point by point, not as a whole. Also in coming into the mind it gets mixed with the mental movement and forms a kind of intuitive mind activity which is not the pure truth, but something in between the higher Truth and the mental seeking. It can lead the consciousness through a sort of transitional stage and that is practically its function.

Mental intuitive knowledge catches directly some aspect of the truth but without any completeness or certitude and the intuition is easily mixed with ordinary mental stuff that may be erroneous; in application it may easily be a half-truth or be so misinterpreted and misapplied as to become an error. Also, the mind easily imitates the intuition in such a way that it is difficult to distinguish between a true or a false intuition. That is the reason why men of intellect distrust the mental intuition and say that it cannot be accepted or followed unless it is tested and confirmed by the intellect. What comes from the overmind intuition has a light, a certitude, an effective force of Truth in it that the mental intuition at its best even has not.

There are mental, vital, subtle physical intuitions as well as intuitions from the higher and the illumined Mind.

**

It [the identification of *buddhi* with *vijñāna* and intuition] is the error that came with the excessive intellectualism of the philosophers and commentators. I don't think *buddhi* includes intuition as something separate in kind from intellect — the intellectualists considered intuition to be only a rapid process of intellectual thought — and they still think that. In the Taittiriya Upanishad the sense of *vijñāna* is very clear — its essence is *ṛtam*, the spiritual Truth; but afterwards the identification with *buddhi* became general.

**

I do not suppose they mean expressly intuition; they regard *buddhi* as the means of knowledge, so they include all knowledge in it, and as the *vijñānamaya koṣa* is the Knowledge sheath, they think it must mean *buddhi*. Obviously it doesn't. The description you have quoted evidently means something much higher than *buddhi*. It is the *satyam ṛtam bṛhat* of the Upanishad — the truth-consciousness of the Veda.

IV

The phrase "central being" in our yoga is usually applied to the portion of the Divine in us which supports all the rest and survives through death and birth. This central being has two forms — above, it is Jivatman, our true being, of which we become aware when the higher self-knowledge comes, — below, it is the psychic being which stands behind mind, body and life. The Jivatman is above the manifestation in life and presides over it; the psychic being stands behind the manifestation in life and supports it.

The natural attitude of the psychic being is to feel itself as the Child, the Son of God, the Bhakta; it is a portion of the

Divine, one in essence, but in the dynamics of the manifestation there is always even in identity a difference. The Jivatman, on the contrary, lives in the essence and can merge itself in identity with the Divine; but it too, the moment it presides over the dynamics of the manifestation, knows itself as one centre of the multiple Divine, not as the Parameshwara. It is important to remember the distinction; for, otherwise, if there is the least vital egoism, one may begin to think of oneself as an Avatar or lose balance like Hridaya with Ramakrishna.

The word Jiva has two meanings in the Sanskritic tongues — "living creatures"[1] and the spirit individualised and upholding the living being in its evolution from birth to birth. In the latter sense the full term is Jivatma — the Atman, spirit or eternal self of the living being. It is spoken of figuratively by the Gita as "an eternal portion of the Divine" — but the word fragmentation (used by you) is too strong, it could be applicable to the forms, but not to the spirit in them. Moreover the multiple Divine is an eternal reality antecedent to the creation here. An elaborate description of the Jivatma would be: "the multiple Divine manifested here as the individualised self or spirit of the created being." The Jivatma in its essence does not change or evolve, its essence stands above the personal evolution; within the evolution itself it is represented by the evolving psychic being which supports all the rest of the nature.

The Adwaita Vedanta (Monism) declares that the Jiva has no real existence, as the Divine is indivisible. Another school attributes a real but not an independent existence to the Jiva — it is, they say, one in essence, different in manifestation, and as the manifestation is real, eternal and not an illusion, it cannot be called unreal. The dualistic schools affirm the Jiva as an independent category or stand on the triplicity of God, soul and Nature.

[1] In Bengal when one is about to kill a small animal, people often protest saying, "Don't kill — it is Krishna's Jiva (his living creature)."

Jīvātmā is not the psychic being — we have fixed on *caitya puruṣa* as the equivalent in Sanskrit of the psychic being. Jivatma is the individual Self — the central being.

The central being is that which is not born, does not evolve, but presides over all the individual manifestation. The psychic is its projection here — for the psychic being is in the evolution and from within supports our whole evolution; it receives the essence of all experience and by that develops the personality Godward.

The Self is at once one in all and many — one in its essence, it manifests also as the individual self which may be described as in Nature an eternal portion of the Divine; in spirit a centre of the manifestation, individual but extending its universality and rising into transcendence.

By Jivatma we mean the individual self. Essentially it is one self with all others, but in the multiplicity of the Divine it is the individual self, an individual centre of the universe — and it sees everything in itself or itself in everything or both together according to its state of consciousness and point of view.

The self, Atman is in its nature either transcendent or universal (Paramatma, Atma). When it individualises and becomes a central being, it is then the Jivatman. The Jivatman feels his oneness with the universal but at the same time his central separateness as a portion of the Divine.

The soul, representative of the central being, is a spark of the Divine supporting all individual existence in Nature; the psychic being is a conscious form of that soul growing in the evolution — in the persistent process that develops first life in Matter, mind in life, until finally mind can develop into overmind and overmind into the supramental Truth. The soul supports the nature in its evolution through these grades, but is itself not any of these things.

The lower Nature, *aparā prakṛti*, is this external objective and superficial subjective apparent Nature which manifests all these minds, lives and bodies. The supreme Nature, *parā prakṛti*, concealed behind it is the very nature of the Divine — a supreme Consciousness-Force which manifests the multiple Divine as the Many. These Many are in themselves eternal selves of the Supreme in his supreme Nature, *parā prakṛti*. Here in relation to this world they appear as the Jivatmas supporting the evolution of the natural existences, *sarva-bhūtāni*, in the mutable Becoming which is the life of the Kshara (mobile or mutable) Purusha. The Jiva (or Jivatma) and the creatures, *sarva-bhūtāni*, are not the same thing. The Jivatmas really stand above the creation even though concerned in it; the natural existences, *sarva-bhūtāni*, are the creatures of Nature. Man, bird, beast, reptile are natural existences, but the individual Self in them is not even for a moment characteristically man, bird, beast or reptile; in its evolution it is the same through all these changes, a spiritual being that consents to the play of Nature.

What is original and eternal for ever in the Divine is the Being, what is developed in consciousness, conditions, forces, forms, etc., by the Divine Power is the Becoming. The eternal Divine is the Being; the universe in Time and all that is apparent in it is a Becoming. The eternal Being in its superior nature, Para Prakriti, is at once One and Many; but the eternal Multiplicity of the Divine when it stands behind the created existences, *sarva-bhūtāni*, appears as (or as we say, becomes) the Jiva, *parā prakṛtir jīvabhūtā*. In the psychic, on the other hand, there are two aspects, the psychic existence or soul behind and in front the form of individuality it takes in its evolution in Nature.

The soul or psyche is immutable only in the sense that it contains all the possibilities of the Divine within it, but it has to evolve them and in its evolution it assumes the form of a developing psychic individual evolving in the manifestation the individual Prakriti and taking part in the evolution. It is the spark of the Divine Fire that grows behind the mind, vital and physical

by means of the psychic being until it is able to transform the
Prakriti of Ignorance into a Prakriti of Knowledge. This evolving psychic being is not therefore at any time all that the soul or
essential psychic existence bears within it; it temporalises and
individualises what is eternal in potentiality, transcendent in
essence, in this projection of the spirit.

The central being is the being which presides over the different births one after the other, but is itself unborn, for it does not
descend into the being but is above it — it holds together the
mental, vital and physical being and all the various parts of the
personality and it controls the life either through the mental
being and the mental thought and will or through the psychic,
whichever may happen to be most in front or most powerful in
nature. If it does not exercise its control, then the consciousness is in great disorder and every part of the personality acts for
itself so that there is no coherence in the thought, feeling or
action.

The psychic is not above but behind — its seat is behind the
heart, its power is not knowledge but an essential or spiritual
feeling — it has the clearest sense of the Truth and a sort of
inherent perception of it which is of the nature of soul-percep-
tion and soul-feeling. It is our inmost being and supports all the
others, mental, vital, physical, but it is also much veiled by them
and has to act upon them as an influence rather than by its
sovereign right of direct action; its direct action becomes normal
and preponderant only at a high stage of development or by
yoga. It is not the psychic being which, you feel, gives you the
intuitions of things to be or warns you against the results of
certain actions; that is some part of the inner being, sometimes
the inner mental, sometimes the inner vital, sometimes, it may be,
the inner or subtle physical Purusha. The inner being — inner
mind, inner vital, inner or subtle physical — knows much
that is unknown to the outer mind, the outer vital, the
outer physical, for it is in a more direct contact with the
secret forces of Nature. The psychic is the inmost being of all;
a perception of truth which is inherent in the deepest substance
of the consciousness, a sense of the good, true, beautiful, the
Divine, is its privilege.

The central being — the Jivatman which is not born nor evolves but presides over the individual birth and evolution — puts forward a representative of himself on each plane of the consciousness. On the mental plane it is the true mental being, *manomaya puruṣa*, on the vital plane the true vital being, *prāṇamaya puruṣa*, on the physical plane the true physical being, *annamaya puruṣa*. Each being, therefore is, so long as the Ignorance lasts, centred round his mental, vital or physical Purusha, according to the plane on which he predominantly lives, and that is to him his central being. But the true representative all the time is concealed behind the mind, vital and physical — it is the psychic, our inmost being.

When the inmost knowledge begins to come, we become aware of the psychic being within us and it comes forward and leads the sadhana. We become aware also of the Jivatman, the undivided Self or Spirit above the manifestation of which the psychic is the representative here.

The true inner being — the true mental, the true vital, the true physical represent each on its plane and answer to the central being, but the whole of the nature and especially the outer nature does not, nor the ordinary mental, vital or physical personality. The psychic being is the central being for the purposes of the evolution — it grows and develops; but there is a central being above of which the mind is not aware, which presides unseen over the existence and of which the psychic being is the representative in the manifested nature. It is what is called the Jivatman.

The psychic is a spark of the Divine — but I do not know that it can be called a portion of the Jivatma — it is the same put forward in a different way.

Well, it is a little difficult to explain. Perhaps the best thing is to break up my answer into a number of separate statements, for the whole thing has got too complicated to do otherwise.

1. It is impossible to equate my conception or experience of the Jivatman with the pure "I" of the Adwaita, by which you mean, I suppose, something which says, "I am He" and by that perception merges itself into the Brahman. According to the Adwaita of the Mayavadins this Jivatman, like the Ishwara himself, is simply an appearance of the Brahman in illusory Maya. There is no Ishwara, Lord of the world, because there is no world — except in Maya; so too there is no Jivatman, only the Paramatman illusorily perceived as an individual self by the lower (illusory) consciousness in Maya. Those, on the other hand, who wish to unite with the Ishwara, regard or experience the Jiva either as a separate being dependent on the Ishwara or as something one in essence with him, yet different, but this difference like the essential oneness is eternal — and there are also other ideas of the Jivatman and its relation to the Divine or Supreme. So this pure "I", if that is how it is to be described, presents itself differently, in different aspects, one may say, to different people. If you ask why, I refer you to my answer to X. The overmind presents the truth of things in all sorts of aspects and mind, even the spiritual mind, fastens on one or the other as the very truth, the one real truth of the matter. It is the mind that makes these differences, but that does not matter, because, through its own way of seeing and experiencing the soul or individualised consciousness or whatever you may like to call it, the mental being goes where it has to go. I hope this much is clear as the first step in the matter.

2. I do not dispute at all the fact that one can realise the Self, the Brahman or the Ishwara without going into the overhead regions, the dynamic spiritual planes, or stationing oneself permanently above the body as happens in this yoga. Even if it is done through the Sahasrara, well, the Sahasrara extends to the spiritualised mind and can be felt in the top of the head, so any ascent above is not indispensable. But, apart from that, one can very well, as you say, realise the Atman if one stands back from the mind and heart, detaches oneself from the parts of

Prakriti, ceases to identify oneself with mind, life and body, falls into an inner silence. One need not even explore the kingdoms of the inner mind or inner vital, still less is it compulsory to spread one's wings in ranges above. The Self is everywhere and by entering into full detachment and silence, or even by either detachment or silence, one can get anywhere some glimpse, some reflection, perhaps even a full reflection, or a sense of the Self's presence or of one's own immergence in that which is free, wide, silent, eternal, infinite. Obviously if it is a pure "I", of whatever nature, which gets the experience, it must be looked on by the consciousness that has the realisation as the individual self of the Being, Jivatman.

3. One can also have the experience of oneself as not the mind but the thinker, not the heart but the self or "I" which supports the feelings, not the life but that which supports life, not the body but that which assumes a body. This self can be obviously dynamic as well as silent; or else you may say that, even though still and immobile, from its silence it originates the dynamism of Nature. One can also feel this to be the Spirit one in all as well as the true "I" in oneself. All depends on the experience. Very usually, it is the experience of the Purusha, often felt first as the Witness silent, upholding all the nature; but the Purusha can also be experienced as the Knower and the Ishwara. Sometimes it is as or through the mental Purusha in one centre or another, sometimes as or through the vital Purusha that one can become aware of one's self or spirit. It is also possible to become aware of the secret psychic being within by itself as the true individual; or one can be aware of the psychic being as the pure "I" with these others standing in mind or vital as representatives in these domains or on these levels. According to one's experience one may speak of any of these as the Jiva or pure "I" (this last is a very dubious phrase) or the true Person or true Individual who knows himself as one with or a portion of or wholly dependent on the universal or transcendent Being and seeks to merge himself in that or ascend to that and be it or live in oneness with it. All these things are quite possible without any need of the overhead experience or of the stable overhead Permanence.

4. One may ask, first, why not then say that the Jivatman which can be realised in this way is the pure "I" of which the lower self has the experience and through which it gets its salvation; and, secondly, what need is there of going into the overhead planes at all? Well, in the first place, this pure "I" does not seem to be absolutely necessary as an intermediary of the liberation whether into the impersonal Self or Brahman or into whatever is eternal. The Buddhists do not admit any soul or self or any experience of the pure "I"; they proceed by dissolving the consciousness into a bundle of Sanskaras, get rid of the Sanskaras and so are liberated into some Permanent which they refuse to describe or some Shunya. So the experience of a pure "I" or Jivatman is not binding on everyone who wants liberation into the Eternal but is content to get it without rising beyond the spiritualised mind into a higher Light above. I myself had my experience of Nirvana and silence in the Brahman, etc. long before there was any knowledge of the overhead spiritual planes; it came first simply by an absolute stillness and blotting out as it were of all mental, emotional and other inner activities — the body continued indeed to see, walk, speak and do its other business, but as an empty automatic machine and nothing more. I did not become aware of any pure "I" nor even of any self, impersonal or other, — there was only an awareness of That as the sole Reality, all else being quite unsubstantial, void, non-real. As to what realised that Reality, it was a nameless consciousness which was not other than That;[1] one could perhaps say this, though hardly even so much as this, since there was no mental concept of it, but not more. Neither was I aware of any lower soul or outer self called by such and such a personal name that was performing this feat of arriving at the consciousness of Nirvana. Well, then what becomes of your pure "I" and lower "I" in all that? Consciousness (not this or that part of consciousness or an "I" of any kind) suddenly emptied itself of all inner contents and remained aware only of unreal surroundings and of Something real but ineffable. You may say that there must have been a consciousness aware of some perceiving existence,

---

[1] Mark that I did not think these things, there were no thoughts or concepts nor did they present themselves like that to any Me; it simply just was so or was self-apparently so.

if not of a pure "I", but, if so, it was something for which these names seem inadequate.

5. I have said the overhead ascension is not indispensable for the usual spiritual purposes, — but it is indispensable for the purposes of this yoga. For its aim is to become aware of and liberate and transform and unite all the being in the light of a Truth-consciousness which is above and cannot be reached if there is no entirely inward-going and no transcending and upward-going movement. Hence all the complexity of my psychological statements as a whole, not new in essence — for much of it occurs in the Upanishads and elsewhere, but new in its fullness of collective statement and its developments directed towards an integral yoga. It is not necessary for anyone to accept it unless he concurs in the aim; for other aims it is unnecessary and may very well be excessive.

6. But when one *has* made the inner exploration and the ascension, when one's consciousness is located above, one cannot be expected to see things precisely as they are seen from below. The Jivatman is for me the Unborn who presides over the individual being and its developments, associated with it but above it and them and who by the very nature of his existence knows himself as universal and transcendent no less than individual and feels the Divine to be his origin, the truth of his being, the master of his nature, the very stuff of his existence. He is plunged in the Divine and one with the Eternal for ever, aware of his own expression and instrumental dynamism which is the Divine's, dependent in love and delight, with adoration on That with which yet through that love and delight he is one, capable of relation in oneness, harmonic in this many-sidedness without contradiction, because this is another consciousness and existence than that of the mind, even of the spiritualised mind; it is an intrinsic consciousness of the Infinite, infinite not only in essence but in capacity, which can be to its own self-awareness all things and yet for ever the same and one. The triune realisation, therefore, full of difficulties for the mind, is quite natural, easy, indisputable to the supramental consciousness or, generally, to the consciousness of the upper hemisphere. It can be seen and felt as knowledge in all the spiritual planes, but the completely indi-

visible knowledge, the full dynamics of it can only be realised through the supramental consciousness itself on its own plane or by its descent here.

7. The description of a pure "I" is quite insufficient to describe the realisation of the Jivatman — it is rather describable as the true Person or Divine Individual, though that too is not adequate. The word "I" always comes with an under-suggestion of ego, of separativeness; but there is no separativeness in this self-vision, for the individual here is a spiritual living centre of action for the One and feels no separation from all that is the One.

8. The Jivatman has its representative power in the individual nature here; this power is the Purusha upholding the Prakriti — centrally in the psychic, more instrumentally in the mind, vital and physical being and nature. It is therefore possible to regard these or any of them as if they were the Jiva here. All the same I am obliged to make a distinction not only for clear thinking but because of the necessity of experience and integral dynamic self-knowledge without which it is difficult to carry through this yoga. It is not indispensable to formulate mentally to oneself all this, one can have the experience and, if one sees clearly with an inner perception, it is sufficient for progress towards the goal. Nevertheless if the mind is clarified without falling into mental rigidity and error, things are easier for the sadhak of the yoga. But plasticity must be preserved, for loss of plasticity is the danger of a systematic intellectual formulation; one must look into the thing itself and not get tied up in the idea. Nothing of all this can be really grasped except by the actual spiritual experience.

I have used the words Jiva and Jivatman in these and all passages in exactly the same sense — it never occurred to me that there could be a difference. If I had so intended it, I would have drawn the distinction — the two words being similar — very clearly and not left it to be gathered by inference.

In the passage from the chapter on the triple status of the supermind I was describing how the supermind working as a force of the highest self-determination of the Divine manifested

it in three poises and what was the consciousness of the Jivatman
in a supramental creation. There is no statement that the place of
the Jivatman is in the supramental plane alone; if that were so,
man could have no knowledge of his individual Self or Spirit
before he rose to the supramental plane; he could not have any
experience of the Self, though he may have the sense of the dissolution of his ego in something Universal. But he can become
aware of his unborn non-evolving Self, a centre of the Divine
Consciousness, long before that; the Self cosmic or individual is
experienced long before rising to supermind. If it were not so,
spiritual experience of that high kind would be impossible to
mental man, liberation would be impossible; he would first have
to become a supramental being. As for the Purusha it is there on
all planes; there is a mental Purusha, *manomaya*, leader of the life
and body, as the Upanishad puts it, a vital, a physical Purusha;
there is the psychic being or Chaitya Purusha which supports and
carries all these as it were. One may say that these are projections
of the Jivatman put there to uphold Prakriti on the various levels
of the being. The Upanishad speaks also of a supramental and a
Bliss Purusha, and if the supramental and the Bliss Nature were
organised in the evolution on earth we could become aware of
them upholding the movements here.

As for the psychic being, it enters into the evolution, enters
into the body at birth and goes out of it at death; but the Jivatman, as I know it, is unborn and eternal although upholding the
manifested personality from above. The psychic being can be
described as the Jivatman entering into birth, if you like, but if
the distinction is not made, then the nature of the Atman is
blurred and a confusion arises. This is a necessary distinction for
metaphysical knowledge and for something that is very important
in spiritual experience. The word 'Atman' like 'spirit' in English
is popularly used in all kinds of senses, but both for spiritual and
philosophical knowledge it is necessary to be clear and precise in
one's use of terms so as to avoid confusion of thought and vision
by confusion in the words we use to express them.

*
**

The Jiva is realised as the individual Self, Atman, the central being above the Nature, calm, untouched by the movements of Nature, but supporting their evolution though not involved in it. Through this realisation silence, freedom, wideness, mastery, purity, a sense of universality in the individual as one centre of this divine universality become the normal experience. The psychic is realised as the Purusha behind the heart. It is not universalised like the Jivatman, but is the individual soul supporting from its place behind the heart-centre the mental, vital, physical, psychic evolution of the being in Nature. Its realisation brings bhakti, self-giving, surrender, turning of all the movements Godward, discrimination and choice of all that belongs to the Divine Truth, Good, Beauty, rejection of all that is false, evil, ugly, discordant, union through love and sympathy with all existence, openness to the Truth of the Self and the Divine.

To live in the consciousness of the Atman is to live in the calm unity and peace that is above things and separate from the world even when pervading it. But for the psychic consciousness there are two things, the world and itself acting in the world. The Jivatman has not come down into the world, it stands above, always the same supporting the different beings, mental, etc., which act here. The psychic is what has come down here — its function is to offer all things to the Divine for transformation.

The true being may be realised in one or both of two aspects — the Self or Atman and the soul or Antaratman, psychic being, Chaitya Purusha. The difference is that one is felt as universal, the other as individual supporting the mind, life and body. When one first realises the Atman one feels it separate from all things, existing in itself and detached, and it is to this realisation that the image of the dry coconut fruit may apply. When one realises the psychic being, it is not like that; for this brings the sense of union with the Divine and dependence upon It and sole consecration to the Divine alone and the power to change the nature and discover the true mental, the true vital, the true physical being in oneself. Both realisations are necessary for this yoga.

The "I" or the little ego is constituted by Nature and is at once a mental, vital and physical formation meant to aid in centralising and individualising the outer consciousness and action. When the true being is discovered, the utility of the ego is over and this formation has to disappear — the true being is felt in its place.

The Spirit is the consciousness above mind, the Atman or Self, which is always in oneness with the Divine — a spiritual conciousness is one which is always in unity or at least in contact with the Divine.

The psychic is a spark come from the Divine which is there in all things and as the individual evolves it grows in him and manifests as the psychic being, the soul, seeking always for the Divine and the Truth and answering to the Divine and the Truth whenever and wherever it meets it.

The Spirit is the Atman, Brahman, Essential Divine.

When the One Divine manifests its ever inherent multiplicity, this essential Self or Atman becomes for that manifestation the central being who presides from above over the evolution of its personalities and terrestrial lives here, but is itself an eternal portion of the Divine and prior to the terrestrial manifestation — *parā prakṛtir jīvabhūtā*.

In this lower manifestation, *aparā prakṛti*, this eternal portion of the Divine appears as the soul, a spark of the Divine Fire, supporting the individual evolution, supporting the mental, vital and physical being. The psychic being is the spark growing into a Fire, evolving with the growth of the consciousness. The psychic being is therefore evolutionary, not like the Jivatman prior to the evolution.

But man is not aware of the self or Jivatman, he is aware only of his ego, or he is aware of the mental being which controls the life and the body. But more deeply he becomes aware of his soul or psychic being as his true centre, the Purusha in the heart; the psychic is the central being in the evolution, it proceeds from and represents the Jivatman, the eternal portion of the Divine. When there is the full consciousness, the Jivatman and the psychic being join together.

The ego is a formation of Nature; but it is not a formation of physical nature alone, therefore it does not cease with the body. There is a mental and vital ego also.

The base of the material consciousness here is not only the Ignorance, but the Inconscience — that is, the consciousness is involved in form of Matter and energy of Matter. It is not only the material consciousness but the vital and the mental too that are separated from the Truth by the Ignorance.

For the most part the Supreme acts through the Jiva and its nature and the Jiva and the nature act through the ego and the ego acts through the outer instruments — that is the play of the Ignorance.

There is no difference between Jiva and Jivatma in this language — so this distinction cannot be made. The Apara Prakriti is Nature which manifests all these minds, lives and bodies. The Para Prakriti is the very nature of the Divine — a supreme Consciousness-Force which manifests the multiple Divine as the Many.

The body is not the individual self — it is the basis of the external personality or of the physical self, if you like so to express it; but that is not the individual self. The individual self is the central being (Jivatma) manifesting in the lower nature as the psychic being — it is directly a portion of the Divine.

The *Jīvātmā* is above all planes. It has no fixed form or colour; though it may represent itself in a form.

(a) It [each Jivatman] is one, yet different [from other Jivatmans]. The Gita puts it that the Jiva is an *aṁśaḥ sanātanaḥ* of the One. It can also be spoken of as one among many centres of the Universal Being and Consciousness.

(b) Essentially one Jiva has the same nature as all — but in manifestation each puts forth its own line of Swabhava.

(c) No. Kutastha is the *akṣara puruṣa* — it is not the Jivatman.

(d) It [the station of the Jivatman] is on the spiritual plane always that is above the mind, but there it is not fixed to any level.

(e) No [one psychic being cannot unite with another]. Affinity, harmony, sympathy, but not union. Union is with the Divine.

[1]The Jivatma, spark-soul and psychic being are three different forms of the same reality and they must not be mixed up together, as that confuses the clearness of the inner experience.

The Jivatma or spirit is self-existent above the manifested or instrumental being — it is superior to birth and death, always the same, it is the individual Self or Atman; the eternal true being of the individual.

The soul is a spark of the Divine in the heart of the living creatures of Nature. It is not seated above the manifested being; it enters into the manifestation of the self, consents to be a part

---

[1] The original version of this letter was subsequently revised by Sri Aurobindo on two occasions. As the two revised versions differ considerably at places, both of them are published here consecutively.

of its natural phenomenal becoming, supports its evolution in the world of material Nature. It carries with it at first an undifferentiated power of the divine consciousness containing all possibilities which have not yet taken form but to which it is the function of evolution to give form. This spark of Divinity, is there in all terrestrial living beings from the earth's highest to its lowest creatures.

The psychic being is a spiritual personality put forward by the soul in its evolution; its growth marks the stage which the spiritual evolution of the individual has reached and its immediate possibilities for the future. It stands behind the mental, the vital, the physical nature, grows by their experiences, carries the consciousness from life to life. It is the psychic Person, *caitya puruṣa*. At first it is veiled by the mental, vital and physical parts, limited in its self-expression by their limitations, bound to the reactions of Nature, but, as it grows, it becomes capable of coming forward and dominating the mind, life and body. In the ordinary man it still depends on them for expression and is not able to take them up and freely use them. The life of the being is animal and human, not divine. When the psychic being can by sadhana become dominant and freely use its instruments, then the impulse towards the Divine becomes complete and the transformation of mind, vital and body, not merely their liberation becomes possible.

As the Self or Atman is free and superior to birth and death, the experience of the Jivatman and its unity with the supreme or universal Self is sufficient to bring the sense of liberation; but for the transformation of the life and nature the full awareness and awakening of our psychic being also is indispensable.

The psychic being realises at this stage its oneness with the true being, the Self, but it does not disappear or change into it; it remains as its instrument for psychic and spiritual self-expression, a divine manifestation in Nature.

The *bindu* seen by you above may be a symbolic way of seeing the Jivatman, the individual self as a drop of the Sea, an individual portion of the universal Divine; the aspiration on that level would naturally be for the opening of the higher consciousness so that the being may dwell there and not in the ignorance.

The Jivatman is already one with the Divine in reality, but its spiritual demand may be for the rest of the consciousness also to realise it.

The aspiration of the psychic being would then translate this demand entirely for the opening of the whole lower nature, mind, vital, body to the Divine, for the love and union with the Divine, for its presence and power within the heart, for the transformation of the mind, life and body by the descent of the higher consciousness into this instrumental being and nature.

Both aspirations are necessary for the fullness of this yoga, the demand of the self on the nature from above, the psychic aspiration of the nature from below. When the psychic imposes its aspiration on the mind, vital and body, then they too aspire and this is what was felt by you as the aspiration from the level of the lower being. The aspiration felt above is that of the Jivatman for the higher consciousness with its realisation of the One to manifest in all the being. Both aspirations help and are necessary to each other. But the seeking of the lower being is at first intermittent and oppressed by the obscurity and limitations of the ordinary consciousness. It has, by sadhana, to become clear, constant, strong and enduring; it then compels realisation, makes it inevitable.

The sense of peace, purity and calm felt by you is brought about by a union or a strong contact of the lower with the higher consciousness; it cannot be permanent at first, but it can become so by an increased frequency and durability of the calm and peace and finally by the full descent of the eternal peace and calm and silence of the higher consciousness into the lower nature.

The Jivatman, spark-soul and psychic being are three different forms of the same reality and they must not be mixed up together, as that confuses the clearness of the inner experience.

The Jivatman or spirit, as it is usually called in English, is self-existent above the manifested or instrumental being — it is superior to birth and death, always the same, the individual

Self or Atman. It is the eternal true being of the individual.

The soul is a spark of the Divine which is not seated above the manifested being, but comes down into the manifestation to support its evolution in the material world. It is at first an undifferentiated power of the Divine Consciousness containing all possibilities which have not yet taken form, but to which it is the function of evolution to give form. This spark is there in all living beings from the lowest to the highest.

The psychic being is formed by the soul in its evolution. It supports the mind, vital, body, grows by their experiences, carries the nature from life to life. It is the psychic or *caitya puruṣa*. At first it is veiled by mind, vital and body, but as it grows, it becomes capable of coming forward and dominating the mind, life and body; in the ordinary man it depends on them for expression and is not able to take them up and freely use them. The life of the being is animal or human and not divine. When the psychic being can by sadhana become dominant and freely use its instruments, then the impulse towards the Divine becomes complete and the transformation of mind, vital and body, not merely their liberation, becomes possible.

The Self or Atman being free and superior to birth and death, the experience of the Jivatman and its unity with the supreme or universal Self brings the sense of liberation, it is this which is necessary for the supreme spiritual deliverance: but for the transformation of the life and nature the awakening of the psychic being and its rule over the nature are indispensable.

The psychic being realises its oneness with the true being, the Jivatman, but it does not change into it.

The *bindu* seen above may be a symbolic way of seeing the Jivatman, the portion of the Divine; the aspiration there would naturally be for the opening of the higher consciousness so that the being may dwell there and not in the Ignorance. The Jivatman is already one with the Divine in reality, but what is needed is that the rest of the consciousness should realise it.

The aspiration of the psychic being is for the opening of the whole lower nature, mind, vital, body to the Divine, for the love and union with the Divine, for its presence and power within the heart, for the transformation of the mind, life and body by the descent of the higher consciousness into this instrumental being and nature.

Both aspirations are essential and indispensable for the fullness of this yoga. When the psychic imposes its aspiration on the mind, vital and body, then they too aspire and this is what was felt as the aspiration from the level of the lower being. The aspiration felt above is that of the Jivatman for the higher consciousness with its realisation of the One to manifest in the being. Therefore both aspirations help each other. The seeking of the lower being is necessarily at first intermittent and oppressed by the ordinary consciousness. It has, by sadhana, to become clear, constant, strong and enduring.

The sense of peace, purity and calm is brought about by the union of the lower with the higher consciousness. It is usually either intermittent or else remains in a deeper consciousness, veiled often by the storms and agitations of the surface; it is seldom permanent at first, but it can become permanent by increased frequency and endurance of the calm and peace and finally by the full descent of the eternal peace and calm and silence of the higher consciousness into the lower nature.

In the experience of yoga the self or being is in essence one with the Divine or at least it is a portion of the Divine and has all the divine potentialities. But in manifestation it takes two aspects, the Purusha and Prakriti, conscious being and Nature. In Nature here the Divine is veiled, and the individual being is subjected to Nature which acts here as the lower Prakriti, a force of Ignorance, Avidya. The Purusha in itself is divine, but exteriorised in the ignorance of Nature it is the individual apparent being imperfect with her imperfection. Thus the soul or psychic essence, which is the Purusha entering into the evolution and supporting it, carries in itself all the divine potentialities; but the individual psychic being which it puts forth as its representative assumes the imperfection of Nature and evolves in it till it has recovered its full psychic essence and united itself with the Self above of which the soul is the individual projection in the evolution. This duality in the being on all its planes — for it is true in different ways not only of the Self and the psychic but of the mental, vital and physical Purushas — has to be grasped and accepted before the experiences of the yoga can be fully understood.

The Being is one throughout, but on each plane of Nature, it is represented by a form of itself which is proper to that plane, the mental Purusha in the mental plane, the vital Purusha in the vital, the physical Purusha in the physical. The Taittiriya Upanishad speaks of two other planes of the being, the Knowledge or Truth plane and the Ananda plane, each with its Purusha, but although influences may come down from them, these are superconscient to the human mind and their nature is not yet organised here.

The individual self is usually described as a portion of the Transcendent and cosmic Self — in the higher and subtler ranges of the consciousness it knows itself as that, but in the lower where the consciousness is more and more clouded it identifies itself with surface forms of personality, creations of Prakriti and becomes unaware of its divine origin. Self when one becomes aware of it is felt as something self-existent and eternal which is not identified with forms of mental, vital and physical personality, — these are only small expressions of its potentialities in Nature. What people call themselves now is only the ego or the mind or the life-force or the body, but that is because they think in the terms of the formations of Prakriti and do not see behind them.

The central being and the soul are both in different ways portions of the Divine. They are in fact two aspects of the same entity, but one is unevolving above Nature, the other evolves a psychic being in Nature.

It is the individual being that is a portion of the Divine. The

universal self or Atman which is the same in all, is not a portion
but an aspect of the Divine.

*
**

The self is the Divine itself in an essential aspect; it is not a portion. There is no meaning in the phrase "not even a portion"
or "only an aspect." An aspect is not something inferior to a
portion.

*
**

Do you not know what "essential" means? There is a difference between the essence of a thing which is always the same
and its formations and developments which vary. There is, for
instance, the essence of gold and there are the many forms which
gold can take.

*
**

Essence can never be defined — it simply is.

*
**

The Divine is more than the Atman. It is Nature also. It
contains everything in Itself.

*
**

In order to get the dynamic realisation it is not enough to rescue
the Purusha from subjection to Prakriti; one must transfer the
allegiance of the Purusha from the lower Prakriti with its play
of ignorant Forces to the Supreme Divine Shakti, the Mother.

It is a mistake to identify the Mother with the lower Prakriti
and its mechanism of forces. Prakriti here is a mechanism only
which has been put forth for the working of the evolutionary
ignorance. As the ignorant mental, vital or physical being is not
itself the Divine, although it comes from the Divine — so the
mechanism of Prakriti is not the Divine Mother. No doubt
something of her is there in and behind this mechanism main-

taining it for the evolutionary purpose; but what she is in herself is not a Shakti of Avidya, but the Divine Consciousness, Power, Light, Para Prakriti to whom we turn for the release and the divine fulfilment.

The realisation of the Purusha consciousness calm, free, observing the play of forces but not attached or involved in them is a means of liberation. The calm, the detachment, a peaceful strength and joy (*ātmarati*) must be brought down into the vital and physical as well as into the mind. If this is established, one is no longer a prey to the turmoil of the vital forces. But this calm, peace, silent strength and joy is only the first descent of the Power of the Mother into the adhar. Beyond that is a Knowledge, an executive Power, a dynamic Ananda which is not that of the ordinary Prakriti even at its best and most sattwic, but Divine in its nature.

First, however, the calm, the peace, the liberation is needed. To try to bring down the dynamic side too soon is not advisable, for then it would be a descent into a troubled and impure nature unable to assimilate it and serious perturbations might be the consequence.

*
**

What is meant by Prakriti or Nature is the outer or executive side of the Shakti or Conscious Force which forms and moves the worlds. This outer side appears here to be mechanical, a play of the forces, Gunas, etc. Behind it is the living Consciousness and Force of the Divine, the divine Shakti. The Prakriti itself is divided into the lower and higher, — the lower is the Prakriti of the Ignorance, the Prakriti of mind, life and Matter separated in consciousness from the Divine; the higher is the Divine Prakriti of Sachchidananda with its manifesting power of supermind, always aware of the Divine and free from Ignorance and its consequences. Man so long as he is in the ignorance is subject to the lower Prakriti, but by spiritual evolution he becomes aware of the higher Nature and seeks to come into contact with it. He can ascend into it and it can descend into him — such an ascent and descent can transform the lower nature of mind, life and Matter.

V

The psychic is not by definition,[1] that part which is in direct touch with the supramental plane, — although, once the connection with the supramental is made, it gives to it the readiest response. The psychic part of us is something that comes direct from the Divine and is in touch with the Divine. In its origin it is the nucleus pregnant with divine possibilities that supports this lower triple manifestation of mind, life and body. There is this divine element in all living beings, but it stands hidden behind the ordinary consciousness, is not at first developed and, even when developed, is not always or often in the front; it expresses itself, so far as the imperfection of the instruments allows, by their means and under their limitations. It grows in the consciousness by Godward experience, gaining strength every time there is a higher movement in us, and, finally, by the accumulation of these deeper and higher movements, there is developed a psychic individuality, — that which we call usually the psychic being. It is always this psychic being that is the real, though often the secret cause of man's turning to the spiritual life and his greatest help in it. It is therefore that which we have to bring from behind to the front in the yoga.

The word 'soul', as also the word 'psychic', is used very vaguely and in many different senses in the English language. More often than not, in ordinary parlance, no clear distinction is made between mind and soul and often there is an even more serious confusion, for the vital being of desire — the false soul or desire-soul — is intended by the words 'soul' and 'psychic' and not the true soul, the psychic being. The psychic being is

---

[1] Someone had asked what the psychic being was, whether it could be defined as that part of the being which is always in direct touch with the supramental. I replied that it could not be so defined. For the psychic being in animals or in most human beings is not in direct touch with the supramental — therefore it cannot be so described, *by definition*.

But once the connection between the supramental and the human consciousness is made, it is the psychic being that gives *the readiest response* — more ready than the mind, the vital or the physical. It may be added that it is also a purer response; the mind, vital and physical can allow other things to mix with their reception of the supramental influence and spoil its truth. The psychic is pure in its response and allows no such mixture.

The supramental change can take place only if the psychic is awake and is made the chief support of the descending supramental power.

quite different from the mind or vital; it stands behind them where they meet in the heart. Its central place is there, but behind the heart rather than in the heart; for what men call usually the heart is the seat of emotion, and human emotions are mental-vital impulses, not ordinarily psychic in their nature. This mostly secret power behind, other than the mind and the life-force, is the true soul, the psychic being in us. The power of the psychic, however, can act upon the mind and vital and body, purifying thought and perception and emotion (which then becomes psychic feeling) and sensation and action and everything else in us and preparing them to be divine movements.

The psychic being may be described in Indian language as the Purusha in the heart or the Chaitya Purusha;[1] but the inner or secret heart must be understood, *hṛdaye guhāyām*, not the outer vital-emotional centre. It is the true psychic entity (distinguished from the vital desire-mind) — the psyche — spoken of in the page of the *Arya* to which you make reference.

The psychic being in the old systems was spoken of as the Purusha in the heart (the secret heart — *hṛdaye guhāyām*) which corresponds very well to what we define as the psychic being behind the heart centre. It was also this that went out from the body at death and persisted — which again corresponds to our teaching that it is this which goes out and returns, linking a new life to former life. Also we say that the psychic is the divine portion within us — so too the Purusha in the heart is described as Ishwara of the individual nature in some place.

[1] The Chitta and the psychic part are not in the least the same. Chitta is a term in a quite different category in which are co-ordinated and put into their place the main functionings of our external consciousness, and to know it we need not go behind our surface or external nature.

'Category' means here another class of psychological factors, *tattva-vibhāga*. The psychic belongs to one class — supermind, mind, life, psychic, physical — and covers both the inner and the outer nature. Chitta belongs to quite another class or category — buddhi, manas, chitta, prana, etc. — which is the classification made by ordinary Indian psychology; it covers only the psychology of the external being. In this category it is the main functions of our external consciousness only that are co-ordinated and put in their place by the Indian thinkers; chitta is one of these main functions of the external consciousness and, therefore, to know it we need not go behind the external nature.

The word soul is very vaguely used in English — as it often refers to the whole non-physical consciousness including even the vital with all its desires and passions. That was why the word psychic being has to be used so as to distinguish this divine portion from the instrumental parts of the nature.

It appears X supposed that by the psychic being I meant the enlightened ego. But people do not understand what I mean by the psychic being, because the word psychic has been used in English to mean anything of the inner mental, inner vital or inner physical or anything abnormal or occult or even the more subtle movements of the outer being, all in a jumble; also occult phenomena are often called psychic. The distinction between these different parts of the being is unknown. Even in India the old knowledge of the Upanishads in which they are distinguished has been lost. The Jivatman, the psychic being (Purusha Antaratman), the Manomaya Purusha, the Pranamaya Purusha are all confused together.

I do not know what is exactly meant by this phrase — it is too vague and limited for a description of the psychic. *Antaḥkaraṇa* usually means the mind and vital as opposed to the body — the body being the outer instrument and *manaḥ-prāṇa* the inner instrument of the soul. By psychic I mean something different from a purified mind and vital. A purified mind and vital are the result of the action of the awakened and liberated psychic being but it is not itself the psychic.

Again, it depends on what is meant by *ahambhāva*. But the psychic is not a *bhāva*. It is a Purusha. *Ahambhāva* is a formation of Prakriti, it is not a being or a Purusha. *Ahambhāva* can disappear and yet the Purusha will be there.

By liberated psychic being I mean that it is no longer obliged to express itself under the conditions of the obscure and ignorant instruments, from behind a veil, but is able to come forward, control and change the action of mind and life and body.

If it is perhaps sometimes spoken of as purified and perfected, what must be meant is the pychic action in the mind, vital and the physical instruments. A purified inner being does not mean a purified psychic, but a purified inner mental, vital and physical. The epithets I used for the psychic were "awakened and liberated".

Spiritual individuality is rather a vague term and might be variously interpreted. I have written about the psychic being that the psychic is the soul or spark of the Divine Fire supporting the individual evolution on the earth and the psychic being is the soul-consciousness developing itself or rather its manifestation from life to life with the mind, vital and body as its instruments until all is ready for the union with the Divine. I don't know that I can add anything to that.

Purusha in Prakriti is the Kshara Purusha — standing back from it is the Akshara Purusha.

Ego-sense and Purusha are two quite different things — ego-sense is a mechanism of Prakriti, Purusha is the conscious being.

The psychic being evolves, so it is not the immutable.

The psychic being is especially the soul of the individual evolving in the manifestation the individual Prakriti and taking part in the evolution. It is that spark of the Divine Fire that grows behind the mind, vital and physical as the psychic being until it is able to transform the Prakriti of Ignorance into Prakriti of knowledge. These things are not in the Gita, but we cannot limit our knowledge by the points in the Gita.

No, the intuitive self is quite different, or rather the intuitive consciousness that is somewhere above the mind. The psychic stands behind the being — a simple and sincere devotion to the Divine, single-hearted and immediate sense of what is right and helps towards the Truth and the Divine, an instinctive withdrawal from all that is the opposite are its most visible characteristics.

[1]A distinction has to be made between the soul in its essence and the psychic being. Behind each and all there is the soul which is the spark of the Divine — none could exist without that. But it is quite possible to have a vital and physical being supported by such a soul essence but without a clearly evolved psychic being behind it.

There is indeed an inner being composed of the inner mental, inner vital, inner physical, — but that is not the psychic being. The psychic is the inmost being of all and quite distinct from these. The word psychic is indeed used in English to indicate anything that is other or deeper than the external mind, life and body or it indicates sometimes anything occult or supraphysical; but that is a use which brings confusion and error and we have almost entirely to discard it.

The psychic being is veiled by the surface movements and expresses itself as best it can through the three outer instruments which are more governed by the outer forces than by the inner being or the psychic entity. But that does not mean that they are entirely isolated from the soul. The soul is in the body in the same way as the mind or vital — but the body is not this gross physical body only, but the subtle body also. When the gross body falls away, the vital and mental sheaths of the body still remain as the soul's vehicle till these too dissolve.

The soul of a plant or an animal is not dormant — only its means of expression are less developed than those of a human being. There is much that is psychic in the plant, much that is psychic in the animal. The plant has only the vital-physical elements evolved in its form; the consciousness behind the form of the plant has no developed or organised mentality capable of expressing itself, — the animal takes a step farther; it has a vital mind and some extent of self-expression, but its consciousness

---

[1] The original version of this letter was subsequently revised by Sri Aurobindo on two occasions. As the two revised versions differ considerably at places, both of them are published here consecutively.

is limited, its mentality limited, its experiences are limited; the psychic essence too puts forward to represent it a less developed consciousness and experience than is possible in man. All the same, animals have a soul and can respond very readily to the psychic in man.

The "ghost" of a man is of course not his soul. It is either the man appearing in his vital body or it is a fragment of his vital structure that is seized on by some force or being of the vital world for its own purpose. For normally the vital being with its personality exists after the dissolution of the physical body for some time only; afterwards it passes away into the vital plane where it remains till the vital sheath dissolves. Next one passes in the mental sheath, to some mental world; but finally the soul leaves its mental sheath also and goes to its place of rest. If the mental is strongly developed, then the mental being can remain and so also can the strongly developed vital, provided they are organised by and centred around the true psychic being — they then share the immortality of the psychic. But ordinarily this does not happen; there is a dissolution of the mental and vital as well as the physical parts and the soul in rebirth assumes a new mind, life and body and not, as is often supposed, a replica of its old nature-self. Such a repetition would be meaningless and useless and would defeat the purpose of rebirth which is a progression of the nature by experience, an evolutionary growth of the soul in nature towards its self-finding. At the same time the soul preserves the impression of what was essential in its past lives and personalities and the new birth and personality are a balance between this past and the soul's need for its future.

P.S. There are cases in which there is a rapid rebirth of the exterior being with a continuation of the old personality and even the memory of its past life, but this is exceptional and happens usually when there is a frustration by premature death and a strong will in the vital to continue its unfinished experience.

A distinction has to be made between the soul in its essence and the psychic being. Behind each and all there is the soul which is the spark of the Divine — none could exist without that. But it is quite possible to have a vital and physical being without a clearly evolved psychic being behind it. Still, one cannot make general statements that no aboriginal has a soul or there is no display of soul anywhere.

The inner being is composed of the inner mental, inner vital, inner physical, — but that is not the psychic being. The psychic is the inmost being and quite distinct from these. The word 'psychic' is indeed used in English to indicate anything that is other or deeper than the external mind, life and body, anything occult or supraphysical, but that is a use which brings confusion and error and we entirely discard it when we speak or write about yoga. In ordinary parlance we may sometimes use the word 'psychic' in the looser popular sense or in poetry, which is not bound to intellectual accuracy, we may speak of the soul sometimes in the ordinary and more external sense or in the sense of the true psyche.

The psychic being is veiled by the surface movements and expresses itself as best it can through these outer instruments which are more governed by the outer forces than by the inner influences of the psychic. But that does not mean that they are entirely isolated from the soul. The soul is in the body in the same way as the mind or vital — but the body it occupies is not this gross physical frame only, but the subtle body also. When the gross sheath falls away, the vital and mental sheaths of the body still remain as the soul's vehicle till these too dissolve.

The soul of a plant or an animal is not altogether dormant — only its means of expression are less developed than those of a human being. There is much that is psychic in the plant, much that is psychic in the animal. The plant has only the vital-physical evolved in its form, so it cannot express itself; the animal has a vital mind and can, but its consciousness is limited and its experiences are limited, so the psychic essence has a less developed consciousness and experience than is present or at least possible in man. All the same, animals have a soul and can respond very readily to the psychic in man.

The ghost is of course not the soul. It is either the man

appearing in his vital body or it is a fragment of his vital that is seized on by some vital force or being. The vital part of us normally exists after the disolution of the body for some time and passes away into the vital plane where it remains till the vital sheath dissolves. Afterwards it passes, if it is mentally evolved, in the mental sheath to some mental world and finally the psychic leaves its mental sheath also and goes to its place of rest. If the mental is strongly developed, then the mental part of us can remain; so also can the vital, provided they are organised by and centred round the true psychic being — for they then share the immortality of the psychic. Otherwise the psychic draws mind and life into itself and enters into an internatal quiescence.

In a mere vampire there is no psychic, for the vampire is a vital being — but in all humans (even if dominated by a vital being or vampire force) there is a psychic veiled behind it all.

The soul is described as a spark of the Divine Fire in life and matter, that is an image. It has not been described as a spark of consciousness.

There is mental, vital, physical consciousness — different from the psychic. The psychic being and consciousness are not identical.

When the soul or "spark of the Divine Fire" begins to develop a psychic individuality, that psychic individuality is called the psychic being.

The soul or spark is there before the development of an organised vital and mind. The soul is something of the Divine that descends into the evolution as a divine Principle within it to support the evolution of the individual out of the Ignorance into the Light. It develops in the course of the evolution a psychic individual or soul individuality which grows from life to life, using the evolving mind, vital and body as its instruments. It is the soul that is immortal while the rest disintegrates; it passes from life to life carrying its experience in essence and the continuity of the evolution of the individual.

It is the whole consciousness, mental, vital, physical also, that has to rise and join the higher consciousness and, once the joining is made, the higher has to descend into them. The psychic is behind all that and supports it.

The supermind is the Truth-consciousness; below it there intervenes the overmind of which the principle is to receive the powers of the Divine and try to work them out separately, each acting in its own right and working to realise a world of its own or, if it has to act with others, enforcing its own principle as much as possible. Souls descending into the overmind act in the same way. The principle of separated Individuality is from here. At first still aware of its divine origin, it becomes as it descends still more and more separated and oblivious of it, governed by the principle of division and ego. For Mind is farther removed from the Truth than overmind, Vital Nature is engrossed in the realisation of ignorant forces, while in Matter the whole passes into what seems an original Inconscience. It is the overmind Maya that governs this world, but in Matter it has deepened into Inconscience out of which consciousness re-emerges and climbs again bringing down into Matter life and mind, and opening in mind to the higher reaches — which are still in some direct connection with the Truth (Intuition, overmind, supermind).

Formed souls enter only into formed organisms — in the protoplasm etc. it is only the spark of the Divine that is there, not the formed soul.

The psychic is the spark of the Divine involved here in the individual existence. It grows and evolves in the form of the psychic being — so obviously it cannot have already the powers of the Divine. Only its presence makes it possible for the individual to open to the Divine and grow towards the Divine Consciousness and when it acts it is always in the sense of the Light and the Truth and with the push towards the Divine.

This is the function of the psychic — it has to work on each plane so as to help each to awaken to the true truth and the Divine Reality.

Every soul is not evolved and active; nor is every soul turned directly to the Divine before practising yoga. For a long time it seeks the Divine through men and things much more than directly.

You do not seem to have understood my answer at all. In the ordinary consciousness in which the mind etc. are *not* awakened the psychic acts as well as it can through them, but according to the laws of the Ignorance.

All belongs to Nature — the soul itself acts under the conditions and by the agency of Nature.

The soul is always pure, but the knowledge and force in it are involved and come out only as the psychic being evolves and grows stronger.

The psychic being is the soul evolving in course of birth and rebirth and the soul is a portion of the Divine — but with the soul there is always the veiled Divine, Hrishikesha.

The Divine is always in the inner heart and does not leave it.

It [the psychic] is constantly in contact with the immanent Divine — the Divine secret in the individual.

They [the psychic being and the Divine Presence in the heart] are quite different things. The psychic being is one's own individual soul-being. It is not the Divine, though it has come from the Divine and develops towards the Divine.

It is the psychic that is in direct relation with the transcendent Divine and leads the nature upwards towards the Supreme.

The psychic is the support of the individual evolution; it is connected with the universal both by direct contact and through the mind, vital and body.

The contribution of the psychic being to the sadhana is: (1) love and bhakti, a love not vital, demanding and egoistic but unconditioned and without claims, self-existent; (2) the contact or the presence of the Mother within; (3) the unerring guidance from within; (4) a quieting and purification of the mind, vital and physical consciousness by their subjection to the psychic influence and guidance; (5) the opening up of all this lower consciousness to the higher spiritual consciousness above for its descent into a nature prepared to receive it with a complete receptivity and right attitude — for the psychic brings in everything, right thought, right perception, right feeling, right attitude.

One can raise up one's consciousness from the mental and vital and bring down the power, Ananda, light, knowledge from above; but this is far more difficult and uncertain in its result, even dangerous, if the being is not prepared or not pure enough. To ascend with the psychic for the purpose is by far the best way. If you are thus rising from the psychic centre, so much the better.

What you say indicates that the psychic and mental centres are in communication and through them you are able to bring down things from the higher consciousness. But you have not changed your head centre for the above-head centre or for the above-head wideness. That usually comes by a gradual rising of the conscious parts to the top of the head and then above it. But this must not be strained after or forced; it will come of itself.

The psychic being is the soul, the Purusha in the secret heart supporting by its presence the action of the mind, life and body. The vital is the *prāṇamaya puruṣa* spoken of in the Taittiriya Upanishad, the being behind the Force of Life; in its outer form in the Ignorance it generates the desire-soul which governs most men and which they mistake often for the real soul.

The Atman is the Self or Spirit that remains above, pure and stainless, unaffected by the stains of life, by desire and ego and ignorance. It is realised as the true being of the individual, but also more widely as the *same being* in all and as the Self in the cosmos; it has also a self-existence above the individual and cosmos and it is then called the Paramatma, the supreme Divine Being. This distinction has nothing to do with the distinction between the psychic and the vital: the vital being is not what is known as the Atman.

The vital as the desire-soul and desire-nature controls the consciousness to a large extent in most men, because men are governed by desire. But even in the surface human nature the proper ruler of the consciousness is the mental being, *manomayaḥ puruṣaḥ prāṇa-śarīra-netā* of the Upanishad. The psychic influences the consciousness from behind, but one has to go out of the ordinary consciousness into the inmost being to find it and make it the ruler of the consciousness as it should be. To do that is one of the principal aims of the yoga. The vital should be an instrument of the consciousness, not its ruler.

The vital being is not the I — the ego is mental, vital, physical. Ego implies the identification of our existence with outer self, the ignorance of our true self above and our psychic being within us.

In a certain sense the various Purushas or beings in us, psychic, mental, vital, physical are projections of the Atman, but that gets its full truth only when we get into our inner being and know the inner truth of ourselves. On the surface, in the Ignorance, it is the mental, vital, physical Prakriti that acts and the Purusha is disfigured, as it were, in the action of the Prakriti. It is not our true mental being, our true vital being, our true physical being even that we are aware of; these remain behind, veiled and silent. It is the mental, vital, physical ego that we take for our being until we get knowledge.

The soul and the life are two quite different powers. The soul is a spark of the Divine Spirit which supports the individual nature; mind, life, body are the instruments for the manifestation of the nature. In most men the soul is hidden and covered over by the action of the external nature; they mistake the vital being for the soul, because it is the vital which animates and moves the body. But this vital being is a thing made up of desires and executive forces, good and bad; it is the desire-soul, not the true thing. It is when the true soul (psyche) comes forward and begins first to influence and then govern the actions of the instrumental nature that man begins to overcome vital desire and grow towards a divine nature.

*
**

1. The soul and the psychic being are practically the same, except that even in things which have not developed a psychic being, there is still a spark of the Divine which can be called the soul. The psychic being is called in Sanskrit the Purusha in the heart or the Chaitya Purusha. (The psychic being is the soul developing in the evolution.)

2. The distinction between Purusha and Prakriti is according to the Sankhya System — the Purusha is the silent witness consciousness which observes the actions of Prakriti — Prakriti is the force of Nature which one feels as doing all the actions, when one gets rid of the sense of the ego as doer. Then there is the realisation of these 2 entities. This is quite different from the psychic being. It is felt in the mind, vital, physical — most easily in the mind where the mental being (Purusha) is seated and controls the others (*manomayaḥ puruṣaḥ prāṇa-śarīra-netā*).

3. Prajna, Taijasa, etc. are a different classification and have to do, not with the different parts of the being, but with three different states (waking, dream, sleep — gross, subtle, causal).

I think one ought not to try to relate these different things to each other — as that may lead to confusion. They belong to different categories — and to a different order of experiences.

The mental being within watches, observes and passes judgment on all that happens in you. The psychic does not watch and observe in this way like a witness, but it feels and knows spontaneously in a much more direct and luminous way, by the very purity of its own nature and the divine instinct within it, and so, whenever it comes to the front it reveals at once what are the right and what the wrong movements in your nature.

The being of man is composed of these elements — the psychic behind supporting all, the inner mental, vital and physical, and the outer, quite external nature of mind, life and body which is their instrument of expression. But above all is the central being (Jivatma) which uses them all for its manifestation: it is a portion of the Divine Self; but this reality of himself is

hidden from the external man who replaces this inmost self and
soul of him by the mental and vital ego. It is only those who
have begun to know themselves that become aware of their true
central being; but still it is always there standing behind the
action of mind, life and body and is most directly represented by
the psychic which is itself a spark of the Divine. It is by the
growth of the psychic element in one's nature that one begins to
come into conscious touch with one's central being above. When
that happens and the central being uses a conscious will to control and organize the movements of the nature, it is then that one
has a real, a spiritual as opposed to a partial and merely mental
or moral self-mastery.

The mental being spoken of by the Upanishad is not part of the
mental nervous physical composite — it is the *manomayaḥ puruṣaḥ
prāṇa-śarīra-netā*, the mental being leader of the life and body.
It could not be so described if it were part of the composite. Nor
can the composite or part of it be the Purusha, — for the composite is composed of Prakriti. It is described as *manomaya* by
the Upanishads because the psychic being is behind the veil and
man being the mental being in the life and body lives in his mind
and not in his psychic, so to him the *manomaya puruṣa* is the leader
of the life and body, — of the psychic behind supporting the
whole he is not aware or dimly aware in his best moments. The
psychic is represented in man by the Prime Minister, the *manomaya*, itself being a mild constitutional king; it is the *manomaya*
to whom Prakriti refers for assent to her actions. But still the
statement of the Upanishads gives only the apparent truth of the
matter, valid for man and the human stage only — for in the
animal it would be rather the *prāṇamaya puruṣa* that is the *netā*,
leader of mind and body. It is one reason why I have not yet
allowed the publication of Rebirth and Karma[1] because this had
to be corrected and the deeper truth put in its place. I had

---

[1] An incomplete series of articles first published in the *Arya* intermittently during 1915-
21 and subsequently reprinted without completion in book-form under the title *The Problem
of Rebirth* (February 1952).

intended to do it later on, but had not the time to finish the remaining articles.

The "tragi-ridiculous" inconsistency you speak of comes from the fact that man is not made up of one piece but of many pieces and each part of him has a personality of its own. That is a thing which people yet have not sufficiently realised — the psychologists have begun to glimpse it, but recognise only when there is a marked case of double or multiple personality. But all men are like that, in reality. The aim should be in yoga to develop (if one has it not already) a strong central being and harmonise under it all the rest, changing what has to be changed. If this central being is the psychic, there is no great difficulty. If it is the mental Being, *manomayaḥ puruṣaḥ prāṇa-śarira-netā*, then it is more difficult — unless the mental being can learn to be always in contact with and aided by the greater Will and Power of the Divine.

I do not understand the question as put. Each part has to be kept clear from the other and do its own work and each has to get the Truth in it from the psychic or above. The Truth descending from above will more and more harmonise their action, though the perfect harmony can come only when there is the supramental fulfilment.

What you experience is the first condition of the yogic consciousness and self-knowledge. The ordinary mind knows itself only as an ego with all the movements of the nature in a jumble and, identifying itself with these movements, thinks "I am doing this, feeling that, thinking, in joy or in sorrow etc." The first beginning of real self-knowledge is when you feel yourself separate from the nature in you and its movements and then you see that there are many parts of your being, many personalities each acting on its own behalf and in its own way. The two different beings you feel are — one, the psychic being which draws you towards the Mother, the other the external being mostly vital which draws you outward and downwards towards the play of the lower nature. There is also in you behind the mind the being who observes, the witness Purusha, who can stand detached from the play of the nature, observing it and able to choose. It has to put itself always on the side of the psychic being and assent to and support its movement and to reject the downward and outward movement of the lower nature, which has to be subjected to the psychic and changed by its influence.

The moral of the condition you describe is not that yoga should not be done but that you have to go steadily healing the rift between the two parts of the being. The division is very usual, almost universal in human nature, and the following of the lower impulse in spite of the contrary will in the higher parts happens to almost everybody. It is the phenomenon noted by Arjuna in his question to Krishna, "Why does one do evil though one wishes not to do it, as if compelled to it by force?", and expressed sententiously by Horace: "*video meliora proboque, Deteriora sequor*".[1] By constant effort and aspiration one can arrive at a turning point when the psychic asserts itself and what seems a very slight psychological change of reversal alters the whole balance of the nature.

You take the outer waking consciousness as if it were the real person or being and conclude that if it is not this but something else that has the realisation or abides in the realisation, then no one has it — for there is no one here except the waking consciousness. That is the very error by which the ignorance lasts and cannot be got rid of. The very first step in getting out of the ignorance is to accept the fact that this outer consciousness is not one's soul, not oneself, not the real person, but only a temporary formation on the surface for the purposes of the surface play. The soul, the person is within, not on the surface — the outer

---

[1] "I see the better and approve of it, I follow the worse."

personality is the person only in the first sense of the Latin word
persona which meant originally a mask.

The psychic has the position you speak of, because the psychic
is in touch with the Divine in the lower nature. But the inner
mind, vital and physical are a part of the universal and open to
the dualities — only they are wider than the external mind, life
and body, and can receive more largely and easily the divine
influence.

***

The word Antaratma is very vaguely used like the word soul in
English — so used, it covers all the inner being, inner mind, inner
vital, inner physical even, as well as the inmost being, the
psychic.

***

The European mind, for the most part, has never been able to go
beyond the formula of soul + body — usually including mind in
soul and everything except body in mind. Some occultists make
a distinction between spirit, soul and body. At the same time
there must be some vague feeling that soul and mind are not quite
the same thing, for there is the phrase "This man has no soul",
or "he is a soul" meaning he has something in him beyond a mere
mind and body. But all that is very vague. There is no clear
distinction between mind and soul and none between mind and
vital and often the vital is taken for the soul.

***

But that[1] is just what is disputed by the Western scientific mind
or was up till yesterday and is still considered as unverifiable today. It is contended that the idea of self is an illusion — apart
from the body. It is the experiences of the body that create the
idea of a self and the desire to live prolongs itself illusorily in the

---

[1] The belief that the body is a temporary residence of the self for one life.

notion that the self outlasts the body. The West is accustomed besides to the Christian idea that the self is created with the body — an idea which the Christians took over from the Jews who believed in God but not in immortality — so the Western mind is dead set against any idea of reincarnation. Even the religious used to believe that the soul was born in the body, God first making the body then breathing the soul into it (Prana?). It is difficult for Europeans to get over this past mental inheritance.

The psychic being is described in the Upanishads as no bigger than the size of one's thumb! That of course is a symbolic image. For usually when one sees anybody's psychic being in a form, it is bigger than that. As for the inner being, one feels it big because the true mental or the true vital or even the true physical being is much wider in consciousness than the external consciousness which is limited by the body. If the external parts seem to occupy the whole consciousness, it is when one comes down into the physical and feels all the activities of Nature playing on it — even the mental and vital movements are then felt through the physical and as things of a separate plane. But when one lives in the inner being then one is aware of a consciousness which begins to spread into the universal and the external is only a surface movement thrown up by the universal forces.

Yes, the psychic being has a form. But that does not appear from the photo; for the psychic has not always or usually a form closely resembling that of the physical body, it is sometimes even quite different. When looking at the photo what is seen is not a form, but something of the consciousness that either is expressed in the body or comes through somehow; one perceives or feels it there through the photo.

The soul is not limited by any form, but the psychic being puts out a form for its expression just as the mental, vital and subtle physical Purushas do — that is to say, one can see or another person can see one's psychic being in such and such a form. But this seeing is of two kinds — there is the standing characteristic form taken by this being in this life and there are symbolic forms such as when one sees the psychic as a new-born child in the lap of the Mother.

If the sadhak in question really saw his psychic in the form of a woman it can only have been a constructed appearance expressing some quality or attribute of the psychic.

VI

There are always two different consciousnesses in the human being, one outward in which he ordinarily lives, the other inward and concealed of which he knows nothing. When one does sadhana, the inner consciousness begins to open and one is able to go inside and have all kinds of experiences there. As the sadhana progresses, one begins to live more and more in this inner being and the outer becomes more and more superficial. At first the inner consciousness seems to be the dream and the outer the waking reality. Afterwards the inner consciousness becomes the reality and the outer is felt by many as a dream or delusion, or else as something superficial and external. The inner consciousness begins to be a place of deep peace, light, happiness, love, closeness to the Divine or the presence of the Divine, the Mother. One is then aware of two consciousnesses, the inner one and the outer which has to be changed into its counterpart and instrument — that also must become full of peace, light, union with the Divine. At present you are moving between the two and in this period all the feelings you have are quite natural. You must not be at all anxious about that, but wait for the full development of the inner consciousness in which you will be able to live.

*
**

I did not mean by the inner being the psychic or inmost being. It is the psychic being that feels love, bhakti and union with the Mother. I was speaking of the inner mental, inner vital, inner physical; in order to reach the hidden seat of the psychic one has first to pass through these things. When one leaves the outer consciousness and goes inside, it is here that one enters — some or most entering into the inner vital first, others into the inner mental or inner physical; the emotional vital is the most direct road, for the seat of the psychic is just behind the emotional in the heart-centre. It is absolutely necessary for our purpose that one should become conscious in these inner regions, for if they are not awake, then the psychic being has no proper and sufficient instrumentation for its activities; it has then only the outer mind, outer vital and body for its means and these are too small and narrow and obscure. You as yet have been able only to enter the outskirts of the inner vital and are still insufficiently conscious there. By becoming more conscious there and going deeper one can reach the psychic — the safe refuge, *nirā-pada sthāna*, of which you speak; then you will not be disturbed by the confused visions and experiences of the inner vital outskirts.

The inner consciousness means the inner mind, inner vital, inner physical and behind them the psychic which is their inmost being. But the inner mind is not the higher mind; it is more in touch with the universal forces and more open to the higher consciousness and capable of an immensely deeper and larger range of action than the outer or surface mind — but it is of the same essential nature. The higher consciousness is that above the ordinary mind and different from it in its workings; it ranges from higher mind through illumined mind, intuition and overmind up to the border line of the supramental.

If the psychic were liberated, free to act in its own way, there would not be all this stumbling in the Ignorance. But the psychic is covered up by the ignorant mind, vital and physical and compelled to act through them according to the law of the Ignorance. If it is liberated from this covering, then it can act according to its own nature with a free aspiration, a direct contact with the higher consciousness and a power to change the ignorant nature.

The true being mental, vital or subtle physical has always the greater qualities of its plane — it is the Purusha and like the psychic, though in another way, the projection of the Divine, therefore in connection with the higher consciousness and reflects something of it, though it is not altogether that — it is also in tune with the cosmic Truth.

There is behind all the vital nature in man his true vital being concealed and immobile which is quite different from the surface vital nature. The surface vital is narrow, ignorant, limited, full of obscure desires, passions, cravings, revolts, pleasures and pains, transient joys and griefs, exultations and depressions. The true vital being, on the contrary, is wide, vast, calm, strong, without limitations, firm and immovable, capable of all power, all knowledge, all Ananda. It is moreover without ego, for it knows itself to be a projection and instrument of the Divine: it is the divine Warrior, pure and perfect; in it is an instrumental Force for all divine realisations. It is the true vital being that has become awake and come in front within you. In the same way there is too a true mental being, a true physical being. When these are manifest, then you are aware of a double existence in you: that behind is always calm and strong, that on the surface alone is troubled and obscure. But if the true being behind remains stable and you live in it, then the trouble and obscurity remain only on the surface; in this condition the exterior parts can be dealt with more potently and they also made free and perfect.

It [the true vital] is capable of receiving the movements of the higher consciousness, and afterwards it can be capable of receiving the still greater supramental power and Ananda. If it is not, then the descent of the higher consciousness would be impossible and supramentalisation would be impossible. It is not meant that it possesses these things itself in its own right and that as soon as one is aware of the true vital, one gets all these things as inherent in the true vital.

The true vital is in the inner consciousness, the external is that which is instrumental for the present play of Prakriti in the surface personality. When the change comes, the true vital rejects what is out of tune with its own truth from the external and makes it a true instrument for its expression, a means of expression of its inner will, not a thing of responses to the suggestions of the lower Nature. The strong distinction between the two practically disappears.

The true vital consciousness is one in which the vital makes full surrender, converts itself into an instrument of the Divine, making no demand, insisting on no desire, answering to the Mother's force and to no other, calm, unegoistic, giving an absolute loyalty and obedience, with no personal vanity or ambition, only asking to be a pure and perfect instrument, desiring nothing for itself but that the Truth may prevail within itself and everywhere and the Divine Victory take place and the Divine Work be done.

It [the illumined vital] is in contact with the Divine Power or the higher Truth and seeks to transform itself and become a true instrument — it rejects the ordinary vital movements.

If the inner being does not manifest or act, the outer will never get transformed.

The outer consciousness is that which usually expresses itself in ordinary life. It is the external mental, vital, physical. It is not connected very much with the inner being except in a few — until one connects them together in the course of the sadhana.

They [the inner mind and the inner vital] exercise an influence and send out their powers or suggestions which the outer sometimes carries out as best it can, sometimes does not follow. How much they work on the outer depends on how far the individual has an inner life. E.g. the poet, musician, artist, thinker, live much from within — men of genius and those who try to live according to an ideal also. But there are plenty of people who have very little inner life and are governed entirely by the forces of Nature.

As one gathers experience from life to life, mental or vital, the inner mind and vital also develop according to the use made of our experiences and the extent to which they are utilised for the growth of the being.

The outer being is a means of expression only, not one's self. One must not identify with it, for what it expresses is a personality formed by the old ignorant nature. If not identified one can change it so as to express the true inner personality of the Light.

They [the outer mind, vital and body] are small, but not unimportant in spite of their apparent insignificance — because they

are a necessary passage of transmission between the soul and the
outer world.

The outer consciousness is shut up in the body limitation and in
the little bit of personal mind and sense dependent on the body
— it sees only the outward, sees only things. But the inner
consciousness can see behind the thing, it is aware of the play of
forces, personal or universal — for it is in conscious touch with
the universal action.

Our inner being is in touch with universal mind, life and Matter;
it is a part of all that, but by that very fact it cannot be in possession of liberation and peace. You are thinking probably of the
Atman and confusing it with the inner being.

The inner being cannot be "located" above, it can only join with
the above, penetrate it and be penetrated by it. If it were located
above, then there would be no inner being.

I do not know what you mean by it (inner being) being "around"
the psychic. It is obviously nearer to the psychic than the outer
mind, vital or physical, but that does not insure its being open
to the psychic only and not to the other universal forces.

The psychic can have peace behind it — but the inner mind, vital
and physical are not necessarily silent — they are full of movements. It is the higher consciousness that has a basis of peace.

The inner being is not usually unquiet but it can be quiet or unquiet like the outer.

The inner parts in everybody remain vulgar or become high according as they are turned to the outward forces of the Ignorance or towards the higher forces from above and the inner impulsion of the psychic. All forces can play there. It is the outer being that is fixed in a certain character, certain tendencies, certain movements.

The inner being has its own time which is sometimes slower, sometimes faster than the physical.

VII

The individual is not limited to the physical body — it is only the external consciousness which feels like that. As soon as one gets over this feeling of limitation, one can feel first the inner consciousness which is connected with the body, but does not belong to it, afterwards the planes of consciousness above the body, also a consciousness surrounding the body, but part of oneself, part of the individual being, through which one is in contact with the cosmic forces and with other beings. The last is what I have called the environmental consciousness.

Each man has his own personal consciousness entrenched in his body and gets into touch with his surroundings only through his body and senses and the mind using the senses.

Yet all the time the universal forces are pouring into him without his knowing it. He is aware only of thoughts, feelings, etc., that rise to the surface and these he takes for his own. Really they come from outside in mind waves, vital waves, waves of feeling and sensation, etc., which take particular form in him and rise to the surface after they have got inside.

But they do not get into his body at once. He carries about with him an environmental consciousness (called by the Theosophists the aura) into which they first enter. If you can become conscious of this environmental self of yours, then you can catch the thought, passion, suggestion or force of illness and prevent it from entering into you. If things in you are thrown out, they often do not go altogether but take refuge in this environmental atmosphere and from there they try to get in again. Or they go to a distance outside but linger on the outskirts or even perhaps far off, waiting till they get an opportunity to attempt entrance.

The environmental is not a world — it is an individual thing.

They [the subconscient and the environmental consciousness] are two quite different things. What is stored in the subconscient — impressions, memories, rise up from there into the conscious parts. In the environmental things are not stored up and fixed, although they move about there. It is full of mobility, a field of vibration or passage of forces.

It [the environmental consciousness] can become silent when there is the wideness. One can become conscious of it and deal with what passes through it. A man without it would be without contact with the rest of the world.

VIII

The consciousness in the individual widens itself into the cosmic consciousness outside and can have any kind of dealing with it, penetrate, know its movements, act upon it or receive from it, even become commensurate with or contain it, which is what was meant in the language of the old yogas by having the Brahmanda within you.

The cosmic consciousness is that of the universe, of the cosmic spirit and cosmic Nature with all the beings and forces within it. All that is as much conscious as a whole as the individual separately is, though in a different way. The consciousness of the individual is part of this, but a part feeling itself as a separate being. Yet all the time most of what he is comes into him from the cosmic consciousness. But there is a wall of separative ignorance between. Once it breaks down he becomes aware of the cosmic Self, of the consciousness of the cosmic Nature, of the forces playing in it, etc. He feels all that as he now feels physical things and impacts. He finds it all to be one with his larger or universal self.

There is the universal mental, the universal vital, the universal physical Nature and it is out of a selection of their forces and movements that the individual mind, vital and physical are made. The soul comes from beyond this nature of mind, life and body. It belongs to the transcendent and because of it we can open to the higher Nature beyond.

The Divine is always One that is Many. The individual spirit is part of the "Many" side of the One, and the psychic being is what it puts forth to evolve here in the earth-nature. In liberation the individual self realises itself as the One (that is yet Many). It may plunge into the One and merge or hide itself in its bosom — that is the *laya* of the Adwaita; it may feel its oneness and yet as part of the Many that is One enjoy the Divine, that is the Dwaitadwaita liberation; it may lay stress on its Many aspect and be possessed by the Divine, the Visishtadwaita or go on playing with Krishna in the eternal Vrindavan, the Dwaita liberation. Or it may, even being liberated, remain in the Lila or manifestation or descend into it as often as it likes. The Divine is not bound by human philosophies — it is free in its play and free in its essence.

There is no difference between the terms "universal" and "cos-

mic" except that "universal" can be used in a freer way than
"cosmic". Universal may mean "of the universe", cosmic in that
general sense. But it may also mean "common to all", e.g.,
"This is a universal weakness" — but you cannot say "This is a
cosmic weakness".

1. The spiritual consciousness is that in which we enter into
the awareness of Self, the Spirit, the Divine and are able to see
in all things their essential reality and the play of forces and
phenomena as proceeding from that essential Reality.

2. The cosmic consciousness is that in which the limits of
ego, personal mind and body disappear and one becomes aware
of a cosmic vastness which is or is filled by a cosmic spirit and
aware also of the direct play of cosmic forces, universal mind
forces, universal life forces, universal energies of Matter, universal
overmind forces. But one does not become aware of all these
together; the opening of the cosmic consciousness is usually
progressive. It is not that the ego, the body, the personal mind
disappear, but one feels them as only a small part of oneself.
One begins to feel others too as part of oneself or varied repetitions of oneself, the same self modified by Nature in other bodies.
Or, at the least, as living in the larger universal self which is
henceforth one's own greater reality. All things in fact begin to
change their nature and appearance; one's whole experience of
the world is radically different from that of those who are shut
up in their personal selves. One begins to know things by a
different kind of experience, more direct, not depending on the
external mind and the senses. It is not that the possibility of
error disappears, for that cannot be so long as mind of any kind
is one's instrument for transcribing knowledge, but there is a
new, vast and deep way of experiencing, seeing, knowing, con-
tacting things; and the confines of knowledge can be rolled back
to an almost unmeasurable degree. The thing one has to be on
guard against in the cosmic consciousness is the play of a magnified ego, the vaster attacks of the hostile forces — for they too
are part of the cosmic consciousness — and the attempt of the

cosmic Illusion (Ignorance, Avidya) to prevent the growth of the soul into the cosmic Truth. These are things that one has to learn from experience; mental teaching or explanation is quite insufficient. To enter safely into the cosmic consciousness and to pass safely through it, it is necessary to have a strong central unegoistic sincerity and to have the psychic being, with its divination of truth and unfaltering orientation towards the Divine, already in front in the nature.

3. The ordinary consciousness is that in which one knows things only or mainly by the intellect, the external mind and the senses and knows forces etc. only by their outward manifestations and results and the rest by inferences from these data. There may be some play of mental intuition, deeper psychic seeing or impulsions, spiritual intimations, etc. — but in the ordinary consciousness these are incidental only and do not modify its fundamental character.

The ordinary man lives in his own personal consciousness knowing things through his mind and senses as they are touched by a world which is outside him, outside his consciousness. When the consciousness subtilises, it begins to come into contact with things in a much more direct way, not only with their forms and outer impacts but with what is inside them, but still the range may be small. But the consciousness can also widen and begin to be first in direct contact with a universe of range of things in the world, then to contain them as it were, — as it is said to see the world in oneself, — and to be in a way identified with it. To see all things in the self and the self in all things — to be aware of one being everywhere, aware directly of the different planes, their forces, their beings — that is universalisation.

Yes, certainly [in the cosmic Mind there is a stratum of the physical mind], there is nothing in the individual that is not in the cosmic Energy. For all ordinary purposes the individual is

only a differentiated centre of the universal forces — although
his soul comes from beyond.

As he [each human being] lives in a separative consciousness,
he makes a mental world of his own out of his experiences of the
common world in which all here live. It is built in the same way
as that of others and he receives into it the thoughts, feelings
of others, without knowing it most often, and uses that too as
material for his separate world.

All life is the play of universal forces. The individual gives a
personal form to these universal forces. But he can choose whether he shall respond or not to the action of a particular force.
Only most people do not really choose — they indulge the play of
the forces. Your illnesses, depressions etc. are the repeated play
of such forces. It is only when one can make oneself free of them
that one can be the true person and have a true life — but one
can be free only by living in the Divine.

It is Prakriti (Nature) that sends these impulses. Nature sends
all kinds of forces and experiences to each. It is for you as a conscious being (Purusha) to choose whether you shall do or not do;
you should reject what you see to be wrong, accept only what is
true and right. In Nature there is the higher and the lower, the
true and the false. What the Divine wants of you is that you
should grow in the Truth and the higher Nature, reject the false
and the lower Nature.

One can not only receive a force, but an impulse, thought or
sensation. One may receive it from others, from beings in

Nature or from Nature herself if she chooses to give her Force a ready-made form of that kind.

⁎⁎⁎

1. There can be a vital without desire. When desire disappears from the being, the vital does not disappear with it.

2. By Prakriti is meant universal Prakriti. Universal Prakriti entering into the vital being creates desires which appear by its habitual response as an individual nature; but if the habitual desires she throws in are rejected and exiled, the being remains but the old individual Prakriti of vital desire is no longer there — a new nature is formed responding to the Truth above and not to the lower Nature.

3. Universal Prakriti determined it [the habit of response] and the soul or Purusha accepted it. In the acceptance lies the responsibility. The Purusha is that which sanctions or refuses. The vital being responds to the ordinary life waves in the animal; man responds to them but has the power of mental control. He has also, as the mental Purusha is awake in him, the power to choose whether he shall have desire or train his being to surmount it. Finally there is the possibility of bringing down a higher nature which will not be subject to desire but act on another vital principle.

⁎⁎⁎

It is not possible for the individual mind, so long as it remains shut up in its personality, to understand the workings of the Cosmic Will, for the standards made by the personal consciousness are not applicable to them. A cell in the body, if conscious, might also think that the human being and its actions are only the resultant of the relations and workings of a number of cells like itself and not the action of a unified self. It is only if one enters into the Cosmic Consciousness that one begins to see the forces at work and the lines on which they work and get a glimpse of the Cosmic Self and the Cosmic Mind and Will.

⁎⁎⁎

There is no ignorance that is not part of the Cosmic Ignorance, only in the individual it becomes a limited formation and movement, while the Cosmic Ignorance is the whole movement of world consciousness separated from the supreme Truth and acting in an inferior motion in which the Truth is perverted, diminished, mixed and clouded with falsehood and error. The Cosmic Truth is the view on things of a cosmic consciousness in which things are seen in their true essence and their true relation to the Divine and to each other.

The cosmic Truth is the truth of things as they are at present expressed in the universe. The Divine Truth is independent of the universe, above it and originates it.

The yogi's experiences are spiritual experiences — experience of the play of the Forces and its relation with the self, the action of the Guide, what is behind the appearance of things, occurrences etc., etc., the actual realities of the workings of Purusha and Prakriti etc. The Divine Truth is the Truth of the Divine Essence, Consciousness, Self, Knowledge, Light, Power, Bliss. It is something from which the cosmos derives with all its movements, but it is more than the cosmos.

IX

The "Mind" in the ordinary use of the word covers indiscriminately the whole consciousness, for man is a mental being and mentalises everything; but in the language of this yoga the words "mind" and "mental" are used to connote specially the part of the nature which has to do with cognition and intelligence, with ideas, with mental or thought perceptions, the reactions of thought to things, with the truly mental movements and formations, mental vision and will, etc., that are part of his intelligence.

The vital has to be carefully distinguished from mind, even though it has a mind element transfused into it; the vital is the Life-nature made up of desires, sensations, feelings, passions, energies of action, will of desire, reactions of the desire-soul in man and of all that play of possessive and other related instincts, anger, fear, greed, lust, etc., that belong to this field of the nature. Mind and vital are mixed up on the surface of the consciousness, but they are quite separate forces in themselves and as soon as one gets behind the ordinary surface consciousness one sees them as separate, discovers their distinction and can with the aid of this knowledge analyse their surface mixtures. It is quite possible and even usual during a time shorter or longer, sometimes very long, for the mind to accept the Divine or the yogic ideal while the vital is unconvinced and unsurrendered and goes obstinately on its way of desire, passion and attraction to the ordinary life. Their division or their conflict is the cause of most of the more acute difficulties of the sadhana.

St. Augustine was a man of God and a great saint, but great saints are not always — or often — great psychologists or great thinkers. The psychology here is that of the most superficial schools, if not that of the man in the street; there are as many errors in it as there are psychological statements — and more, for several are not expressed but involved in what he writes. I am aware that these errors are practically universal, for psychological enquiry in Europe (and without enquiry there can be no sound knowledge) is only beginning and has not gone very far, and what has reigned in men's minds up to now is a superficial statement of the superficial appearances of our consciousness as they look to us at first view and nothing more. But knowledge only begins when we get away from the surface phenomena and look behind them for their true operations and causes. To the superficial view of the outer mind and senses the sun is a little fiery ball circling in mid air round the earth and the stars twinkling little things stuck in the sky for our benefit at night. Scientific enquiry comes and knocks this infantile first-view to pieces. The sun is a huge affair (millions of miles away from our air) around which the small earth circles, and the stars are huge members of huge systems indescribably distant which have nothing apparently to do with the tiny earth and her creatures. All Science is like that, a contradiction of the sense-view or superficial appearances of things and an assertion of truths which are unguessed by the common and the uninstructed reason. The same process has to be followed in psychology if we are really to know what our consciousness is, how it is built and made and what is the secret of its functionings or the way out of its disorder.

There are several capital and common errors here:—

1. That mind and spirit are the same thing.
2. That all consciousness can be spoken of as "mind".
3. That all consciousness therefore is of a spiritual substance.
4. That the body is merely Matter, not conscious, therefore something quite different from the spiritual part of the nature.

First, the spirit and the mind are two different things and should not be confused together. The mind is an instrumental entity or instrumental consciousness whose function is to think and perceive — the spirit is an essential entity or consciousness which does not need to think or perceive either in the mental or the sensory way, because whatever knowledge it has is direct or essential knowledge, *svayamprakāśa.*

Next, it follows that all consciousness is not necessarily of a spiritual make and it need not be true and is not true that the thing commanding and the thing commanded are the same, are not at all different, are of the same substance and therefore are bound or at least ought to agree together.

Third, it is not even true that it is the mind which is commanding the mind and finds itself disobeyed by itself. First, there are many parts of the mind, each a force in itself with its formations, functionings, interests, and they may not agree. One part of the mind may be spiritually influenced and like to think of the Divine and obey the spiritual impulse, another part may be rational or scientific or literary and prefer to follow the formations, beliefs or doubts, mental preferences and interests which are in conformity with its education and its nature. But quite apart from that, what was commanding in St. Augustine may very well have been the thinking mind or reason while what was commanded was the vital, and mind and vital, whatever anybody may say, are not the same. The thinking mind or *buddhi* lives, however imperfectly in man, by intelligence and reason. Vital, on the other hand, is a thing of desires, impulses, force-pushes, emotions, sensations, seekings after life-fulfilment, possession and enjoyment; these are its functions and its nature; — it is that part of us which seeks after life and its movements for their own sake and it does not want to leave hold of them if they bring it suffering as well as or more than pleasure; it is even capable of luxuriating in tears and suffering as part of the drama of life. What then is there in common between the thinking intelligence and the vital and why should the latter obey the mind and not follow its own nature? The disobedience is perfectly normal instead of being, as Augustine suggests, unintelligible. Of course, man can establish a mental control over his vital and in so far as he does it he is a man, — because the thinking mind is a nobler and more enlightened entity and consciousness than the vital and ought, therefore, to rule and, if the mental will is strong, *can* rule. But this rule is precarious, incomplete and held only by much self-discipline. For if the mind is more enlightened, the vital is nearer to earth, more intense, vehement, more directly able to touch the body. There is too a vital mind which lives by imagination, thoughts of desire, will to act and enjoy from its own impulse and this is able to seize on the reason itself and make it its auxiliary and its justifying counsel and supplier of pleas and excuses. There is also the sheer force of Desire in man which is the vital's principal support and strong enough to sweep off the reason, as the Gita says, "like a boat on stormy waters", *nāvamivāmbhasi*.

Finally, the body obeys the mind automatically in those things in which it is formed or trained to obey it, but the relation of the body to the mind is not in all things that of an automatic perfect instrument. The body also has a consciousness of its own and, though it is a submental instrument or servant consciousness, it can disobey or fail to obey as well. In many things, in

matters of health and illness for instance, in all automatic functionings, the body acts on its own and is not a servant of the mind.
If it is fatigued, it can offer a passive resistance to the mind's
will. It can cloud the mind with *tamas*, inertia, dullness, fumes of
the subconscient so that the mind cannot act. The arm lifts,
no doubt, when it gets the suggestion, but at first the legs do not
obey when they are asked to walk; they have to learn how to
leave the crawling attitude and movement and take up the erect
and ambulatory habit. When you first ask the hand to draw a
straight line or to play music, it can't do it and won't do it. It
has to be schooled, trained, taught, and afterwards it does automatically what is required of it. All this proves that there is a
body-consciousness which can do things at the mind's order, but
has to be awakened, trained, made a good and conscious instrument. It can even be so trained that a mental will or suggestion
can cure the illness of the body. But all these things, these relations of mind and body, stand on the same footing in essence as
the relation of mind to vital and it is not so easy or primary a
matter as Augustine would have it.

This puts the problem on another footing with the causes
more clear and, if we are prepared to go far enough, it suggests
the way out, the way of yoga.

P.S. All this is quite apart from the contributing and very
important factor of plural personality of which psychological
enquiry is just beginning rather obscurely to take account. That
is a more complex affair.

When the mind is turned towards the Divine and the Truth and
feels and responds to that only or mainly, it can be called a psychic mind — it is something formed by the influence of the psychic being on the mental plane.

The spiritual mind is a mind which, in its fullness, is aware
of the Self, reflecting the Divine, seeing and understanding the
nature of the Self and its relations with the manifestation, living
in that or in contact with it, calm, wide and awake to higher

knowledge, not perturbed by the play of the forces. When it gets its full liberated movement, its central station is very usually felt above the head, though its influence can extend downward through all the being and outward through space.

*
* *

Spiritual capacity means simply a natural capacity for true spiritual experience and development. It can be had on any plane, but the natural result is that one gets easily into touch with the Self and the higher planes.

Psychic mind and mental psychic are the same thing practically — when there is a movement of the mind in which the psychic influence predominates, it is called the psychic in the mind or the psychic mind.

*
* *

Higher Mind is one of the planes of the spiritual mind, the first and lowest of them; it is above the normal mental level. Inner mind is that which lies behind the surface mind (our ordinary mentality) and can only be directly experienced (apart from its *vrttis* in the surface mind such as philosophy, poetry, idealism, etc.) by sadhana, by breaking down the habit of being on the surface and by going deeper within.

Larger mind is a general term to cover the realms of mind which become our field whether by going within or widening into the cosmic consciousness.

The true mental being is not the same as the inner mental — true mental, true vital, true physical being means the Purusha of that level freed from the error and ignorant thought and will of the lower Prakriti and directly open to the knowledge and guidance above.

Higher vital usually refers to the vital mind and emotive being as opposed to the middle vital which has its seat in the navel and is dynamic, sensational and passionate and the lower which is made up of the smaller movements of human life-desire and life-reactions.

Everything here that belongs strictly to the earth plane is evolved out of the Inconscient, out of Matter — but the essential mental being exists already, not involved, in the mental plane. It is only the personal mental that is evolved here by something rising out of the Inconscient and developing under a pressure from above.

The tendency to inquire and know is in itself good, but it must be kept under control. What is needed for progress in sadhana is gained best by increase of consciousness and experience and of intuitive knowledge.

Above the head is the universal or Divine Consciousness and Force. The Kundalini is the latent power asleep in the chakras.

The mind proper is divided into three parts — thinking Mind, dynamic Mind, externalising Mind — the former concerned with ideas and knowledge in their own right, the second with the putting out of mental forces for realisation of the idea, the third with the expression of them in life (not only by speech, but by any form it can give). The word "physical mind" is rather ambiguous, because it can mean this externalising Mind and the mental in the physical taken together.

Vital Mind proper is a sort of a mediator between vital emotion, desire, impulsion, etc. and the mental proper. It expresses the desires, feelings, emotions, passions, ambitions, possessive and active tendencies of the vital and throws them into mental forms (the pure imaginations or dreams of greatness, happiness, etc. in which men indulge are one peculiar form of the vital-mind activity). There is still a lower stage of the mental in the vital which merely expresses the vital stuff without subjecting it to any play of intelligence. It is through this mental vital that the vital passions, impulses, desires rise up and get into the Buddhi and either cloud or distort it.

As the vital Mind is limited by the vital view and feeling of things (while the dynamic Intelligence is not, for it acts by the idea and reason), so the mind in the physical or mental physical is limited by the physical view and experience of things, it mentalises the experiences brought by the contacts of outward life and things, and does not go beyond that (though it can do that much very cleverly), unlike the externalising mind which deals with them more from the reason and its higher intelligence. But in practice these two usually get mixed together. The mechanical mind is a much lower action of the mental physical which, left to itself, would only repeat customary ideas and record the natural reflexes of the physical consciousness to the contacts of outward life and things.

The lower vital as distinguished from the higher is concerned only with the small greeds, small desires, small passions, etc. which make up the daily stuff of life for the ordinary sensational man — while the vital-physical proper is the nervous being giving vital reflexes to contacts of things with the physical consciousness.

It is quite usual for the dynamic and formative part of the mind to be more quick to action than the reflective and discriminate part to control it. It is a question of getting a kind of balance and harmony between them.

The thinking mind does not lead men, does not influence them the most — it is the vital propensities and the vital mind that predominate. The thinking mind with most men is, in matters of life, only an instrument of the vital.

The true thinking mind does not belong to the physical, it is a separate power. The physical mind is that part of the mind which is concerned with the physical things only — it depends on the sense-mind, sees only objects, external actions, draws its ideas from the data given by external things, infers from them only and knows no other Truth until it is enlightened from above.

***

The physical mind can deal only with outward things. One has to think and decide in other things with the mind itself (Buddhi), not with the physical part of it.

That part of the being [the physical mind] has no reason except its whims, its habits or an inclination to be tamasic.

It is the physical mind that would like everything made easy.

The physical mind is in the habit of observing things with or without use.

Repetition is the habit of the mental physical — it is not the true thinking mind that does like that, it is the mental physical or else the lowest part of the physical mind.

But the main error here is in your description of the physical part of the mind — what you have described there is the mechanical mental physical or body-mind which when left to itself simply goes on repeating the past customary thoughts and movements or at the most adds to them such further mechanical reactions to things and reflexes as are in the round of life. The true physical mind is the receiving and externalising intelligence which has two functions — first, to work upon external things and give them a mental order with a way of practically dealing with them and, secondly, to be the channel of materialising and putting into effect whatever the thinking and dynamic mind sends down to it for the purpose.

The mechanical mind is a sort of engine — whatever comes to it it puts into the machine and goes on turning it round and round no matter what it is.

That is the nature of the mental physical to go on repeating without use the movement that has happened. It is what we call the mechanical mind — it is strong in childhood because the thinking mind is not developed and has besides a narrow range of interests. Afterwards it becomes an undercurrent in the mental activities. It must now have risen up with the other characteristics of the mental physical because it is in the physical that the action has come down. Sometimes also when there is silence of the mind, these things come up till they also are quieted down.

From what you describe it seems that you have got into contact with the mechanical mind whose nature is to go on turning round in a circle on the thoughts that come into it. This sometimes happens when the thinking mind is quiet. This is part of the physical mind and you should not be disturbed or alarmed by its rising up, but see what it is and quiet it down or get control of its movements.

The vital mind is usually energetic and creative even in its more mechanical rounds, so it must be the physical that is turning. It is that and the mechanical that last longest, but these too fall silent when the peace and silence become massive and complete. Afterwards knowledge begins to come from the higher planes — the Higher Mind to begin with, and this creates a new action of thought and perception which replaces the ordinary mental. It does that first in the thinking mind, but afterwards also in the vital mind and physical mind, so that all these begin to go through a transformation. This kind of thought is not random and restless, but precise and purposeful — it comes only when needed or called for and does not disturb the silence. Moreover

the element of what we call thought there is secondary and what
might be called a seeing perception (intuition) takes its place.
But so long as the mind does not become capable of a complete
silence, this higher knowledge, thought, perception either does
not come down or, if partially it does, it is liable to get mixed
up with or imitated by the lower, and that is a bother and a hindrance. So the silence is necessary.

When the higher consciousness takes hold of the mechanical
mind, it ceases to be mechanical.

The terms Manas, etc. belong to the ordinary psychology applied
to the surface consciousness. In our yoga we adopt a different
classification — based on the yogic experience. What answers to
this movement of the Manas there would be two separate things
— a part of the physical mind communicating with the physical-
vital. It receives from the physical senses and transmits to the
Buddhi — i.e., to some part or other of the Thought-Mind. It
receives back from the Buddhi and transmits idea and will to the
organs of sensation and action. All that is indispensable in the
ordinary action of the consciousness. But in the ordinary consciousness everything gets mixed up together and there is no
clear order or rule. In the yoga one becomes aware of the
different parts and their proper action, and puts each in its place
and to its proper action under the control of the higher Consciousness or else under the control of the Divine Power. Afterwards all gets surcharged with the spiritual consciousness and
there is an automatic right perception and right action of the
different parts because they are controlled entirely from above
and do not falsify or resist or confuse its dictates.

In physical mind there can be an action of intelligent reasoning and coordination which is a delegation from the Buddhi and would perhaps not be attributed to the Manas by the old psychology. Still the larger part of the action of physical mind corresponds to that of Manas, but it comprises also much of what we would attribute to vital mind and to the nervous being. It is a little difficult to equate this old nomenclature with that of this yoga, for the former takes the mixed action of the surface and tries to analyse it — while in this yoga what is mixed together on the surface gets separated and seen in the light of the deeper working behind which is hidden from the surface awareness. So we have to adopt a different classification.

The physical mind has first to open to the higher consciousness — its limitations are then removed and it admits what is supraphysical and begins to see things in harmony with the higher knowledge. It becomes an instrument for externalising that knowledge in the pragmatic perceptions and actions of the physical life. It sees things as they are and deals with them according to the larger Truth with an automatic rightness of perception and will and reaction to impacts.

I don't use these terms [Manas, etc.] myself as a rule — they are the psychological phraseology of the old yoga.

[The function of Manas:] To sense things and react mentally to objects and convey impressions to the Buddhi etc.

The Chitta is the general stuff of mental consciousness which supports Manas and everything else — it is an indeterminate consciousness which gets determined into thoughts and memories and desires and sensations and perceptions and impulses and feelings (*cittavṛtti*).

The Chitta is the consciousness out of which all is formed, but the formation is made by the mind or vital or other force — which are, as it were, the instruments of the Chitta for self-expression.

It is both ways — The Chitta receives these things, gives them for formation to the vital and mind and all is transmitted to the Buddhi, but also it receives thoughts from the Buddhi and turns these into desires and sensations and impulses.

Yes. But the Chitta does not receive desires and sensations from the Buddhi. It takes thoughts from the Buddhi and turns them into desires.

There is always or generally at least a modifying reaction [to thoughts, etc. received from outside] in the Chitta — except when it simply receives and stores without passing over to the instruments.

Yes, certainly, but as its [the Chitta's] whole business is to receive from above or below or around it cannot stop doing it, it cannot of itself determine what it shall or shall not receive. It has to be assisted by the Buddhi, vital will or some higher power. Afterwards when the higher consciousness descends it begins to be transformed and capable of an automatic rejection of what is not true or right or divine or helpful to the growth of the divine in the being.

Chitta really means the ordinary consciousness including the mind, vital and physical — but practically it can be taken to mean something central in the consciousness. If that is centred in the Divine, the rest follows more or less quickly as a natural result.

*
**

The Chitta is not near the heart — if you mean the substance of the lower consciousness, it has no particular place. All things of this life are there in this stuff of the consciousness but the memory of past lives is wrapped up and involved elsewhere. The heart is the main centre of this consciousness for most men, of course, so you may feel its activities centred in that level.

*
**

The same as with any part of the being — there is a subconscient part of the Chitta which keeps the past impression of things and sends up forms of them to the consciousness in dream or else keeps the habit of old movements and sends up these whenever it finds an opportunity.

*
**

If the word *vāsanā* is used in the original,[1] it does not mean "desire". It means usually the idea or mental feeling rising from the *citta*, imaginations, impressions, memories etc., impressions of liking and disliking, of pain and pleasure. What Vasistha wants to say is that while the ideas, impressions, impulsions, that lead to action in an ordinary man rise from the *citta*, those that rise in the Jivanmukta come straight from the *sattva* — from the essential consciousness of the being — in other words they are not mental but spiritual formations. As one might say, instead of *cittavṛtti* they are *sattvapreraṇā*, direct indications from the inner being of what is to be thought, felt or done. When the *citta* is no longer active and the mind silent — which happens when the *mukti* comes and no one can be Jivanmukta without that, then what remains and perceives and does things is felt as an essential consciousness, the consciousness of the true self or true being.

*
**

---

[1] *Yoga-vāsiṣṭha.*

Mahat is, I suppose, the essential and original matrix of consciousness (involved not evolved) in Prakriti out of which individuality and formation come.

Tanmatra is only the basis of matter. In the Sankhya the basis is Pradhana (of Prakriti) out of which come Buddhi and everything else. In the Vedanta it is spiritual substance out of which all comes.

X

There are four parts of the vital being — first, the mental vital which gives a mental expression by thought, speech or otherwise to the emotions, desires, passions, sensations and other movements of the vital being; the emotional vital which is the seat of various feelings, such as love, joy, sorrow, hatred, and the rest; the central vital which is the seat of the stronger vital longings and reactions, e.g. ambition, pride, fear, love of fame, attractions and repulsions, desires and passions of various kinds and the field of many vital energies; last, the lower vital which is occupied with small desires and feelings, such as make the greater part of daily life, e.g. food desire, sexual desire, small likings, dislikings, vanity, quarrels, love of praise, anger at blame, little wishes of all kinds — and a numberless host of other things. Their respective seats are: (1) the region from the throat to the heart, (2) the heart (it is a double centre, belonging in front to the emotional and vital and behind to the psychic), (3) from the heart to the navel, (4) below the navel.

There is a part of the nature which I have called the vital mind; the function of this mind is not to think and reason, to perceive, consider and find out or value things, for that is the function of the thinking mind proper, *buddhi*, — but to plan or dream or imagine what can be done. It makes formations for the future which the will can try to carry out if opportunity and circumstances become favourable or even it can work to make them favourable. In men of action this faculty is prominent and a leader of their nature; great men of action always have it in a very high measure. But even if one is not a man of action or practical realisation or if circumstances are not favourable or one can do only small and ordinary things, this vital mind is there. It acts in them on a small scale, or if it needs some sense of largeness, what it does very often is to plan in the void, knowing that it cannot realise its plans or else to imagine big things, stories, adventures, great doings in which oneself is the hero or the creator. What you describe as happening in you is the rush of this vital mind or imagination making its formations; its action is not peculiar to you but works pretty much in the same way in most people — but in each according to his turn of fancy, interest, favourite ideas or desires. You have to become master of its action and not to allow it to seize your mind and carry it away when and where it wants. In sadhana when the experiences begin to come, it is exceedingly important not to allow this power to do what it likes with you; for it then creates false experiences according to its nature and persuades the sadhak that these experiences are true or it builds unreal formations and persuades him that this is what he has to do. Some have been taken away by this misleading force used by powers of Falsehood who persuaded them through it that they had a great spiritual, political or social work to do in the world and led them away to disappointment and failure. It is rising in you in order that you may understand what it is and reject it. For there are several things you had to get out of the vital plane before the deeper or greater spiritual experiences could safely begin or safely continue.

The descent of the peace is often one of the first major positive experiences of the sadhana. In this state of peace the normal thought-mind (*buddhi*) is apt to fall silent or abate most of its activity and when it does, very often either this vital mind can rush in, if one is not on one's guard, or else a kind of mechanical physical or random subconscient mind can begin to come up and act; these are the chief disturbers of the silence. Or else the lower vital mind can try to disturb; that brings up the ego and passions and their play. All these are signs of elements that have to be got rid of, because if they remain and other of the higher powers begin to descend, Power and Force, Knowledge, Love or Ananda, those lower things may come across with the result that either the higher consciousness retires or its descent is covered up and the stimulation it gives is misused for the purposes of the lower nature. This is the reason why many sadhaks after having big experiences fall into the clutch of a magnified ego, upheavals, ambition, exaggerated sex or other vital passions or distortions. It is always well therefore if a complete purification of the vital can either precede or keep pace with the positive experience — at least in natures in which the vital is strongly active.

It [the vital mind] is a mind of dynamic (not rationalising) will, action, desire — occupied with force and achievement and satisfaction and possession, enjoyment and suffering, giving and taking, growth, expansion, success and failure, good fortune and ill fortune etc. etc.

Vital thought expresses vital movements, the play of vital forces — it does not think freely and independently of them as the thinking mind can do. The true thinking mind can stand above the vital movements, watch and observe and judge them freely as it would observe and judge outside things. In most men however the thinking mind (reason) is invaded by the vital mind and not free.

That is the ordinary activity of the vital mind which is always imagining and thinking and planning what to do about this and how to arrange about that. It has obviously its utility in human nature and human action, but acts in a random and excessive way without discipline, economy of its powers or concentration on the things that have really to be done.

The things which come to you in this way in sleep or waking are of the nature of vital mind imaginations and activities about things and work and whatever presents itself to the mind. On all things that present themselves to the mind, the vital imagination in man is able to work, imagining, speculating, building ideas or plans for the future etc. etc. It has its utility for the consciousness in ordinary life, but must quiet down and be replaced by a higher action in yoga. In sleep it is also the vital plane into which you enter. If properly seen and coordinated, what is experienced in the vital plane has its value and gives knowledge which is useful and control over the vital self and vital plane. But all that is coming to you through the subconscient in an incoherent way — this is the cause of the trouble. The whole thing has to be quieted down and we shall try to get that done. When I spoke of your opening yourself, I meant simply that you should fix it in your mind that the help is coming and have the will to receive it — not necessarily that you should open yourself by an effort.

The source from which these imaginations come has nothing to do with reason and does not care for any rational objections. They are either from the vital mind, the same source from which come all the fine imaginations and long stories which men tell themselves in which they are the heroes and do great things or they come from little entities attached to the physical mind which pick up any random suggestion anywhere and present it to the mind just to see whether it will be accepted. If one watches oneself closely one can find the most queer and extraordinary or nonsensical things crossing the mind or peeping in on it in this way. Usually one laughs or hardly notices and the thing falls back to the world of incoherent thought from which it came.

It is again the vital mind. It has no sense of proportion or measure and is eager to be or achieve something big at once.

[Day-dreaming:] All that is the vital mind; it lies in everybody, the habit of such imaginations. It is not very important, but of course it has to be got rid of, as the basis is ego.

The vital mind in the ordinary nature cannot get on without these imaginations — so the habit remains for a long time. To be detached and indifferent is the best, then after a time it may get disgusted and drop the habit.

That kind of talking [talking mentally to another person] is very common with the vital mind. It is a way it has of acting on the subtle plane on things in which it is interested, especially if the physical action is stopped or restricted.

The point about the emotional and the higher vital is a rather difficult one. In the classification in which the mind is taken as something more than the thinking, perceiving and willing intelligence, the emotional can be reckoned as part of the mind, the vital in the mental. In another classification it is rather the most mentalised part of the vital nature. In the first case, the term 'higher vital' is confined to that larger movement of the conscious life-force which is concerned with creation, with power and force and conquest, with giving and self-giving and gathering from the world for further action and expenditure of power, throwing it-self out in the wider movements of life, responsive to the greater objects of Nature. In the second arrangement, the emotional being stands at the top of the vital nature and the two together make the higher vital. As against them stands the lower vital which is concerned with the pettier movements of action and desire and stretches down into the vital physical where it sup-ports the life of the more external activities and all physical sen-sations, hungers, cravings, satisfactions. The term 'lower' must not be considered in a pejorative sense; it refers only to the position in the hierarchy of the planes. For although this part of the nature in earthly beings tends to be very obscure and is full of perversions, — lust, greed of all kinds, vanity, small ambi-tions, petty anger, envy, jealousy are its ordinary guests, — still there is another side to it which makes it an indispensable mediator between the inner being and the outer life.

It is not a fact that every psychic experience embodies itself in a purified and rightly directed vital current; it does that when it has to externalise itself in action. Psychic experience is in itself a quite independent thing and has its own characteristic forms. The psychic being stands behind all the others; its force is the true soul-power. But if it comes to the front, it can suffuse all the rest; mind, vital, the physical consciousness can take its stamp and be transformed by its influence. When the nature is properly developed, there is a psychic in the mental, a psychic in the vital, a psychic in the physical. It is when that is there and strong, that we can say of someone that he evidently has a soul. But there are some in whom this element is so lacking that we have to use faith in order to believe that they have a soul at all. The centre of the psychic being is behind the centre of the emotional being; it is the emotional that is nearest dynamically to the psychic and in most men it is through the emotional centre that the psychic can be most easily reached and through the psychicised emotion that it can be most easily expressed. Many therefore mistake the one for the other; but there is a world of difference between the two. The emotions normally are vital in their character and not part of the psychic nature.

It must be remembered that while this classification is indis-

pensable for psychological self-knowledge and discipline and
practice, it can be used best when it is not made too rigid and
cutting a formula. For things run very much into each other
and a synthetical sense of these powers is as necessary as the
analysis. Mind, for instance, is everywhere. The physical mind
is technically placed below the vital and yet it is a prolongation
of the mind proper and one that can act in its own sphere by
direct touch with the higher mental intelligence. And there is too
an obscure mind of the body, of the very cells, molecules, cor-
puscles. Haeckel, the German materialist, spoke somewhere
of the will in the atom, and recent science, dealing with the incalculable individual variation in the activity of the electrons, comes
near to perceiving that this is not a figure but the shadow thrown
by a secret reality. This body-mind is a very tangible truth;
owing to its obscurity and mechanical clinging to past movements
and facile oblivion and rejection of the new, we find in it one of
the chief obstacles to permeation by the supermind Force and the
transformation of the functioning of the body. On the other
hand, once effectively converted, it will be one of the most pre-
cious instruments for the stabilisation of the supramental Light
and Force in material Nature.

It is not possible to say with any precision what the resistance in
the higher vital parts will be, what form it takes, because it may
take different forms with different natures. It is quite normal
that there should be some resistance almost at every point to the
descent of the higher consciousness; for the different parts of
the present nature are each more or less attached to their own
established way of seeing, acting, feeling, reacting to things and
to the habitual movements and formations of their own domain
which each individual has made for himself in the past or in his
present life. What is needed is a general plasticity of the mind,
the vital, the physical consciousness, a readiness to give up all
attachment to these things, to accept whatever the higher consciousness brings down with it however contrary to one's own
received ideas, feelings, habits of nature. The greater the plasti-

city in any part of the nature, the less the resistance there.

By the higher vital parts of the nature I mean the vital mind, the emotional nature, the life-force dynamis in the being. The vital mind is that part of the vital being which builds, plans, imagines, arranges things and thoughts according to the life-pushes, desires, will to power or possession, will to action, emotions, vital ego reactions of the nature. It must be distinguished from the reasoning will which plans and arranges things according to the dictates of the thinking mind proper, the discriminating reason or according to the mental intuition or a direct insight and judgment. The vital mind uses thought for the service not of reason but of life-push and life-power and when it calls in reasoning it uses that for justifying the dictates of these powers, imposes their dictates on the reason instead of governing by a discriminating will the action of the life-forces. This higher vital with all its parts is situated in the chest and has the cardiac centre as its main stronghold governing all this part down to the navel. I need not say anything about the emotional nature, for its character and movements are known to all. From the navel downwards is the reign of the vital passions and sensations and all the small life-impulses that constitute the bulk of the ordinary human life and character. This is what we call the lower vital nature. The Muladhara is the main support of the physical consciousness and the material parts of the nature.

The *antarātman* is the soul, the portion of the Divine that is at the inmost basis of the evolving individual and supports the mind and life and body which are the instrumental parts of nature and through which it tries to grow from the material Inconscience towards the divine Light and Immortality which are its proper being. The limitations of its instruments impose upon it an acceptance of the lower movements and a compromise between soul and nature which retard this movement even while it gets its means of advance from that interchange. The psychic being is the soul-form or soul personality developing through this evolution and passing from life to life till all is ready for the higher evolution beyond the Ignorance.

The realisation of the psychic being, its awakening and the bringing of it in front depend mainly on the extent to which

one can develop a personal relation with the Divine, a relation of
Bhakti, love, reliance, self-giving, rejection of the insistences of
the separating and self-asserting mental, vital and physical ego.

I can say little about the last question. Sanatkumar is, I
believe, one of the four mind-born sons of Brahma; he cannot
therefore be identical with Skanda who is a son of Shiva.

The emotional being is itself a part of the vital.

The heart is the centre of the emotional being and the emotions
are vital movements. When the heart is purified, the vital emotions change into psychic feelings or else psychicised vital movements.

Pure and true thoughts and emotions and impulses can rise
from the human mind, heart and vital, because all is not evil
there. The heart may be unpurified but that does not mean that
everything in it is impure.

Above the heart is the vital mind, but the rising of sensation is
lower than the emotion, not higher.

Sensation is much nearer the physical than emotion.

The place of desire is below the heart in the central vital
(navel) and in the lower vital, but it moves the emotion and the
vital mind.

I make the distinction [between the lower vital movements and
the emotions of the heart] by noting where these things rise from.
Anger, fear, jealousy touch the heart no doubt just as they touch
the mind but they rise from the navel region and entrails (i.e.

the lower or at highest the middle vital). Stevenson has a striking passage in "Kidnapped" where the hero notes that his fear is felt primarily not in the heart but the stomach. Love, hope have their primary seat in the heart, so with pity etc.

Joy is a vital feeling, like its opposite, sorrow.

But is it true that even anger which is of the lower vital and therefore close to the body, invariably produces these effects?[1] Of course the psychologist can't know that another man is angry unless he shows physical signs of it, but also he can't know what a man is thinking unless the man speaks or writes — does it follow that the state of thought cannot be "fancied" without its sign in speaking or writing? A Japanese who is accustomed to control all his "emotions" and give no sign (if he is angry the first sign you will have of it is a knife in your stomach from a calm or smiling assailant) will have none of these things when he is angry, — not even the "ebullition" in the chest, — in its place there will be a settled fire that will burn till his anger achieves itself in action.

A strong vital is one that is full of life-force, has ambition, courage, great energy, a force for action or for creation, a large expansive movement whether for generosity in giving or for possession and lead and domination, a power to fulfil and materialise — many other forms of vital strength there are also. It is often difficult for such a vital to surrender itself because of this sense of its own powers — but if it can do so, it becomes an admirable instrument for the Divine Work.

---

[1] Physical signs like ebullition in the chest, flushing of the face, etc.

No, a weak vital has not the strength to turn spiritually — and being weak, more easily falls under a wrong influence and even when it wants, finds it difficult to accept anything beyond its own habitual nature. The strong vital, when the will is there, can do it much more easily — its one central difficulty is the pride of the ego and the attraction of its powers.

The chest has more connection with the psychic than the vital. A strong vital may have a good physique, but as often it has not — it draws too much on the physical, eats it up as it were.

*
**

I think I said it [an old desire] was left in the subconscient part of the physical vital. As there is a physical mind, so there is a physical vital — a vital turned entirely upon physical things, full of desires and greeds and seekings for pleasure on the physical plane.

*
**

The physical-vital is the being of small desires and greeds, etc. — the vital-physical is the nervous being; they are closely connected together.

*
**

The vital-physical governs all the small daily reactions to outward things — reactions of the nerves and the body consciousness and the reflex emotions and sensations; it motives much of the ordinary actions of man and joins with the lower parts of the vital proper in producing lust, jealousy, anger, violence etc. In its lowest parts (vital-material) it is the agent of pain, physical illness etc.

*
**

Yes — they [the lower vital, the physical vital and the most material vital] become very clear to the increasing consciousness. And the distinctions are necessary — otherwise one may influence or control the lower vital or a part of the physical vital and then be astonished to find that something intangible but apparently invincible still resists — it is the material vital with so much of the rest as it can influence by its resistance.

The nervous part of the being is a portion of the vital — it is the vital-physical, the life-force closely enmeshed in the reactions, desires, needs, sensations of the body. The vital proper is the life-force acting in its own nature, impulses, emotions, feelings, desires, ambitions, etc., having as their highest centre what we may call the outer heart of emotion, while there is an inner heart where are the higher or psychic feelings and sensibilities, the emotions or intuitive yearnings and impulses of the soul. The vital part of us is, of course, necessary to our completeness, but it is a true instrument only when its feelings and tendencies have been purified by the psychic touch and taken up and governed by the spiritual light and power.

I do not know about subtle vital. One says subtle physical to distinguish from gross material physical, because to our normal experience all physical is gross, *sthūla*. But the vital is in its nature non-material, so that the adjective is superfluous. By material vital we mean the vital so involved in Matter as to be bound by its movements and gross physical character; the action is to support and energise the body and keep in it the capacity of life, growth, movement, etc., also of sensitiveness to outside impacts.

This question has no practical meaning — for the vital physical forces can be received from anywhere by the body, from around, below or above. The order of the planes is in reference to each other, not in reference to the body. In reference to each other, the vital physical is below the physical mind, but above the material: but at the same time these powers interpenetrate each other.

The body-energy is a manifestation of material forces supported by vital-physical energy which is the vital energy precipitated into matter and conditioned by it.

Vitality means life-force — wherever there is life, in plant or animal or man, there is life-force — without the vital there can be no life in matter and no living action. The vital is a necessary force and nothing can be done or created in the bodily existence, if the vital is not there as an instrument. Even sadhana needs the vital force.

But if the vital is unregenerated and enslaved to desire, passion and ego, then it is as harmful as it can otherwise be helpful. Even in ordinary life the vital has to be controlled by the mind and mental will, otherwise it brings disorder or disaster. When people speak of a vital man, they mean one under the domination of vital force not controlled by the mind or the spirit. The vital can be a good instrument, but it is a bad master.

The vital has not to be killed or destroyed, but purified and transformed by the psychic and spiritual control.

The physical depends on the vital, at every step — it could not do anything without the help of the vital — so it is quite natural that it should receive its suggestions.

The physical life cannot last without the body nor can the body live without the life-force, but the life in itself has a separate existence and a separate body of its own, the vital body, just as the mind has a separate existence and can exist on its own plane.

All the organisation is held together by the psychic which is the support of all.

XI

Each plane of our being — mental, vital, physical — has its own consciousness, separate though interconnected and interacting; but to our outer mind and sense, in our waking experience, they are all confused together. The body, for instance, has its own consciousness and acts from it, even without any mental will of our own or even against that will, and our surface mind knows very little about this body-consciousness, feels it only in an imperfect way, sees only its results and has the greatest difficulty in finding out their causes. It is part of the yoga to become aware of this separate consciousness of the body, to see and feel its movements and the forces that act upon it from inside or outside and to learn how to control and direct it even in its most hidden and (to us) subconscient processes. But the body-consciousness itself is only part of the individualised physical consciousness in us which we gather and build out of the secretly conscious forces of universal physical Nature.

There is the universal physical consciousness of Nature and there is our own which is a part of it, moved by it, and used by the central being for the support of its expression in the physical world and for a direct dealing with all these external objects and movements and forces. This physical consciousness-plane receives from the other planes their powers and influences and makes formations of them in its own province. Therefore we have a physical mind as well as a vital mind and the mind proper; we have a vital-physical part in us — the nervous being — as well as the vital proper; and both are largely conditioned by the gross material bodily part which is almost entirely subconscient to our experience.

The physical mind is that which is fixed on physical objects and happenings, sees and understands these only, and deals with them according to their own nature, but can with difficulty respond to the higher forces. Left to itself, it is sceptical of the existence of supraphysical things, of which it has no direct experience and to which it can find no clue; even when it has spiritual experiences, it forgets them easily, loses the impression and result and finds it difficult to believe. To enlighten the physical mind by the consciousness of the higher spiritual and supramental planes is one object of this yoga, just as to enlighten it by the power of the higher vital and higher mental elements of the being is the greatest part of human self-development, civilisation and culture.

The vital physical, on the other hand, is the vehicle of the nervous responses of our physical nature; it is the field and instrument of the smaller sensations, desires, reactions of all kinds to the impacts of the outer physical and gross material life. This vital physical part (supported by the lowest part of the vital proper) is therefore the agent of most of the lesser movements of our external life; its habitual reactions and obstinate pettinesses are the chief stumbling-block in the way of transformation of the outer consciousness by the yoga. It is also largely responsible for most of the suffering and disease of mind or body to which the physical being is subject in Nature.

As to the gross material part, it is not necessary to specify its place, for that is obvious; but it must be remembered that this too has a consciousness of its own, the obscure consciousness proper to the limbs, cells, tissues, glands, organs. To make this obscurity luminous and directly instrumental to the higher planes and to the divine movement is what we mean in our yoga by making the body conscious, — that is to say, full of a true, awake and responsive awareness instead of its own obscure, limited half-subconscience.

There is an inner as well as an outer consciousness all through our being, upon all its levels. The ordinary man is aware only of his surface self and quite unaware of all that is concealed by the surface. And yet what is on the surface, what we know or think we know of ourselves and even believe that that is all we are, is only a small part of our being and by far the larger part of us is below the surface. Or, more accurately, it is behind the frontal consciousness, behind the veil, occult and known only by an occult knowledge. Modern psychology and psychic science have begun to perceive this truth just a little. Materialistic psychology calls this hidden part the Inconscient, although practically admitting that it is far greater, more powerful and profound than the surface conscious self, — very much as the Upanishads called the superconscient in us the Sleep-self, although this Sleep-self is said to be an infinitely greater Intelligence, omniscient, omnipotent, Prajna, the Ishwara. Psychic science calls this hidden consciousness the subliminal self, and here too it is seen that this subliminal self has more powers, more knowledge, a freer field of movement than the smaller self that is on the surface. But the truth is that all this that is behind, this sea of which our waking consciousness is only a wave or series of waves, cannot be described by any one term, for it is very complex. Part of it is subconscient, lower than our waking consciousness, part of it is on a level with it but behind and much larger than it; part is above and superconscient to us. What we call our mind is only an outer mind, a surface mental action, instrumental for the partial expression of a larger mind behind of which we are not ordinarily aware and can only know by going inside ourselves. So too what we know of the vital in us is only the outer vital, a surface activity partially expressing a larger secret vital which we can only know by going within. Equally, what we call our physical being is only a visible projection of a greater and subtler invisible physical consciousness which is much more complex, much more aware, much wider in its receptiveness, much more open and plastic and free.

If you understand and experience this truth, then only you will be able to realise what is meant by the inner mental, the inner vital, the inner physical consciousness. But it must be noted that this term 'inner' is used in two different senses. Sometimes it denotes the consciousness behind the veil of the outer being, the mental or vital or physical within, which is in direct touch with the universal mind, the universal life-forces, the universal physical forces. Sometimes, on the other hand, we mean an inmost mental, vital, physical, more specifically called the true mind, the true vital, the true physical consciousness which is nearer to the soul and can most easily and directly respond to the Divine Light and Power. There is no real yoga possible, still less any integral yoga, if we do not go back from the outer self and become aware of all this inner being and inner nature. For then alone can we break the limitations of the ignorant external self which receives consciously only the outer touches and knows things indirectly through the outer mind and senses, and become directly aware of the universal consciousness and the universal forces that play through us and around us. And then only too can we hope to be directly aware of the Divine in us and directly in touch with the Divine Light and the Divine Force. Otherwise we can feel the Divine only through external signs and external results and that is a difficult and uncertain way and very occasional and inconstant, and it leads only to belief and not to knowledge, not to the direct consciousness and awareness of the constant presence.

As for instances of the difference, I may give you two from the opposite poles of experience, one from the most external phenomena showing how the inward opens to the awareness of the universal forces, one of spiritual experience indicating how the inward opens to the Divine. Take illness. If we live only in the outward physical consciousness, we do not usually know that we are going to be ill until the symptoms of the malady declare themselves in the body. But if we develop the inward physical consciousness, we become aware of a subtle environmental physical atmosphere and can feel the forces of illness coming towards us through it, feel them even at a distance and, if we have learnt how to do it, we can stop them by the will or otherwise. We sense too around us a vital physical or nervous envelope which radiates from the body and protects it, and we can feel the adverse forces trying to break through it and can interfere, stop them or reinforce the nervous envelope. Or we can feel the symptoms of illness, fever or cold, for instance, in the subtle physical sheath before they are manifest in the gross body and destroy them there, preventing them from manifesting in the body. Take now the call for the Divine Power, Light, Ananda. If we live only in the outward physical consciousness, it may descend and work behind the veil, but we shall feel nothing and only see certain results after a long time. Or at most we feel a certain clarity and peace in the mind, a joy in the vital a happy state in the physical and infer the touch of the Divine. But if we are awake in the physical, we shall feel the light, power or Ananda flowing through the body, the limbs, nerves, blood, breath and, through the subtle body, affecting the most material cells and making them conscious and blissful and we shall sense directly the Divine Power and Presence. These are only two instances out of a thousand that are possible and can be constantly experienced by the sadhak.

Everything has a physical part — even the mind has a physical part; there is a mental physical, a mind of the body and the material. So the emotional being has a physical part. It has no location separate from the rest of the emotional. One can only distinguish that when the consciousness becomes sufficiently subtle to do so.

It [the material] is the most physical grade of the physical — there is the mental physical, the vital physical, the material physical.

Yes — or at least [the material consciousness] is a separate part of the physical consciousness. Physical mind for instance is narrow and limited and often stupid, but not inert. Matter consciousness is on the contrary inert as well as largely sub-conscious — active only when driven by an energy, otherwise inactive and immobile. When one first falls into direct contact with this level, the feeling in the body is that of inertia and immobility, in the vital-physical exhaustion or lassitude, in the physical mind absence of *prakāśa* and *pravṛtti* or only the most ordinary thoughts and impulses. It took me a long time to get down any kind of light or power into this level. But when once it is illumined, the advantage is that the subconscient becomes conscient and this removes a very fundamental obstacle from the sadhana.

By the gross physical is meant the earthly and bodily physical —
as experienced by the outward sense-mind and senses. But that
is not the whole of Matter. There is a subtle physical also with a
subtler consciousness in it which can, for instance, go to a distance from the body and yet feel and be aware of things in a not
merely mental or vital way. As for mind and vital, they are everywhere — there is an obscure mind and life even in the cells of the
body, the stones or in molecules and atoms.

The physical nerves are part of the material body but they are
extended into the subtle body and there is a connection between
the two.

Yes, there are nerves in the subtle body.
    Yes — sheaths is simply a term for bodies, because each is
superimposed on the other and acts as a covering and can be cast
off. Thus the physical body itself is called the food sheath and its
throwing off is what is called death.

This is what is called nervous envelope surrounding the body.
You are probably seeing the *sūkṣma* and nervous envelope in one
view. The *sūkṣma deha* contains the *sthūla deha*, only it is not
bound to its limitations.

You can only distinguish the different sheaths either by intuition
or by experience and then you have established direct knowledge
of the different sheaths.

The appearance of the being in other planes is not the same
necessarily as that of the physical body. Very often the form
taken by the vital or psychic or mental being is very different

from the physical form. Even when they resemble on the whole, there is always some difference.

XII

In our yoga we mean by the subconscient that quite submerged part of our being in which there is no wakingly conscious and coherent thought, will or feeling or organized reaction, but which yet receives obscurely the impressions of all things and stores them up in itself and from it too all sorts of stimuli, of persistent habitual movements, crudely repeated or disguised in strange forms can surge up into dream or into the waking nature. For if these impressions rise up most in dream in an incoherent and disorganized manner, they can also and do rise up into our waking consciousness as a mechanical repetition of old thoughts, old mental, vital and physical habits or an obscure stimulus to sensations, actions, emotions which do not originate in or from our conscious thought or will and are even often opposed to its perceptions, choice or dictates. In the subconscient there is an obscure mind full of obstinate Sanskaras, impressions, associations, fixed notions, habitual reactions formed by our past, an obscure vital full of the seeds of habitual desires, sensations and nervous reactions, a most obscure material which governs much that has to do with the condition of the body. It is largely responsible for our illnesses; chronic or repeated illnesses are indeed mainly due to the subconscient and its obstinate memory and habit of repetition of whatever has impressed itself upon the body-consciousness. But this subconscient must be clearly distinguished from the subliminal parts of our being such as the inner or subtle physical consciousness, the inner vital or inner mental; for these are not at all obscure or incoherent or ill-organized, but only veiled from our surface consciousness. Our surface constantly receives something, inner touches, communications or influences, from these sources but does not know for the most part whence they come.

**

No, subliminal is a general term used for all parts of the being which are not on the waking surface. Subconscient is very often used in the same sense by European psychologists because they do not know the difference. But when I use the word, I mean always what is *below* the ordinary physical consciousness, not what is behind it. The inner mental, vital, physical, the psychic are not subconscious in this sense, but they can be spoken of as subliminal.

The subconscient is below the waking physical consciousness — it is an automatic, obscure, incoherent, half-unconscious realm into which light and awareness can with difficulty come. The inner vital and physical are quite different — they have a larger plastic, subtler, freer and richer consciousness than the surface vital and physical, much more open to the Truth and in direct touch with the universal.

The subconscient is universal as well as individual like all the other main parts of the Nature. But there are different parts or planes of the subconscient. All upon earth is based on the Inconscient as it is called, though it is not really inconscient at all, but rather a complete "sub"-conscience, a suppressed or involved consciousness, in which there is everything but nothing is formulated or expressed. The subconscient lies between this Inconscient and the conscious mind, life and body. It contains the potentiality of all the primitive reactions to life which struggle out to the surface from the dull and inert strands of Matter and form by a constant development a slowly evolving and self-formulating consciousness; it contains them not as ideas, perceptions or conscious reactions but as the fluid substance of these things. But also all that is consciously experienced sinks down into the subconscient, not as precise though submerged memories but as obscure yet obstinate impressions of experience, and these can come up at any time as dreams, as mechanical repetitions of past thought, feelings, action, etc., as "complexes"

exploding into action and event, etc., etc. The subconscient is the main cause why all things repeat themselves and nothing ever gets changed except in appearance. It is the cause why people say character cannot be changed, the cause also of the constant return of things one hoped to have got rid of for ever. All seeds are there and all Sanskaras of the mind, vital and body, — it is the main support of death and disease and the last fortress (seemingly impregnable) of the Ignorance. All too that is suppressed without being wholly got rid of sinks down there and remains as seed ready to surge up or sprout up at any moment.

The subconscient is not the whole foundation of the nature; it is only the lower basis of the Ignorance and affects mostly the lower vital and physical exterior consciousness and these again affect the higher parts of the nature. While it is well to see what it is and how it acts, one must not be too preoccupied with this dark side or this apparent aspect of the instrumental being. One should rather regard it as something not oneself, a mask of false nature imposed on the true being by the Ignorance. The true being is the inner with all its vast possibilities of reaching and expressing the Divine and especially the inmost, the soul, the psychic Purusha which is always in its essence pure, divine, turned to all that is good and true and beautiful. The exterior being has to be taken hold of by the inner being and turned into an instrument no longer of the upsurging of the ignorant subconscient Nature, but of the Divine. It is by remembering always that and opening the nature upwards that the Divine Consciousness can be reached and descend from above into the whole inner and outer existence, mental, vital, physical, the subconscient, the subliminal, all that we overtly or secretly are. This should be the main preoccupation. To dwell solely on the subconscient and the aspect of imperfection creates depression and should be avoided. One has to keep a right balance and stress on the positive side most, recognising the other but only to reject and change it. This and a constant faith and reliance on the Mother are what is needed for the transformation to come.

P.S. It is certainly the abrupt and decisive breaking that is the easiest and best way for these things — vital habits.

The subconscient is a concealed and unexpressed inarticulate consciousness which works below all our conscious physical activities. Just as what we call the superconscient is really a higher consciousness above from which things descend into the being, so the subconscient is below the body-consciousness and things come up into the physical, the vital and the mind-nature from there.

Just as the higher consciousness is superconscient to us and supports all our spiritual possibilities and nature, so the subconscient is the basis of our material being and supports all that comes up in the physical nature.

Men are not ordinarily conscious of either of these planes of their own being, but by sadhana they can become aware.

The subconscient retains the impressions of all our past experiences of life and they can come up from there in dream forms: most dreams in ordinary sleep are formations made from subconscient impressions.

The habit of strong recurrence of the same things in our physical consciousness, so that it is difficult to get rid of its habits, is largely due to a subconscient support. The subconscient is full of irrational habits.

When things are rejected from all other parts of the nature, they go either into the environmental consciousness around us through which we communicate with others and with universal Nature and try to return from there or they sink into the subconscient and can come up from there even after lying long quiescent so that we think they are gone.

When the physical consciousness is being changed, the chief resistance comes from the subconscient. It is constantly maintaining or bringing back the inertia, weakness, obscurity, lack of intelligence which afflict the physical mind and vital or the obscure fears, desires, angers, lusts of the physical vital, or the illnesses, dullnesses, pains, incapabilities to which the body-nature is prone.

If light, strength, the Mother's Consciousness is brought down into the body, it can penetrate the subconscient also and convert its obscurity and resistance.

When something is erased from the subconscient so completely that it leaves no seed and thrown out of the circumconscient so completely that it can return no more, then only can we be sure that we have finished with it for ever.

The Muladhar is the centre of the physical consciousness proper, and all below in the body is the sheer physical, which as it goes downward becomes increasingly subconscient, but the real seat of the subconscient is below the body, as the real seat of the higher consciousness (superconscient) is above the body. At the same time, the subconscient can be felt anywhere, felt as something below the movement of the consciousness and, in a way, supporting it from beneath or else drawing the consciousness down towards itself. The subconscient is the main support of all habitual movements, especially the physical and lower vital movements. When something is thrown out of the vital or physical, it very usually goes down into the subconscient and remains there as if in seed and comes up again when it can. That is the reason why it is so difficult to get rid of habitual vital movements or to change the character; for, supported or refreshed from this source, preserved in this matrix your vital movements, even when suppressed or repressed, surge up again and recur. The action of the subconscient is irrational, mechanical, repetitive. It does not listen to reason or the mental will. It is only by bringing the higher Light and Force into it that it can change.

The subconscient is the support of habitual action — it can support good habits as well as bad.

The sub-conscious is the evolutionary basis in us, it is not the whole of our hidden nature, nor is it the whole origin of what we are. But things can rise from the subconscient and take shape in the conscious parts and much of our smaller vital and physical instincts, movements, habits, character-forms has this source.

There are three occult sources of our action — the super-conscient, the subliminal, the subconscient, but of none of them are we in control or even aware. What we are aware of is the surface being which is only an instrumental arrangement. The source of all is the general Nature, — universal Nature individualising itself in each person; for this general Nature deposits certain habits of movement, personality, character, faculties, dispositions, tendencies in us, and that, whether formed now or before our birth, is what we usually call ourselves. A good deal of this is in habitual movement and use in our known conscious parts on the surface, a great deal more is concealed in the other unknown three which are below or behind the surface.

But what we are on the surface is being constantly set in motion, changed, developed or repeated by the waves of the general Nature coming in on us either directly or else indirectly through others, through circumstances, through various agencies or channels. Some of this flows straight into the conscious parts and acts there, but our mind ignores its source, appropriates it and regards all that as its own; a part comes secretly into the subconscient or sinks into it and waits for an opportunity of rising up into the conscious surface; a good deal goes into the subliminal and may at any time come out — or may not, may rather rest there as unused matter. Part passes through and is rejected, thrown back or thrown out or spilt into the universal sea. Our nature is a constant activity of forces supplied to us out of which (or rather out of a small amount of it) we make what we will or can. What we make seems fixed and formed for good, but in reality it is all a play of forces, a flux, nothing fixed or stable; the appearance of stability is given by constant repetition and recurrence of the same vibrations and formations. That is why our nature can be changed in spite of Vivekananda's

saying and Horace's adage and in spite of the conservative
resistance of the subconscient, but it is a difficult job because
the master mode of Nature is this obstinate repetition and
recurrence.

As for the things in our nature that are thrown away from
us by rejection but come back, it depends on where you throw
them. Very often there is a sort of procedure about it. The
mind rejects its mentalities, the vital its vitalities, the physical
its physicalities — these usually go back into the corresponding
domain of general Nature. It all stays at first, when that happens,
in the environmental consciousness which we carry about with
us, by which we communicate with the outside Nature, and
often it persistently rushes back from there — until it is so
absolutely rejected, or thrown far away as it were, that it cannot
return upon us any more. But when what the thinking and
willing mind rejects is strongly supported by the vital, it leaves
the mind indeed but sinks down into the vital, rages there
and tries to rush up again and reoccupy the mind and compel
or capture our mental acceptance. When the higher vital too
— the heart or the larger vital dynamis rejects it, it sinks from
there and takes refuge in the lower vital with its mass of small
current movements that make up our daily littleness. When
the lower vital too rejects it, it sinks into the physical consciousness and tries to stick by inertia or mechanical repetition.
Rejected even from there it goes into the subconscient and
comes up in dreams, in passivity, in extreme *tamas*. The Inconscient is the last resort of the Ignorance.

As for the waves that recur from the general Nature, it is
the natural tendency of the inferior forces there to try and
perpetuate their action in the individual, to rebuild what he has
unbuilt of their deposits in him; so they return on him, often
with an increased force, even with a stupendous violence, when
they find their influence rejected. But they cannot last long
once the environmental consciousness is cleared — unless the
"Hostiles" take a hand. Even then these can indeed attack,
but if the sadhak has established his position in the inner self,
they can only attack and retire.

It is true that we bring most of ourselves, — or rather

most of our predispositions, tendencies of reaction to the universal Nature, from past lives. Heredity only affects strongly the external being; besides, all the effects of heredity are not accepted even there, only those that are in consonance with what we are to be or not preventive of it at least.

What he has written about the subconscient and the outer nature is true. But the role of subliminal forces cannot be said to be small, since from there come all the greater aspirations, ideals, strivings towards a better self and better humanity without which man would be only a thinking animal — as also most of the art, poetry, philosophy, thirst for knowledge which relieve, if they do not yet dispel, the ignorance.

The role of the superconscient has been to evolve slowly the spiritual man out of the mental half-animal. That also cannot be called an insignificant role.

About the subconscient — it is the sub-mental base of the being and is made up of impressions, instincts, habitual movements that are stored there. Whatever movement is impressed in it, it keeps. If one impresses the right movement in it, it will keep and send up that. That is why it has to be cleared of old movements before there can be a permanent and total change in the nature. When the higher consciousness is once established in the waking parts, it goes down into the subconscient and changes that also, makes a bedrock of itself there also. Then no further trouble from the subconscient will be possible. But even before that one can minimise the trouble by putting the right will and the right habit of reaction in the subconscient parts.

The subconscient is a thing of habits and memories and repeats persistently or whenever it can old suppressed reactions, reflexes, mental, vital or physical responses. It must be trained by a still more persistent insistence of the higher parts of the being to give up its old responses and take on the new and true ones.

Just as one can concentrate the thought on an object or the vision on a point, so one can concentrate will on a particular part or point of the body and give an order to the consciousness there. That order reaches the subconscient.

The human like the animal mind lives largely in impressions rising up from the subconscient.

You do not realise how much of the ordinary natural being lives in the subconscient physical. It is there that habitual movements, mental and vital, are stored and from there they come up into the waking mind. Driven out of the upper consciousness, it is in this cavern of the Panis that they take refuge. No longer allowed to emerge freely in the waking state, they come up in sleep as dreams. It is when they are cleared out of the subconscient, their very seeds killed by the enlightening of these hidden layers, that they cease for good. As your consciousness deepens inwardly and the higher light comes down into those inferior covered parts, the things that now recur in this way will disappear.

You had asked the other day about the subconscient, what it was. In the vision you describe you were shown the universal subconscient in the figure of Patala, a place without light of consciousness and, because universal therefore without bounds or end — the dark unconscious infinite out of which this material universe has arisen — it is walled with darkness on all sides, it seems also to have no bottom. The Light comes from above from the higher consciousness and coming down through the mind and heart and vital and physical has to pour down into this subconscient and make it luminous.

Patala is evidently here a name for the subconscient — the beings there have "no heads", that is to say, there is there no mental consciousness; men have all of them such a subconscient plane in their own being and from there rise all sorts of irrational and ignorant (headless) instincts, impulsions, memories, etc., which have an effect upon their acts and feelings without their detecting the real source. At night many incoherent dreams come from this world or plane. The world above is the super-conscient plane of being — above the human consciousness — there are many worlds of that kind; these are divine worlds.

The dark wells of the subconscient are deep and until they are altogether cleared some gushing up of the old sources is always possible.

The subconscient has many more fears in it than those admitted or acknowledged by the waking consciousness.

All that our consciousness meets in day-to-day experience is registered in subconscient memory and from there can be brought up to the mind or come of itself. But what we call memory is when the thing registered is kept in the conscious mind at its back and brought forward at will — that is con-scious memory.

The clear memory of words, images and thoughts is an action of the conscious mind, not the unconscious. Of course the memory goes behind, so to speak, in the back part of the mind, but it can be brought out. Also the memory can be lost or defaced, so that one remembers wrongly or forgets altogether, but that is still an imperfect action of the conscious mind, not an action of the subconscious. What the subconscious keeps is a mass of impressions, not of clear or exact images and these can come up as in dreams in an incoherent jumble distorted altogether or else in the waking state as a mechanical recurrence or repetition of the same suggestions, impulses (subconscient vital) or sensations. There is a recognisable difference between the two functionings.

Exact images are retained by the subliminal memory. All that is subliminal is described by ordinary psychology as subconscient; but in our psychology that cannot be done, for the consciousness that held them is as precise and far wider and fuller than our waking or surface consciousness, so how can it be called subconscient? Conscious memory is that which can bring up at any moment we like the memory of a thing, it is under our control. Subliminal memory can hold all things, even those which the mind cannot understand, e.g. if you hear somebody talking Hebrew, the subliminal memory can hold that and bring it up accurately in some abnormal state, e.g. the hypnotic. Subconscient memory is a memory of impressions; when they come up as in dream, either the result is something incoherent or fancifully rearranged or it is only the essence of the thing, its psychological deposit that comes up, e.g. sex, fear, some particular libido as the psychoanalysts call it, but the expression given to the latter need not be the same as memory would give, — it may repeat the same forms if it gets hold of the mechanical mind in the physical to help its expression, but also it may be quite different from anything in real life.

*
**

No — that ["The Record of Chitragupta"] is quite different [from the cosmic subconscient], since it belongs to something where the records are precise and accurate. The subconscient is a suppressed and obscure seed state where things are emerging out of the indeterminate inconscience of original Nature but are yet fluent and imprecise, having all the potentiality of determination in them, but not yet determinate. The past things fall back into it not as memories, but as impressions which is a quite different thing. When they come up from there it is in all sorts of queer forms with variations and mixtures.

The submind is always supplying associations from the past life or the earth life in general to experiences of the vital or other planes. One has to get rid of these intrusions in order to get at the true experience.

I don't know that there is any [term corresponding to the subconscient in the traditional books], — this plane was spoken of more as inconscient than subconscient, — it is practically the indiscriminate or *jaḍa prakṛti*, perhaps — or the seed state. In the Veda it is symbolised by the cave of the Panis. Perhaps by looking through books like the *Yoga-vāsiṣṭha* one could find something about the subconscient in fact though not in express terms.

XIII

The centres or Chakras are seven in number:—

1. The thousand-petalled lotus on the top of the head.
2. In the middle of the forehead — the Ajna Chakra — (will, vision, dynamic thought).
3. Throat centre — externalising mind.
4. Heart-lotus — emotional centre. The psychic is behind it.

5. Navel — higher vital (proper).
6. Below navel — lower vital.
7. Muladhara — physical.

All these centres are in the middle of the body; they are supposed to be attached to the spinal cord; but in fact all these things are in the subtle body, *sūkṣma deha*, though one has the feeling of their activities as if in the physical body when the consciousness is awake.

In the process of our yoga the centres have each a fixed psychological use and general function which base all their special powers and functionings. The *mūlādhāra* governs the physical down to the subconscient; the abdominal centre — *svādhiṣṭhāna* — governs the lower vital; the navel centre — *nābhipadma* or *maṇipūra* — governs the larger vital; the heart centre — *hṛtpadma* or *anāhata* — governs the emotional being; the throat centre — *viśuddha* — governs the expressive and externalising mind; the centre between the eye-brows — *ājñācakra* — governs the dynamic mind, will, vision, mental formation; the thousand-petalled lotus — *sahasradala* — above commands the higher thinking mind, houses the still higher illumined mind and at the highest opens to the intuition through which or else by an overflooding directness the overmind can have with the rest communication or an immediate contact.

I never heard of two lotuses in the heart centre; but it is the seat of two powers, in front the higher vital or emotional being, behind and concealed the soul or psychic being.

The colours of the lotuses and the numbers of petals are respectively, from bottom to top:— (1) the Muladhara or physical consciousness centre, four petals, red; (2) the abdominal centre, six petals, deep purple red; (3) the navel centre, ten petals, violet; (4) the heart centre, twelve petals, golden pink; (5) the throat centre, sixteen petals, grey; (6) the forehead centre between the eye-brows, two petals, white; (7) the thousand-

petalled lotus above the head, blue with gold light around.
The functions are, according to our yoga, — (1) commanding
the physical consciousness and the subconscient; (2) commanding the. small vital movements, the little greeds, lusts,
desires, the small sense-movements; (3) commanding the larger
life-forces and the passions and larger desire-movements;
(4) commanding the higher emotional being with the psychic
deep behind it; (5) commanding expression and all externalisation of the mind movements and mental forces; (6) commanding
thought, will, vision; (7) commanding the higher thinking
mind and the illumined mind and opening upwards to the
intuition and overmind. The seventh is sometimes or by some
identified with the brain, but that is an error — the brain is only
a channel of communication situated between the thousand-
petalled and the forehead centre. The former is sometimes called
the void centre, *śūnya*, either because it is not in the body, but in
the apparent void above or because rising above the head one
enters first into the silence of the self or spiritual being.

When we speak of concentrating in the heart in yoga, we are
speaking of the emotional centre and that like all the others is in
the middle of the body in a line corresponding to the spinal cord.
The planes he refers to are four centres: (1) crown of head or
higher mental centre, (2) between the eye-brows or centre of will
and vision, (3) throat or centre of externalising mind, and (4)
heart, i.e. mental-vital, emotional centre with the psychic behind
it (the soul, Purusha in the heart).

Chitta as opposed to Chit or Vijnana is only the basic mind-
life consciousness out of which rises the stuff of (ordinary)
thoughts, feelings, sensations etc. The Force which he feels is
something quite different; it is the larger force exceeding the
individual, and when one feels it in its fullness, it is experienced
as the cosmic force or something of the cosmic force or else the
Divine Force from above, according to its nature.

His mind is not yet ready for the action of the greater force,
because it is full of mental notions and activities and it is for

this reason that heat is generated in the friction between the two; when the other force withdraws and no longer tries to lay hold of the brain, then the personal mind-action feels released (that is the reason for the sense of coolness) and goes about its ordinary notions. It is only in a silent (quiet, not necessarily empty) mind that the greater force can be received and work upon the system without too much reaction and resistance.

It is good that you were able to overcome the difficulty and have a good meditation. Your observation that the difficulty is only in the head and throat and mainly in the latter is very significant. These are the mental centres and it is evident therefore that the difficulty comes from the physical mind. The higher part of the mind belongs to the thinking mind proper, the buddhi, that which understands and observes and guides; the throat is the centre of the externalising mind, that which deals with outer and physical things and responds to them. Its activity is always one of the chief difficulties of the sadhana. If it is quiet it is easier, as you have seen, for the whole being to be quiet.

The last of the four experiences, that of the being within arranged in layers one into the other like the steps of a ladder is also very significant and very true. It is so that the inner consciousness is arranged. There are five main divisions of this ladder. At the top above the head are layers (or as we call them planes) of which we are not conscious and which become conscious to us only by sadhana — those above the human mind — that is the higher consciousness. Below from the crown of the head to the throat are the layers (they are many of them) of the mind, the three principal being one at the top of the head communicating with the higher consciousness, another between the eye-brows where is the thought, sight and will, a third in the throat which is the externalising mind. A second division is from the shoulders to the navel, these are the layers of the higher vital presided over by the heart centre where is the emotional being with the psychic hidden behind it. From the navel downwards is the rest of the vital being containing several layers. From the bottom of the spine downward are the layers of the physical consciousness proper, the material, and below the feet is the subconscient which has also many levels.

The experience of the splitting of the forehead from the middle and the pouring out of light signified the opening of the centre of sight, will and vision there. When this opens, there is the opening of the inner mind consciousness through which the light of the higher can pour out — here it is the Mother's white light that was pouring out through the opening.

The lights you saw were the many lights (powers, forces, full of light) of the higher consciousness, the Truth-consciousness or divine consciousness. Their pouring down was preceded and made possible by the appearance of the moon, the spiritual light. It is when the spiritual light is there that the presence of the Mother is revealed and her action brings down the powers of the Truth, the Divine and she gives them to the sadhak.

When we speak of Purusha in the head, heart, etc., we are using a figure. The Muladhara from which the Kundalini rises is not in the physical body, but in the subtle body (the subtle body is that in which the being goes out in deep trance or more radically, at the time of death); so also are all the centres. But as the subtle body penetrates and is interfused with the gross body, there is a certain correspondence between these chakras and certain centres in the physical proper. So figuratively we speak of the Purusha in this or that centre of the body. Owing to this correspondence, again, when the Ananda or anything else comes down into the being, it is the subtle body that it pervades, but it communicates itself through it to the gross body and its consciousness, so that it is felt as if pervading the body. But all that is very different from saying that the spirit is lodged in a gland. The gross body is an engine, a means of communication and action of the spirit upon the world and it is only a small part of the instrumentation. It is absurd to make so much of it as all that. It is a sort of false materialism intended to placate minds that have a scanty knowledge of Science. But what is the use of that? Everybody now knows that Science is not a statement of the truth of things, but only a language expressing a certain experience of objects, their structure, their mathematics, a coordinated and utilisable impression of their processes — it is nothing more. Matter itself is something (a formation of energy perhaps?) of which we know superficially the structure as it appears to our mind and senses and to certain examining instruments (about which it is now suspected that they largely determine their own results, Nature adapting its replies to the instrument used) but more than that no Scientist knows or can know.

How can a spirit entity be enclosed in a material gland? So far as I know the self or spirit is not enclosed in the body, rather the body is in the self. When we have the full experience of the self, we feel it as a wide consciousness in which the body is a very small thing, an adjunct or a thing contained, not a container.

One can speak of the chakras only in reference to yoga. In ordinary people the chakras are not open, it is only when they do sadhana that the chakras open. For the chakras are the centres of the inner consciousness and belong originally to the subtle body. So much as is active in ordinary people is very little — for in them it is the outer consciousness that is active.

The centres of consciousness, the chakras. It is by their opening that the yogic or inner consciousness develops — otherwise you are bound to the ordinary outer consciousness.

This must be the psychicised higher mental being — the position above the head points to that. In other words, you have become aware of your higher mental being which is in contact at once with the Divine above and with the psychic behind the heart and is aware of the Truth and has the psychic and spiritual insight and view into things.

Above the head extends the higher consciousness centre, *sahasradala padma*. But usually there is partial working of the forehead centre also when the *sahasradala* opens.

The ordinary mind is at its highest the free intelligence, receiving perhaps intuitions and intimations from above which it intellectualises. It is on the surface and sees things from outside except in so far as it is helped by intuition and other powers to see a little deeper. When this ordinary mind opens within to inner mind and psychic and above to higher mind and higher consciousness generally, then it begins to be spiritualised and its highest ranges merge into the spiritual mind-consciousness of which this higher mind can be a beginning. This merging is part of the spiritual transformation.

For the mind there are many centres: (1) the *sahasradala* which centralises spiritual mind, higher mind, intuitive mind and acts as a receiving station for the intuition proper and overmind, (2) the centre in the forehead for inner thought, will and vision, (3) the throat centre for the externalising or physical mind.

The thousand-petalled lotus is above the head. It is the seventh and highest centre.

Usually those who take the centres in the body only, count six centres, the *sahasrāra* being excluded.

It is evidently the *sahasradala padma* through which the higher intuition, illumined mind and overmind all pass their rays.

The supramental is not organised in the body, so there is no separate centre for it; but all that comes from above the Mind uses the *sahasrāra* for its transit and so opens something there.

The centre at the crown must be part of the *sahasradala*, the centre of communication direct between the individual being and the infinite Consciousness above. There is not supposed to be any other main centre of dynamism between that and the *ājñācakra*. But there can be many nerve-centres in various parts of the body, apart from the six or rather seven main centres.

The crown is the place of passage between the body-consciousness with all it contains of mind and life and the higher being above the body. It is there that the two consciousnesses begin to meet.

The crown centre open removes the difficulty of the lid between the ordinary mind and the higher consciousness above. If the *ājñācakra* also is open, then it is possible to have a clear communication between the higher consciousness and the inner mind and the outer mind (throat centre) also. That is the condition for the realisation of knowledge and the mental illumination and transformation. The heart centre commands the psychic and vital — that opening enables the psychic influence to work in the vital and ends in the coming forward of the psychic being.

The brain is only a centre of the physical consciousness. One feels stationed there so long as one dwells in the physical mind or is identified with the body-consciousness, then one receives through the *sahasrāra* into the brain. When one ceases to be stationed in the body, then the brain is not a station but only a passive and silent transmitting channel.

*
**

In the forehead between the eyes but a little above is the *ājñā-cakra*, the centre of the inner will, also of the inner vision, the dynamic mind, etc. (This is not the ordinary outer mental will and sight, but something more powerful, belonging to the inner being.) When this centre opens and the Force there is active, then there is the opening of a greater will, power of decision, formation, effectiveness, beyond what the ordinary mind can achieve.

The centre of vision is between the eyebrows in the centre of the forehead. When it opens one gets the inner vision, sees the inner forms and images of things and people and begins to understand things and people from within and not only from outside, develops a power of will which also acts in the inner (yogic) way on things and people etc. Its opening is often the beginning of the yogic as opposed to the ordinary mental consciousness.

The centre [*ājñācakra*] is in the place I indicated, but the pressure can be felt in all the forehead and the eyebrows also or anywhere there. It radiates from the centre.

Yes. A third eye does open there [in the centre of the forehead] — it represents the occult vision and the occult power which goes with that vision — it is connected with the *ājñācakra*.

If the forehead centre opens, it is fairly certain that the crown centre must have opened sufficiently at least to allow the passage of the higher force which is above it. The psychic is a different matter — it stands behind the centres and the time of its opening varies with different people — in fact it is not so much the opening of a centre as the coming forward of the psychic being.

The usual rule in this yoga is from above downwards. There may be variations in the preparatory stage. There may for instance be a partial opening first of the heart centre. The higher vital centre may become active first also, but that means much struggle and difficulty.

Do you not know that the inner being means the inner mind, inner vital, inner physical with the psychic behind as the inmost? How can there be one centre for all that?

Yes, the centre in the throat is the centre of the physical mind. It is the centre of externalisation — in speech, expression, the power to deal mentally with physical things etc. Its opening brings the power to open the physical mind to the light of the divine consciousness instead of remaining in the ordinary outward-going mentality.

The neck and throat and the lower part of the face belong to the externalising mind, the physical mental. The forehead to the inner Mind. Above the head are the higher planes of Mind.

The nose is connected with the vital dynamic part of the mental, — a man with a strong nose is supposed to have a strong will or a strong mental personality, — though I don't know whether it is invariably true. But the vital physical? Of course the nose is the passage of the Prana and the Prana is the support of the vital physical.

It cannot be anything physical but only a subtle physical sensation. The ear is the passage of communion between the inner mind centre and the thought-forces or thought-waves of the universal Nature. It sounds like a sensation of opening and enlarging of this passage.

It is the physical mind that acts like that. The centre of the physical mind or externalising mind is in the subtle body in the throat and connected strongly with the speech — but it acts by connection with the brain. All forces that want to cover the consciousness rise up to do it by environing and acting on the mind centres if they can — environing because otherwise the covering is not complete.

The organ of speech is an instrument of the physical-mental or expressive externalising mind.

Speech comes from the throat centre, but it is associated with whatever is the governing centre or level of the consciousness — wherever one thinks from. If one rises above the head, then thought takes place above the head and one can speak from there, that is to say, the direction of the speech is from there.

Pashyanti is evidently speech with the vision of Truth in it — Para is probably the revelatory and inspired speech. I am not certain about the exact nature of the others [Vaikhari and Madhyama].

The Tantriks locate these forms of speech in different chakras. Speech may be internal or external, either may have the stamp of the same power. But if it is to be measured by withdrawal from externality, then Para ought to mean something of the causal realm beyond mind.

The throat centre is the externalising (physical) mind, the heart is the emotional mind and beginning of the higher vital. If the heart centre is dominated by the physical mind to any extent it will necessarily be open to the outer attacks that affect the physical and nervous consciousness. The heart has to be in connection with the psychic and the higher consciousness.

The physical heart is in the left side, but the heart centre of yoga is in the middle of the chest — the cardiac centre.

The apex of the psychic and emotional centre (like the apex of all centres) is in the backbone, the base in front in middle of the sternum.

The heart is the centre of the being and commands the rest, as the psychic being or *caitya puruṣa* is there. It is only in that sense that all flows from it, for it is the psychic being who each time creates a new mind, vital and body for himself.

The psychic being (which is the soul) does not make centres for itself in the Adhar. The centres are there. The psychic being can take control of the centres that are already there — the heart and the navel centre and the two below the navel. Also the mind and vital are not abolished — they are brought under the psychic influence and psychicised, or they are occupied by the higher consciousness from above and transformed into its instruments.

One does not pass through the psychic centre or any centre. The centres open under the pressure of the sadhana. You can say that the Force descends or ascends into a centre.

The navel is the chief vital centre below the emotional, — there is another centre of small vital movements below it, — between the navel and Muladhara.

It is the lower vital energy that rushes to the brain and either confuses it and prevents mental self-control or else makes the mind its slave and uses reason to justify the passions.

The physical mind centre is in the throat and mouth — the vital physical is between the two lowest centres — the material consciousness is in the *mūlādhāra*.

The nerves are distributed all over the body, but the vital-physical action is concentrated in its origin between the Muladhara and the centre just above it.

Yogically, psycho-physically, etc., etc., stomach, heart and intestine lodge the vital movements, not the physical consciousness — it is there that anger, fear, love, hate and all other psychological privileges of the animal tumble about and upset physical and moral digestion. The Muladhara is the seat of the physical consciousness proper.

It [the end of the spine] is the place of the physical centre which is also the sex-centre. The apex of it is at the end of the spine and it projects forward from there — commanding the organ and its action.

The lowest centre at the bottom of the spine. It contains many other things but also it is in its front the support of the sexual movements.

No, the subconscient is too vague to have a centre. It has a level — below the feet as the superconscient is above, but from there it can surge up anywhere.

Yes, it [the cerebellum] has some connection with the subconscient.

SECTION SIX

THE DIVINE AND THE HOSTILE POWERS

The Divine and the Hostile Powers

1. FALSEHOOD AND IGNORANCE[1]

IGNORANCE means Avidya, the separative consciousness and the egoistic mind and life that flow from it and all that is natural to the separative consciousness and the egoistic mind and life. This Ignorance is the result of a movement by which the cosmic Intelligence separated itself from the light of the supermind (the divine Gnosis) and lost the Truth, — truth of being, truth of divine consciousness, truth of force and action, truth of Ananda. As a result, instead of a world of integral truth and divine harmony created in the light of the divine Gnosis, we have a world founded on the part truths of an inferior cosmic Intelligence in which all is half-truth, half-error. It is this that some of the ancient thinkers like Shankara, not perceiving the greater Truth-Force behind, stigmatised as Maya and thought to be the highest creative power of the Divine. All in the consciousness of this creation is either limited or else perverted by separation from the integral Light; even the Truth it perceives is only a half-knowledge. Therefore it is called the Ignorance.

Falsehood, on the other hand, is not this Avidya, but an extreme result of it. It is created by an Asuric power which intervenes in this creation and is not only separated from the Truth and therefore limited in knowledge and open to error, but in revolt against the Truth or in the habit of seizing the Truth only to pervert it. This Power, the dark Asuric Shakti or Rakshasic Maya, puts forward its own perverted consciousness as true knowledge and its wilful distortions or reversals of the Truth as the verity of things. It is the powers and personalities of this perverted and perverting consciousness that we call hostile beings, hostile forces. Whenever these perversions created by them out of the stuff of the Ignorance are put forward as the

---

[1] This letter was written to explain certain terms occurring in the book *The Mother* by Sri Aurobindo.

Truth of things, that is the Falsehood, in the yogic sense, *mithyā*, *moha*.

2. POWERS AND APPEARANCES

These are the forces and beings that are interested in maintaining the falsehoods they have created in the world of the Ignorance and in putting them forward as the Truth which men must follow. In India they are termed Asuras, Rakshasas, Pishachas (beings respectively of the mentalised vital, middle vital and lower vital planes) who are in opposition to the Gods, the Powers of Light. These too are Powers, for they too have their cosmic field in which they exercise their function and authority and some of them were once divine Powers (the former gods, *pūrve devāḥ*, as they are called somewhere in the Mahabharata) who have fallen towards the darkness by revolt against the divine Will behind the cosmos. The word "appearances" refers to the forms they take in order to rule the world, forms often false and always incarnating falsehood, sometimes pseudo-divine.

3. POWERS AND PERSONALITIES

The use of the word Power has already been explained — it can be applied to whatever or whoever exercises a conscious power in the cosmic field and has authority over the world-movement or some movement in it. But the Four[1] of whom you speak are also Shaktis, manifestations of different powers of the Supreme Consciousness and Force, the Divine Mother, by which she rules or acts in the universe. And they are at the same time divine personalities; for each is a being who manifests different qualities and personal consciousness-forms of the Godhead. All the greater Gods are in this way personalities of the Divine — one Consciousness playing in many personalities, *ekam sat bahudhā*. Even in the human being there are many personalities and not only one, as used formerly to be imagined; for all consciousness can be at once one and multiple. "Powers and Personalities" simply describe different aspects of the same being; a Power is not necessarily impersonal and certainly it is not *avyaktam*, as you suggest, — on the contrary, it is a manifesta-

[1] Maheshwari, Mahakali, Mahalakshmi, Mahasaraswati.

tion acting in the worlds of the divine Manifestation.

4. EMANATIONS

Emanations correspond to your description of the Matrikas of whom you speak in your letters. An emanation of the Mother is something of her consciousness and power put forth from her which, so long as it is in play, is held in close connection with her and, when its play is no longer required, is withdrawn back into its source, but can always be put out and brought into play once more. But also the detaining thread of connection can be severed or loosened and that which came forth as an emanation can proceed on its way as an independent divine being with its own play in the world. All the Gods can put forth such emanations from their being, identical with them in essence of consciousness and power though not commensurate. In a certain sense the universe itself can be said to be an emanation from the Supreme. In the consciousness of the sadhak an emanation of the Mother will ordinarily wear the appearance, form and characteristics with which he is familiar.

In a sense the four Powers of the Mother may be called, because of their origin, her Emanations, just as the Gods may be called Emanations of the Divine, but they have a more permanent and fixed character; they are at once independent beings allowed their play by the Adya Shakti and yet portions of the Mother, the Mahashakti, and she can always either manifest through them as separate beings or draw them together as her own various Personalities and hold them in herself, sometimes kept back, sometimes at play, according to her will. In the supramental plane they are always in her and do not act independently but as intimate portions of the supramental Mahashakti and in close union and harmony with each other.

5. GODS

These four Powers are the Mother's cosmic Godheads, permanent in the world-play; they stand among the greater cosmic Godheads to whom allusion is made when it is said that the Mother as the Mahashakti of this triple world "stands there (in the overmind plane) above the Gods." The Gods, as has already been said, are in origin and essence permanent Emanations of the Divine put forth from the Supreme by the Transcendent Mother, the Adya Shakti; in their cosmic action they are Powers and Personalities of the Divine each with his independent cosmic standing, function and work in the universe. They are not impersonal entities but cosmic Personalities, although they can and do ordinarily veil themselves behind the movement of impersonal forces. But while in the overmind and the triple world they appear as independent beings, they return in the supermind into the One and stand there united in a single harmonious action as multiple personalities of the One Person, the Divine Purushottama.

6. PRESENCE

It is intended by the word Presence to indicate the sense and perception of the Divine as a Being, felt as present in one's existence and consciousness or in relation with it, without the necessity of any further qualification or description. Thus, of the "ineffable Presence" it can only be said that it is there and nothing more can or need be said about it, although at the same time one knows that all is there, personality and impersonality, Power and Light and Ananda and everything else, and that all these flow from that indescribable Presence. The word may be used sometimes in a less absolute sense, but that is always the fundamental significance, — the essential perception of the essential Presence supporting everything else.

7. THE TRANSCENDENT MOTHER

This is what is termed the Adya Shakti; she is the Supreme Consciousness and Power above the universe and it is by her that all the Gods are manifested, and even the supramental Ishwara comes into manifestation through her — the supramental Purushottama of whom the Gods are Powers and Personalities.

*
**

Of course, the gods exist — that is to say, there are Powers that stand above the world and transmit the divine workings. It is the physical mind which believes only what is physical that denies them. There are also beings of other worlds — gods and Asuras, etc.

There are gods everywhere on all the planes.

The dynamic aspect of the Divine is the Supreme Brahman, not the Gods. The Gods are Personalities and Powers of the dynamic Divine. You speak as if the evolution were the sole creation; the creation or manifestation is very vast and contains many planes and worlds that existed before the evolution, all different in character and with different kinds of beings. The fact of being prior to the evolution does not make them undifferentiated. The world of the Asuras is prior to the evolution, so are the worlds of the mental, vital or subtle physical Devas — but these beings are all different from each other. The great Gods belong to the overmind plane; in the supermind they are unified as aspects of the Divine, in the overmind they appear as separate personalities. Any godhead can descend by emanation to the physical plane and associate himself with the evolution of a human being with whose line of manifestation he is in affinity. But these are things which cannot be very easily understood by the mind, because the mind has too rigid an idea of personality — the difficulty only disappears when one enters into a more flexible consciousness above where one is nearer to the experience of One in all and All in one.

The Formateurs of the overmind have shaped nothing evil — it is the lower forces that receive from the overmind and distort its forms.

In the descent it [the falsehood] begins with Mind, in the evolutionary ascent it is difficult to say where it begins — for here the beginning is Inconscience and Ignorance; but I suppose we may say that conscious falsehood begins with the beginnings of mind still involved in Life or appearing out of it.

The Gods are in the universal Self — if indentified with the universal Self one can feel their presence there. Also there is the experience of microcosm (the universe in oneself) in which all that is in the macrocosm (the larger universe) is present. All these things are for experience, for knowledge and must be taken as such. No merely personal turn should be given to them.

Again, what do you mean by a soul? My proposition simply meant that there is no existence which has not the support of something of the Divine behind it. But the word soul has various meanings according to the context; it may mean the Purusha supporting the formation of Prakriti, which we call a being, though the proper word would be rather a becoming; it may mean, on the other hand, specifically the psychic being in an evolutionary creature like man; it may mean the spark of the Divine which has been put into Matter by the descent of the Divine into the material world and which upholds all evolving formations here. There is and can be no psychic being in a non-evolutionary creature like the Asura; there can be none in a god who does not need one for his existence. But what the god has is a Purusha and a Prakriti or Energy of nature of that Purusha. If any being of the typal worlds wants to evolve, he has to come down to earth and take a human body and accept to share in the evolution. It is because they do not want to do this that the vital beings try to possess men so that they may enjoy the materialities of physical life without having the burden of the evolution or the process of conversion in which it culminates. I hope this is clear and solves the difficulty.

The three stages you speak of are stages not of evolution but of the involution of the Divine in Matter. The Devas and Asuras are not evolved in Matter; for the typal being only a Purusha with its Prakriti is necessary — this Purusha may put out a mental and vital Purusha to represent it and according as it is centred in one or another it belongs to the mental or vital world. That is all.

There is no essential difference anywhere, for all is fundamentally the essential Divine, the difference is in the manifestation. Practically we may say that the Jivatman is one of the Divine Many and dependent on the One; the Atman is the One supporting the Many. The psychic being does not merge in the Jivatman, it becomes united with it so that there is no difference between the eternal being supporting the manifestation from above and the same being supporting the manifestation from within it, because the psychic being has become fully aware of the play of the Divine through it. What is called merging takes place in the Divine Consciousness when the Jivatman feels itself so one with the Divine that there is nothing else.

While the Gods cannot be transformed, for they are typal and not evolutionary beings, they can come for conversion — that is to say, to give up their own ideas and outlook on things and conform themselves to the higher Will and supramental Truth of the Divine.

Where do you find in "The Life Heavens"[1] that I say or anybody says the conditions on the earth are glorious and suited to the Divine Life? There is not a word to that effect there! The Life Heavens are the heavens of the vital gods and there is there a perfect harmony but a harmony of the sublimated satisfied senses and vital desires only. If there is to be a Harmony, it must be of all the powers raised to their highest and harmonised together.

[1] A poem by Sri Aurobindo. See *Collected Poems* (Cent. Ed. Vol. 5), pp. 574-75.

All the non-evolutionary worlds are worlds limited to their own
harmony like the Life Heavens. The Earth, on the other hand, is
an evolutionary world, not at all glorious or harmonious even as
a material world (except in certain appearances), but rather most
sorrowful, disharmonious, imperfect. Yet in that imperfection is
the urge towards a higher and more many-sided perfection. It
contains the last finite which yet yearns to the supreme Infinite,
(it is not satisfied by sense-joys precisely because in the conditions of the earth it is able to see their limitations). God is pent in
the mire (mire is not glorious, so there is no claim to glory or
beauty here), but that very fact imposes a necessity to break
through that prison to a consciousness which is ever rising towards the heights. And so on. That *is* "a deeper power", though
not a greater actual glory or perfection. All that may be true or
not to the mind, but it is the traditional attitude of Indian spiritual experience. Ask any yogin, he will tell you that the Life
Heavens are childish things; even the gods, says the Purana, must
come down to earth and be embodied there if they want *mukti*,
giving up the pride of their limited perfection; they must enter
into the last finite if they want to reach the last infinite. A poem
is not a philosophical treatise or a profession of religious faith
— it is the expression of a vision or an experience of some kind,
mundane or spiritual. Here it is the vision of the Life Heavens,
its perfection, its limitation and the counter-claim of the Earth or
rather the Spirit or Power behind the earth-consciousness. It has
to be taken at that, as an expression of a certain aspect of things,
an expression of a certain kind of experience, not of a mental
dogma. There is a deep truth behind it, though it may not be the
whole truth of the matter. In the poem, also, there is no question
of a divine life here, though that is hinted at as the inexpressed
possible result of the ascent — because the Earth is not put aside
("Earth's heart was felt beating below me still"); nevertheless the
poem expresses only the ascent towards the Highest, far beyond
the Life Heavens, and the Earth-Spirit claims that power and
does not speak of any descent of a divine life.

*
**

The Gods have their own enjoyments though they may not be of a material character.

The higher beings are not likely to be in disharmony with each other, as they are not subject to the lower ignorance.

There are no planes of manifestation without forms — for without form creation or manifestation cannot be complete. But the supraphysical planes are not bound to the forms like the physical. The forms there are expressive, not determinative. What is important in the vital plane is the force or feeling and the form expresses it. A vital being has a characteristic form but he can vary it or mask his true form under others. What is primary on the mental plane is the perception, the idea, the mental significance and the form expresses that and these mental forms too can vary — there can be many forms expressing an idea in different ways or on different sides of the idea. Form exists but it is more plastic and variable than in physical nature.

As to the gods, man can build forms which they will accept but these forms too are inspired into man's mind from the planes to which the god belongs. All creation has the two sides, the formed and the formless, — the gods too are formless and yet have forms, but a godhead can take many forms, here Maheshwari, there Pallas Athene. Maheshwari herself has many forms in her lesser manifestation, Durga, Uma, Parvati, Chandi, etc. The gods are not limited to human forms — man also has not always seen them in human forms only.

The lion with Durga on it is the symbol of the Divine Consciousness acting through a divinised physical-vital and vital-emotional force.

The lion is the attribute of the Goddess Durga, the conquering and protecting aspect of the Universal Mother.

The Death's Head is the symbol of the Asura (the adversary of the gods) vanquished and killed by the Divine Power.

Mahakali and Kali are not the same. Kali is a lesser form. Mahakali in the higher planes appears usually with the golden colour.

I indicate the psychological powers which they bring with them.

Mitra—Harmony.
Varuna—Wideness.
Aryaman—Power—Tapasya.
Brihaspati—Wisdom (Word and Knowledge).
Vishnu — Cosmic Consciousness.
Vayu — Life.

Yes, Mitra is rather a combination of two powers [Mahalakshmi and Mahasaraswati].

Vayu and Indra are cosmic godheads presiding over the action of cosmic principles — they are not the *manomaya puruṣa* or *prāṇamaya puruṣa* in each man.

The Purusha is an essential being supporting the play of Prakriti; the godhead (Indra, Vayu, etc.) is a dynamic being manifested in Prakriti for the works of the plane to which he belongs.

Brahma, Vishnu, Shiva are only three Powers and Personalities of the One Cosmic Godhead.

Brahma is the Power of the Divine that stands behind formation and the creation.

As for Vishnu being the creator, all the three gods are often spoken of as creating the universe — even Shiva who is by tradition the Destroyer.

There is no particular connection between Shiva and the overmind — the overmind is the higher station of all the Gods. It is better not to call it the overmind until the action of it is clear and there can be no mistake.

Mahashiva means a greater manifestation than that ordinarily worshipped as Shiva — the creative dance of a greater Divine manifesting Power.

It is probably the realm of the dynamic creative spirit from the highest mental plane which you saw as the world of Parvati-Shankara.

Shiva is the Lord of Tapas. The power is the power of Tapas. Krishna as a godhead is the Lord of Ananda, Love and Bhakti; as an incarnation, he manifests the union of wisdom (Jnana) and works and leads the earth-evolution through this towards union with the Divine by Ananda, Love and Bhakti.

The Devi is the Divine Shakti — the Consciousness and Power of the Divine, the Mother and Energy of the worlds. All powers are hers. Sometimes Devi-power may mean the power of the universal World-Force; but this is only one side of the Shakti.

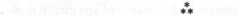

It is, I suppose, the image of Sri Krishna as Lord of the divine love and Ananda — and his flute calls the physical being to awake out of the attachments of the physical world and turn to that love and Ananda.

The boy with the flute is Sri Krishna, the Lord descended into the world-play from the divine Ananda; his flute is the music of the call which seeks to transform the lower ignorant play of mortal life and bring into it and establish in its place the Lila of his divine Ananda. It was the psychic being in you that heard the call and followed after it.

This is the Krishna of the Gita (the boy Krishna is the Krishna of Brindaban), Krishna bringing the spiritual Knowledge, Will, bhakti — and not love and bhakti alone.

The eye indicates the vision of the higher spiritual consciousness and the blue expanse indicates that consciousness.

Buddha stands for the conquest over the Ignorance of the lower nature.

Narada stands for the expression of the Divine Love and Knowledge.

Ganesha is the Power that removes obstacles by the force of Knowledge; Kartikeya represents victory over the hostile Powers. Of course, the names given are human, but the gods exist.

Ganesha (among other things) is the Devata of spiritual Knowledge — so, as you are getting this Knowledge you saw yourself in this form identified with Ganesha.

*
**

The peacock is the bird of Victory and Kartikeya the leader of the divine forces.

II

The hostile forces exist and have been known to yogic experience ever since the days of the Veda and Zoroaster in Asia (and the mysteries of Egypt and the Cabbala) and in Europe also from old times. These things, of course, cannot be felt or known so long as one lives in the ordinary mind and its ideas and perceptions; for there, there are only two categories of influences recognisable, the ideas and feelings and actions of oneself and others and the play of environment and physical forces. But once one begins to get the inner view of things, it is different. One begins to experience that all is an action of forces, forces of Prakriti psychological as well as physical, which play upon our nature — and these are conscious forces or are supported by a consciousness or consciousnesses behind. One is in the midst of a big universal working and it is impossible any longer to explain everything as the result of one's own sole and independent personality. You yourself have at one time written that your crises of despair etc. came upon you as if thrown on you and worked themselves out without your being able to determine or put an end to them. That means an action of universal forces and not merely an independent action of your own personality, though it is something in your nature of which they make use. But you are not conscious, and others also, of this intervention and pressure at its source for the reason I state. Those who have developed the inner view of things on the vital plane have plenty of experience of the hostile forces. However, you need not personally concern yourself with them so long as they remain incognito.

One may have the experiences on the mental plane without this knowledge coming; for there mind and idea predominate and one does not feel the play of Forces — it is only in the vital that that becomes clear. In the mind plane they manifest at most as mental suggestions and not as concrete Powers. Also, if one looks at things with the mind only (even though it be the inner mind), one may see the subtle play of Nature-forces but without recognising the conscious intention which we call hostile.

There are two kinds of Asuras — one kind were divine in their origin but have fallen from their divinity by self-will and opposition to the intention of the Divine: they are spoken of in the Hindu scriptures as the former or earlier gods; these can be converted and their conversion is indeed necessary for the ultimate purposes of the universe. But the ordinary Asura is not of this character, is not an evolutionary but a typal being and represents a fixed principle of the creation which does not evolve or change and is not intended to do so. These Asuras, as also the other hostile beings, Rakshasas, Pishachas and others resemble the devils of the Christian tradition and oppose the divine intention and the evolutionary purpose in the human being: they don't change the purpose in them for which they exist which is evil; but have to be destroyed like the evil. The Asura has no soul, no psychic being which has to evolve to a higher state; he has only an ego and usually a very powerful ego; he has a mind, sometimes even a highly intellectualised mind; but the basis of his thinking and feeling is vital and not mental, at the service of his desire and not of truth. He is a formation assumed by the life-principle for a particular kind of work and not a divine formation or a soul.

The Asuras and Rakshasas etc. do not belong to the earth, but to supraphysical worlds; but they act upon the earth-life and dispute the control of human life and character and action with the Gods. They are the Powers of Darkness combating the Powers of Light.

Sometimes they possess men in order to act through them, sometimes they take birth in a human body. When their use in the play is over, they will either change or disappear or no longer seek to intervene in the earth-play.

The Asuras are really the dark side of the mental, or more strictly, of the vital mind plane. This mind is the very field of the Asuras. Their main characteristic is egoistic strength and struggle, which refuse the higher law. The Asura has self-control, *tapas* and intelligence, but all that for the sake of his ego. On the lower vital plane the corresponding forces we call the Rakshasas which represent violent passions and influences. There are also other kinds of beings on the vital plane which are called the Pishachas and Pramathas. They manifest more or less in the physico-vital.

On the physical plane the corresponding forces are obscure beings, more forces than beings, what the Theosophists call the elementals. They are not strongly individualised beings like the Rakshasas and Asuras, but ignorant and obscure forces working in the subtle physical plane. What we in Sanskrit call the Bhutas mostly come under this class. But there are two kinds of elementals, the one mischievous and the other not.

There are no Asuras on the higher planes where the Truth prevails, except in the Vedic sense — "the Divine in its strength". The mental and vital Asuras are only a deviation of that power.

Yes, some kinds of Asuras are very religious, very fanatical about their religion, very strict about rules of ethical conduct. Others of course are just the opposite. There are others who use spiritual ideas without believing in them to give them a perverted twist and delude the sadhak. It is what Shakespeare described as the Devil quoting scripture for his own purpose.

At present what they are most doing is to try to raise up the obscurity and weakness of the most physical mind, vital, material parts to prevent the progress or fulfilment of the sadhana.

The Gandharvas are of the vital plane but they are vital Gods, not Asuras. Many Asuras are beautiful in appearance and can carry even a splendour or light with them. It is the Rakshasas, Pishachas, etc. who are ugly or evil in appearance.

Hostile Forces. The purpose they serve *in the world* is to give a full chance to the possibilities of the Inconscience and Ignorance — for this world was meant to be a working out of these possibilities with the supramental harmonisation as its eventual outcome. The life, the work developing here in the Ashram has to deal with the world problem and has therefore to meet — it could not avoid — the conflict with the working of the hostile Powers in the human being.

The universe is certainly or has been up to now in appearance a rough and wasteful game with the dice of chance loaded in favour of the Powers of darkness, the Lords of obscurity, falsehood, death and suffering. But we have to take it as it is and find out — if we reject the way out of the old sages — the way to conquer. Spiritual experience shows that there is behind it all a wide terrain of equality, peace, calm, freedom, and it is only by getting into it that we can have the eye that sees and hope to gain the power that conquers.

If there were no hostile forces and there were still the evolutionary world, there could be ignorance still but not perversity in the ignorance. All would be a partial truth acting through imperfect instruments but for the best purposes of this or that stage in a progressive manifestation.

They are not hostile forces, they are simply the forces of the ordinary Nature. The hostile forces are those which try to pervert everything and are in revolt against the Divine and opposed to the yoga.

The lesser forces of Light are usually too much insistent on seeking for Truth to make effectivity their logic or their rule — the hostiles are too pragmatic to care for Truth, they want only success. As for the greater Forces (e.g. overmind) they are dynamic and try always to make consciousness effective, but they insist on consciousness, while the hostiles care nothing for that — the more unconscious you are and their automatic tool, the better they are pleased — for it is unconsciousness that gives them their chance.

About the contact with the world and the hostile forces, that is of course always one of the sadhak's chief difficulties, but to transform the world and the hostile forces is too big a task and the personal transformation cannot wait for it. What has to be done is to come to live in the Power that these things, these disturbing elements cannot penetrate, or, if they penetrate, cannot disturb, and to be so purified and strengthened by it that there is in oneself no response to anything hostile. If there is a protecting envelopment, an inner purifying descent and, as a result, a settling of the higher consciousness in the inner being and finally, its substitution even in the most external outwardly active parts in place of the old ignorant consciousness, then the world and the hostile forces will no longer matter — for one's own soul at least; for there is a larger work not personal in which of course they will have to be dealt with; but that need not be a main preoccupation at the present stage.

It is the movements of the lower nature that get purified. The Asuras are not so easily transformed.

As to Asuras, not many of them have shown signs of repentance or possibility of conversion up to now. It is not surprising that they should be powerful in a world of ignorance for they have only to persuade people to follow the established bent of their lower nature, while the Divine calls always for a change of nature. It is not to be wondered at that the Asura has an easier task and more momentary success in his combinations. But that temporary success does not bind the future.

Some of the vital beings are very intelligent but they do not make friends with the Light - - they only try to avoid destruction and wait their time.

The evil forces are perversions of the Truth by the Ignorance — in any complete transformation they must disappear and the Truth behind them be delivered. In this way they can be said to be transformed by destruction.

THE PURPOSE OF AVATARHOOD

The Purpose of Avatarhood

SURELY for the earth-consciousness the very fact that the Divine manifests himself is the greatest of all splendours. Consider the obscurity here and what it would be if the Divine did not directly intervene and the Light of Lights did not break out of the obscurity — for that is the meaning of the manifestation.

An incarnation is the Divine Consciousness and Being manifesting through the body. It is possible from any plane.

It is the omnipresent cosmic Divine who supports the action of the universe; if there is an Incarnation, it does not in the least diminish the cosmic Presence and the cosmic action in the three or thirty million universes.

The Descending Power (Avatar) chooses its own place, body, time for the manifestation.

The Avatar is necessary when a special work is to be done and in crises of the evolution. The Avatar is a special manifestation while for the rest of the time it is the Divine working within the ordinary human limits as a Vibhuti.

Avatarhood would have little meaning if it were not connected with the evolution. The Hindu procession of the ten Avatars is itself, as it were, a parable of evolution. First the Fish Avatar, then the amphibious animal between land and water, then the land animal, then the Man-Lion Avatar, bridging man and animal, then man as dwarf, small and undeveloped and physical but containing in himself the godhead and taking possession of existence, then the rajasic, sattwic, nirguna Avatars, leading the human development from the vital rajasic to the sattwic mental man and again the overmental superman. Krishna, Buddha and Kalki depict the last three stages, the stages of the spiritual development — Krishna opens the possibility of overmind, Buddha tries to shoot beyond to the supreme liberation but that liberation is still negative, not returning upon earth to complete positively the evolution; Kalki is to correct this by bringing the Kingdom of the Divine upon earth, destroying the opposing Asura forces. The progression is striking and unmistakable.

As for the lives in between the Avatar lives, it must be remembered that Krishna speaks of many lives in the past, not only a few supreme ones, and secondly that while he speaks of himself as the Divine, in one passage he describes himself as a Vibhuti, *vrsninām vāsudevah*. We may therefore fairly assume that in many lives he manifested as the Vibhuti veiling the fuller Divine Consciousness. If we admit that the object of Avatarhood is to lead the evolution, this is quite reasonable, the Divine appearing as Avatar in the great transitional stages and as Vibhutis to aid the lesser transitions.

It [the overmind liberation] can't be supreme if there is something beyond it — but there is a liberation even in higher Mind. But in speaking of supreme liberation I was simply taking the Buddhist-Adwaita view for granted and correcting it by saying that this Nirvana view is too negative. Krishna opened the possibility of overmind with its two sides of realisation, static and dynamic. Buddha tried to shoot from mind to Nirvana in the Supreme, just as Shankara did in another way after him. Both agree in overleaping the other stages and trying to get at a nameless and featureless Absolute. Krishna on the other hand was leading by the normal course of evolution. The next normal step is not a featureless Absolute, but the supermind. I consider that in trying to overshoot, Buddha like Shankara made a mistake, calling away the dynamic side of the liberation. Therefore there has to be a correction by Kalki.

I was of course dealing with the ten Avatars as a "parable of the evolution", and only explaining the interpretation we can put on it from that point of view. It was not my own view of the thing that I was giving.

Too much importance need not be attached to the details about Kalki — they are rather symbolic than an attempt to prophesy details of future history. What is expressed is something that has to come, but it is symbolically indicated, no more.

So too, too much weight need not be put on the exact figures about the Yugas in the Purana. Here again the Kala and the Yugas indicate successive periods in the cyclic wheel of evolution, — the perfect state, decline and disintegration of successive ages of humanity followed by a new birth — the mathematical calculations are not the important element. The argument of the end of the Kali Yuga already come or coming and a new Satya Yuga coming is a very familiar one and there have been many who have upheld it.

*
**

I only took the Puranic list of Avatars and interpreted it as a parable of evolution, so as to show that the idea of evolution is implicit behind the theory of Avatarhood. As to whether one accepts Buddha as an Avatar or prefers to put others in his place (in some lists Balaram replaces Buddha), is a matter of individual feeling. The Buddhist Jatakas are legends about the past incarnations of the Buddha, often with a teaching implied in them, and are not a part of the Hindu system. To the Buddhists Buddha was not an Avatar at all, he was the soul climbing up the ladder of spiritual evolution till it reached the final stage of emancipation

— although Hindu influence did make Buddhism develop the idea of an eternal Buddha above, that was not a universal or fundamental Buddhistic idea. Whether the Divine in manifesting his Avatarhood could choose to follow the line of evolution from the lowest scale, manifesting on each scale as a Vibhuti is a question again to which the answer is not inevitably in the negative. If we accept the evolutionary idea, such a thing may have its place.

If Buddha taught something different from Krishna, that does not prevent his advent from being necessary in the spiritual evolution. The only question is whether the attempt to scale the heights of an absolute Nirvana through negation of cosmic existence was a necessary step or not, having a view to the fact that one can make the attempt to reach the Highest on the *neti neti* as well as the *iti iti* line.

He [Buddha] affirmed practically something unknowable that was Permanent and Unmanifested. Adwaita does the same. Buddha never said he was an Avatar of a Personal God but that he was the Buddha. It is the Hindus who made him an Avatar. If Buddha had looked upon himself as an Avatar at all, it would have been as an Avatar of the impersonal Truth.

I don't know that historically there could have been any other Buddha. It is the Vaishnava Puranas, I think, that settled the list of Avatars, for they are all Avatars of Vishnu according to the Purana. The final acceptance by all may have come later than Shankara, after the Buddhist-Brahminic controversy had ceased to be an actuality. For some time there was a tendency to substitute Balarama's name for Buddha's or to say that Buddha was an Avatar of Vishnu, but that he came to mislead the Asuras. He is evidently aimed at in the story of Mayamoha in the Vishnu Purana.

If a Divine Consciousness and Force descended and through the personality we call Buddha did a great work for the world, then Buddha can be called an Avatar — the tapasya and arriving at knowledge are only an incident of the manifestation.

If on the other hand Buddha was only a human being like many others who arrived at some knowledge and preached it, then he was not an Avatar — for of that kind there have been thousands and they cannot be all Avatars.

Krishna is not the supramental Light. The descent of Krishna would mean the descent of the overmind Godhead preparing, though not itself actually, the descent of supermind and Ananda. Krishna is the Anandamaya; he supports the evolution through the overmind leading it towards the Ananda.

One can be the head of a spiritual organisation or the Messiah of a religion or an Avatar without in this life reaching the supermind and beyond.

Yuge yuge[1] may be used in a general sense, as in English "from age to age" and not refer technically to the *yuga* proper according to the Puranic computation. But the *bahūni*[2] has an air of referring to very numerous lives especially when coupled with *tava ca*. In that case all these many births could not be full incarnations, — many may have been merely Vibhuti births carrying on the thread from incarnation to incarnation. About Arjuna's accompanying him in each and every birth, nothing is said, but it would not be likely — many, of course.

[1] About his many births Krishna says in the Gita, *sambhavāmi yuge yuge*. See Gita, Ch. IV, 8.
[2] *Bahūni me vyatītāni janmāni tava cārjuna.* Gita, Ch. IV, 5.

But each being in a new birth prepares a new mind, life and body — otherwise John Smith would always be John Smith and would have no chance of being Piyusha Kanti Ghose. Of course inside there are old personalities contributing to the new life — but I am speaking of the new visible personality, the outer man, mental, vital, physical. It is the psychic being that keeps the link from birth to birth and makes all the manifestations of the same person. It is therefore to be expected that the Avatar should take on a new personality each time, a personality suited for the new times, work, surroundings. In my own view of things, however, the new personality has a series of Avatar births behind him, births in which the intermediate evolution has been followed and assisted from age to age.

I suppose very few recognised him [Krishna] as an Avatar, — certainly it was not at all a general recognition. Among the few those nearest him do not seem to have counted — it was less prominent people like Vidura etc.

Those who were with Krishna were in all appearance men like other men. They spoke and acted with each other as men with men and were not thought of by those around them as gods. Krishna himself was known by most as a man — only a few worshipped him as the Divine.

An Avatar, roughly speaking, is one who is conscious of the presence and power of the Divine born in him or descended into him and governing from within his will and life and action; he feels identified inwardly with this divine power and presence.

A Vibhuti is supposed to embody some power of the Divine and is enabled by it to act with great force in the world, but that is all that is necessary to make him a Vibhuti: the power may be very great, but the consciousness is not that of an inborn or indwelling Divinity. This is the distinction we can gather from the Gita which is the main authority on this subject. If we follow this distinction, we can confidently say from what is related of them that Rama and Krishna can be accepted as Avatars; Buddha figures as such although with a more impersonal consciousness of the Power within him. Ramakrishna voiced the same consciousness when he spoke of Him who was Rama and who was Krishna being within him. But Chaitanya's case is peculiar; for according to the accounts he ordinarily felt and declared himself a bhakta of Krishna and nothing more, but in great moments he manifested Krishna, grew luminous in mind and body and was Krishna himself and spoke and acted as the Lord. His contemporaries saw in him an Avatar of Krishna, a manifestation of the Divine Love.

Shankara and Vivekananda were certainly Vibhutis; they cannot be reckoned as more, though as Vibhutis they were very great.

*
**

It was not my intention to question in any degree Chaitanya's position as an Avatar of Krishna and the Divine Love. That character of the manifestation appears very clearly from all the accounts about him and even, if what is related about the appearance of Krishna in him from time to time is accepted, these outbursts of the splendour of the Divine Being are among the most remarkable in the story of the Avatar. As for Sri Ramakrishna, the manifestation in him was not so intense but more many-sided and fortunately there can be no doubt about the authenticity of the details of his talk and action since they have been recorded from day to day by so competent an observer as Mahendranath Gupta. I would not care to enter into any comparison as between these two great spiritual personalities: both exercised an extraordinary influence and did something supreme in their own sphere.

*
**

He [Ramakrishna] never wrote an autobiography — what he said was in conversation with his disciples and others. He was certainly quite as much an Avatar as Christ or Chaitanya.

Mahomed would himself have rejected the idea of being an Avatar, so we have to regard him only as the prophet, the instrument, the Vibhuti. Christ realised himself as the Son who is one with the Father — he must therefore be an *aṁśāvatāra*, a partial incarnation.

What Leonardo da Vinci held in himself was all the new age of Europe on its many sides. But there was no question of Avatarhood or consciousness of a descent or pressure of spiritual forces. Mysticism was no part of what he had to manifest.

II

There are two sides of the phenomenon of Avatarhood, the Divine Consciousness and the instrumental personality. The Divine Consciousness is omnipotent but it has put forth the instrumental personality in Nature under the conditions of Nature and it uses it according to the rules of the game — though also sometimes to change the rules of the game. If Avatarhood is only a flashing miracle, then I have no use for it. If it is a coherent part of the arrangement of the omnipotent Divine in Nature, then I can understand and accept it.

I have said that the Avatar is one who comes to open the Way for humanity to a higher consciousness — if nobody can follow the Way, then either our conception of the thing, which is also that of Christ and Krishna and Buddha also, is all wrong or the whole life and action of the Avatar is quite futile. X seems to say that there is no way and no possibility of following, that the struggles and sufferings of the Avatar are unreal and all humbug, — there is no possibility of struggle for one who represents the Divine. Such a conception makes nonsense of the whole idea of Avatarhood; there is then no reason in it, no necessity in it, no meaning in it. The Divine being all-powerful can lift people up without bothering to come down on earth. It is only if it is a part of the world-arrangement that he should take upon himself the burden of humanity and open the Way that Avatarhood has any meaning.

The Avatar is not supposed to act in a non-human way — he takes up human action and uses human methods with the human consciousness in front and the Divine behind. If he did not his taking a human body would have no meaning and would be of no use to anybody. He could just as well have stayed above and done things from there.

As for the Divine and the human, that also is a mind-made difficulty. The Divine is there in the human, and the human fulfilling and exceeding its highest aspirations and tendencies becomes the Divine. That is what your depression could not understand — that when the Divine descends, he takes upon himself the burden of humanity in order to exceed it — he becomes human in order to show humanity how to become Divine. But that cannot be if there is only a weakling without any divine Presence within or divine Force behind him — he has to be strong in order to put his strength into all who are willing to receive it. There is therefore in him a double element — human in front, Divine behind — and it is that which gives the impression of unfathomableness of which you complained. If you look upon the human alone, looking with the external eye only and not willing or ready to see anything else, you will see a human being only — if you look for the Divine, you will find the Divine.

It is true that it is impossible for the limited human reason to judge the way or purpose of the Divine, — which is the way of the Infinite dealing with the finite.

It is not by your mind that you can hope to understand the Divine and its action, but by the growth of a true and divine consciousness within you. If the Divine were to unveil and reveal itself in all its glory, the mind might feel a Presence, but it would not understand its action or its nature. It is in the measure of your own realisation and by the birth and growth of that greater consciousness in yourself that you will see the Divine and understand its action even behind its terrestrial disguises.

An Avatar or Vibhuti have the knowledge that is necessary for their work, they need not have more. There was absolutely no reason why Buddha should know what was going on in Rome. An Avatar even does not manifest all the Divine omniscience and omnipotence; he has not come for any such unnecessary display; all that is behind him but not in the front of his consciousness. As for the Vibhuti, the Vibhuti need not even know that he is a power of the Divine. Some Vibhutis like Julius Caesar for instance have been atheists. Buddha himself did not believe in a personal God, only in some impersonal and indescribable Permanent.

Men's way of doing things well is through a clear mental connection; they see things and do things with the mind and what they want is a mental and human perfection. When they think of a manifestation of Divinity, they think it must be an extraordinary perfection in doing ordinary human things — an extraordinary business faculty, political, poetic or artistic faculty, an accurate memory, not making mistakes, not undergoing any defeat or failure. Or else they think of things which they call superhuman like not eating food or telling cotton-futures or sleeping on nails or eating them. All that has nothing to do with manifesting the Divine.... These human ideas are false.

The Divinity acts according to another consciousness, the consciousness of the Truth above and the Lila below and It acts according to the need of the Lila, not according to man's ideas of what It should or should not do. This is the first thing one must grasp, otherwise one can understand nothing about the manifestation of the Divine.

If the Divine were not in essence omnipotent, he could not be omnipotent anywhere — whether in the supramental or anywhere else. Because he chooses to limit or determine his action by conditions, it does not make him less omnipotent. His self-limitation is itself an act of omnipotence....

Why should the Divine be tied down to succeed in all his operations? What if failure suits him better and serves better the ultimate purpose? What rigid primitive notions are these about the Divine!

Certain conditions have been established for the game and so long as those conditions remain unchanged certain things are not done, — so we say they are impossible, can't be done. If the conditions are changed then the same things are done or at least become licit — allowable, legal according to the so-called laws of Nature, and then we say they can be done. The Divine also acts according to the conditions of the game. He may change them, but he has to change them first, not proceed, while maintaining the conditions, to act by a series of miracles.

If the Avatars are shams, they have no value for others nor any true effect, Avatarhood becomes perfectly irrational and unreal and meaningless. The Divine does not need to suffer or struggle for himself; if he takes on these things, it is in order to bear the world-burden and help the world and men; and if the sufferings and struggles are to be of any help, they must be real. A sham or

falsehood cannot help. They must be as real as the struggles and
sufferings of men themselves — the Divine bears them and at the
same time shows the way out of them. Otherwise, his assumption
of human nature has no meaning and no utility and no value.
What is the use of admitting Avatarhood if you take all the meaning out of it?

If your argument is that the life-actions, struggles of the Avatar
(e.g. Rama's, Krishna's) are unreal because the Divine is there
and knows it is all a Maya, in man also there is a self, a spirit that
is immortal, untouched, divine; you can say that man's sufferings
and ignorance are only put on, sham, unreal. But if man feels
them as real and if the Avatar feels his work and the difficulties
to be serious and real?

    If the existence of the Divinity is of no practical effect, what
is the use of a theoretical admission? The manifestation of the
Divine in the Avatar is of help to man because it helps him to
discover his own divinity and find the way to realise it. If the
difference is so great that the humanity by its very nature prevents all possibility of following the way opened by the Avatar,
it merely means that there is no divinity in man that can respond
to the Divinity in the Avatar.

I repeat, the Divine when he takes on the burden of terrestrial
nature, takes it fully, sincerely and without any conjuring tricks
or pretence. If he has something behind him which emerges
always out of the coverings, it is the same thing in essence, even
if greater in degree, that is behind others — and it is to awaken
that that he is there....

    The psychic being does the same for all who are intended
for the spiritual way — men need not be extraordinary beings to
follow it. That is the mistake you are making — to harp on greatness as if only the great can be spiritual.

I am rather perplexed by your strictures on Rama. Cowardice is the last thing that can be charged against Valmiki's Rama; he has always been considered as a warrior and it is the "martial races" of India who have made him their god. Valmiki everywhere paints him as a great warrior. His employment of ruse against an infrahuman enemy does not prove the opposite — for that is always how the human (even great warriors and hunters) has dealt with the infrahuman. I think it is Madhusudan who has darkened Valmiki's hero in Bengali eyes and turned him into a poor puppet, but that is not the authentic Rama who, say what one will, was a great epic figure, — Avatar or no Avatar. As for conventional morality, all morality is a convention — man cannot live without conventions, mental and moral, otherwise he feels himself lost in the rolling sea of the anarchic forces of the vital Nature. Even the Russells and Bernard Shaws can only end by setting up another set of conventions in the place of those they have skittled over. Only by rising above mind can one really get beyond conventions — Krishna was able to do it because he was not a mental human being but an overmental godhead acting freely out of a greater consciousness than man's. Rama was not that, he was the Avatar of the sattwic mind — mental, emotional, moral — and he followed the Dharma of the age and race. That may make him temperamentally congenial to Gandhi and the reverse to you; but just as Gandhi's temperamental recoil from Krishna does not prove Krishna to be no Avatar, so your temperamental recoil from Rama does not establish that he was not an Avatar. However, my main point will be that Avatarhood does not depend upon these questions at all, but has another basis, meaning and purpose.

I have no intention of entering into a supreme defence of Rama — I only entered into the points about Bali etc. because these are usually employed nowadays to belittle him as a great personality on the usual level. But from the point of view of Avatarhood I would no more think of defending his moral perfection according to modern standards than I would think of defending Napo-

leon or Caesar against the moralists or the democratic critics or
the debunkers in order to prove that they were Vibhutis. Vibhuti,
Avatar are terms which have their own meaning and scope, and
they are not concerned with morality or immorality, perfection or
imperfection according to small human standards or setting an
example to men or showing new moral attitudes or giving new
spiritual teachings. These may or may not be done, but they are
not at all the essence of the matter.

Also, I do not consider your method of dealing with the
human personality of Rama to be the right one. It has to be
taken as a whole in the setting that Valmiki gave it (not treated
as if it were the story of a modern man) and with the significance
that he gave to his hero's personality, deeds and works. If it is
pulled out of its setting and analysed under the dissecting knife of
a modern ethical mind, it loses all its significance at once. Krishna
so treated bacomes a debauchee and trickster who no doubt
did great things in politics — but so did Rama in war. Achilles
and Odysseus pulled out of their setting become, one a furious
egoistic savage, and the other a cruel and cunning savage. I consider myself under an obligation to enter into the spirit, significance, atmosphere of the Mahabharata, Iliad, Ramayana and
identify myself with their time-spirit before I can feel what their
heroes were in themselves apart from the details of their outer
action.

As for the Avatarhood, I accept it for Rama because he fills
a place in the scheme — and seems to me to fill it rightly — and
because when I read the Ramayana I feel a great afflatus which I
recognise and which makes of its story — mere faery-tale though
it seems — a parable of a great critical transitional event that
happened in the terrestrial evolution and gives to the main
character's personality and action a significance of the large
typical cosmic kind which these actions would not have had if
they had been done by another man in another scheme of events.
The Avatar is not bound to do extraordinary actions, but he is
bound to give his acts or his work or what he is — any of these
or all — a significance and an effective power that are part of
something essential to be done in the history of the earth and
its races.

All the same, if anybody does not see as I do and wants to eject Rama from his place, I have no objection — I have no particular partiality for Rama — provided somebody is put in who can worthily fill up the gap his absence leaves. There was somebody there, Valmiki's Rama or another Rama or somebody not Rama.

Also I do not mean that I admit the validity of your remarks about Rama, even taken as a piecemeal criticism, but that I have no time for today. I maintain my position about the killing of Bali and the banishment of Sita in spite of Bali's preliminary objection to the procedure, afterwards retracted, and in spite of the opinion of Rama's relatives, necessarily from the point of view of the antique dharma — not from that of any universal moral standard — which besides does not exist, since the standard changes according to clime or age.

No, certainly not — an Avatar is not at all bound to be a spiritual prophet — he is never in fact merely a prophet, he is a realiser, an establisher — not of outward things only, though he does realise something in the outward also, but, as I have said, of something essential and radical needed for the terrestrial evolution which is the evolution of the embodied spirit through successive stages towards the Divine. It was not at all Rama's business to establish the spiritual stage of that evolution — so he did not at all concern himself with that. His business was to destroy Ravana and to establish the Rama-rajya — in other words, to fix for the future the possibility of an order proper to the sattwic civilised human being who governs his life by the reason, the finer emotions, morality, or at least moral ideals, such as truth, obedience, co-operation and harmony, the sense of domestic and public order, — to establish this in a world still occupied by anarchic forces, the Animal mind and the powers of the vital Ego making its own satisfaction the rule of life, in other words, the Vanara and Rakshasa. This is the meaning of Rama and his life-work and it is according as he fulfilled it or not that he must be judged as Avatar or no Avatar. It was not his business to play the comedy of the chivalrous Kshatriya with the formidable brute beast that was Bali, it was his business to kill him and get the Animal under his control. It was his business to be not necessarily a perfect, but a largely representative sattwic Man, a faithful husband and a lover, a loving and obedient son, a tender and perfect brother, father, friend — he is friend of all kinds of people, friend of the outcast Guhaka, friend of the Animal leaders, Sugriva, Hanuman, friend of the vulture Jatayu, friend of even Rakshasa Vibhishana. All that he was in a brilliant, striking but above all spontaneous and inevitable way, not with forcing of this note or that like Harishchandra or Shivi, but with a certain harmonious completeness. But most of all, it was his business to typify and establish the things on which the social idea and its stability depend, truth and honour, the sense of Dharma, public spirit and the sense of order. To the first, to truth and honour, much more than to his filial love and obedience to his father — though to that also — he sacrificed his personal rights as the elect of the King and the assembly and fourteen of the best years of his life and went into exile in the forests. To his public spirit and his sense of public order (the great and supreme civic virtue in the eyes of the ancient Indians, Greeks, Romans, for at that time the maintenance of the ordered community, not the separate development and satisfaction of the individual was the pressing need of the human evolution) he sacrificed his own happiness and domestic life and the happiness of Sita. In that he was at one with the moral sense of all the antique races, though at variance with the later romantic individualistic sentimental morality of the modern man who can afford to have that less stern morality just because the ancients sacrificed the individual in order to make the world safe for the spirit of social order. Finally, it was Rama's business to make the world safe for the ideal of the sattwic human being by destroying the sovereignty of Ravana, the Rakshasa menace. All this he did with such a divine afflatus in his personality and action that his figure has been stamped for more than two millenniums on the mind of Indian culture, and what he stood for has dominated the reason and idealising mind of man in all countries, and in spite of the constant revolt of the human vital, is likely to continue to do so until a greater ideal arises. And you say in spite of all these that he was no Avatar? If you like — but at any rate he stands among the few greatest Vibhutis. You may dethrone him now — for man is no longer satisfied with the sattwic ideal and is seeking for something more — but his work and meaning remain stamped on the past of the earth's evolving race. When I spoke of the gap that would be left by his absence, I did not mean a gap among the prophets and intellectuals, but a gap in the scheme of Avatarhood — there was somebody who was the Avatar of the sattwic Human as Krishna was the Avatar of the overmental Superman — I can see no one but Rama who can fill the place. Spiritual teachers and prophets (as also intellectuals, scientists, artists, poets, etc.) — these are at the greatest Vibhutis but they are not Avatars. For at that rate all religious founders would be Avatars — Joseph Smith (I think that is his name) of the Mormons, St. Francis of Assisi, Calvin, Loyola and a host of others as well as Christ, Chaitanya or Ramakrishna.

For faith, miracles, Bijoy Goswami, another occasion. I wanted to say this much more about Rama — which is still only a hint and is not the thing I was going to write about the general principle of Avatarhood.

Nor, may I add, is it a complete or supreme defence of Rama. For that I would have to write about what the story of the Ramayana meant, appreciate Valmiki's presentation of his chief characters (they are none of them copy-book examples, but great men and women with the defects and merits of human nature, as all men even the greatest are), and show also how the Godhead, which was behind the frontal and instrumental personality we call Rama, worked out every incident of his life as a necessary step in what had to be done. As to the weeping Rama, I had answered that in my other unfinished letter. You are imposing the colder and harder Nordic ideal on the Southern temperament which regarded the expression of emotions, not its suppression, as a virtue. Witness the weeping and lamentations of Achilles, Ulysses and other great heroes, Persian and Indian — the latter especially as lovers.

*
**

Why should not Rama have *kāma* (lust) as well as *prema* (love)? They were supposed to go together as between husband and wife in ancient India. The performances of Rama in the *viraha* of Sita are due to Valmiki's poetic idea which was also Kalidasa's and everybody else's in those far-off times about how a complete lover should behave in such a quandary. Whether the actual Rama bothered himself to do all that is another matter.

As for the unconscious Avatar, why not? Chaitanya is supposed to be an Avatar by the Vaishnavas, yet he was conscious of the Godhead behind only when that Godhead came in front and possessed him on rare occasions. Christ said "I and my father are one", but yet he always spoke and behaved as if there were a difference. Ramakrishna's earlier period was that of one seeking God, not aware from the first of his identity. These are the reputed religious Avatars who ought to be more conscious than a man of action like Rama. And supposing the full and permanent consciousness, why should the Avatar proclaim himself except on rare occasions to an Arjuna or to a few bhaktas or disciples? It is for others to find out what he is; though he does not deny when others speak of him as That, he is not always saying and perhaps never may say or only in moments like that of the Gita, "I am He."

No time for a full answer to your renewed remarks on Rama tonight. You are intrigued only because you stick to the modern standard, modern measuring-rods of moral and spiritual perfection (introduced by Seely and Bankim) for the Avatar — while I start from another standpoint altogether and resolutely refuse these standard human measures. The ancient Avatars except Buddha were not either standards of perfection or spiritual teachers in spite of the Gita which was spoken, says Krishna, in a moment of supernormal consciousness which he lost immediately afterwards. They were, if I may say so, representative cosmic men who were instruments of a divine Intervention for fixing certain things in the evolution of the earth-race. I stick to that and refuse to submit myself in this argument to any other standard whatever.

I did not admit that Rama was a blind Avatar, but offered you two alternatives of which the latter represents my real view founded on the impression made on me by the Ramayana that Rama knew very well but refused to be talkative about it — his business being not to disclose the Divine but to fix mental, moral and emotional man (not to originate him, for he was there already) on the earth as against the Animal and Rakshasa forces. My argument from Chaitanya (who was for most of the time to his own outward consciousness first a pandit and then a bhakta, but only occasionally the Divine himself) is perfectly rational and logical, if you follow my line and don't insist on a high specifically spiritual consciousness for the Avatar. I shall point out what I mean in my next.

By sattwic man I do not mean a moral or an always self-controlled one, but a predominantly mental (as opposed to a vital or merely physical man) who has rajasic emotions and passions, but lives predominantly according to his mind and its will and ideas. There is no such thing, I suppose, as a purely sattwic man — since the three gunas go always together in a state of unstable equilibrium — but a predominantly sattwic man is what I have described. My impression of Rama from Valmiki is such — it is quite different from yours. I am afraid your picture of him is quite out of focus — you efface the main lines of the characters, belittle and brush out all the lights to which Valmiki gave so much value and prominence and hammer always at some details and some parts of shadow which you turn into the larger part of Rama. That is what the debunkers do — but a debunked figure is not the true figure.

By the way, a sattwic man can have a strong passion and strong anger — and when he lets the latter loose, the normally vicious fellow is simply nowhere. Witness the outbursts of anger of Christ, the indignation of Chaitanya — and the general evidence of experience and psychology on the point.

The trait of Rama which you give as that of an undeveloped man, viz., his decisive spontaneous action according to the will and the idea that came to him, is a trait of the cosmic man and many Vibhutis, men of action of the large Caesarian or Napoleonic type.

When I said, "Why not an unconscious Avatar?" I was taking your statement (not mine) that Rama was unconscious and how could there be an unconscious Avatar. My own view is that Rama was not blind, not unconscious of his Avatarhood, only uncommunicative about it. But I said that even taking your statement to be correct, the objection was not insuperable. I instanced the case of Chaitanya and the others, because there the facts are hardly disputable. Chaitanya for the first part of his life was simply Nimai Pandit and had no consciousness of being anything else. Then he had his conversion and became the bhakta Chaitanya. This bhakta at times seemed to be possessed by the presence of Krishna, knew himself to be Krishna, spoke, moved and appeared with the light of the Godhead — none around him could think of or see him as anything else when he was in this glorified and transfigured condition. But from that he fell back to the ordinary consciousness of the bhakta and, as I have read in his biography, refused then to consider himself as anything more. These, I think, are the facts. Well, then what do they signify? Was he only Nimai Pandit at first? It is quite conceivable that he was so and the descent of the Godhead into him only took place after his conversion and spiritual change. But also afterwards when he was in his normal bhakta-consciousness, was he then no longer the Avatar? An intermittent Avatarhood? Krishna coming down for an afternoon call into Chaitanya and then going up again till the time came for the next visit? I find it difficult to believe in this phenomenon. The rational explanation is that in the phenomenon of Avatarhood there is a Consciousness behind, at first veiled or sometimes perhaps half-veiled, which is that of the Godhead and a frontal consciousness, human or apparently human or at any rate with all the appearance of terrestriality which is the instrumental personality. In that case, it is possible that the secret Consciousness was all along there, but waited to manifest until after the conversion and it manifested intermittently because the main work of Chaitanya was to establish the type of a spiritual and psychic bhakti and love in the emotional vital part of man, preparing the vital in us in that way to turn towards the Divine — at any rate, to fix that possibility in the earth-nature. It was not that there had not been the emotional type of bhakti before; but the completeness of it, the *élan*, the vital's rapture in it had never manifested as it manifested in Chaitanya. But for that work it would never have done if he had always been in the Krishna consciousness; he would have been the Lord to whom all gave bhakti, but not the supreme example of the divine ecstatic bhakta. But still the occasional manifestation showed who he was and at the same time evidenced the mystic law of the Immanence.

Voilà — for Chaitanya. But, if Chaitanya, the frontal consciousness, the instrumental personality, was all the time the Avatar, yet except in his highest moments was unconscious of it and even denied it, that pushed a little farther would establish the possibility of what you call an unconscious Avatar, that is to say, of one in which the veiled consciousness might not come in front but always move the instrumental personality from behind. The frontal consciousness might be aware in the inner parts of its being that it was only an instrument of something Divine which was its real Self, but outwardly would think, speak and behave as if it were only the human being doing a given work with a peculiar power and splendour. Whether there was such an Avatar or not is another matter, but logically it is possible.

The question was if certain perfections must not be demanded of the Divine Manifestation which seemed to me quite irrelevant to the reality. I put forward two propositions which appear to me indispensable unless we are to reverse all spiritual knowledge in favour of modern European ideas about things: first, the Divine Manifestation, even when it manifests in mental and human ways, has behind it a consciousness greater than the mind and not bound by the petty mental and moral conventions of this very ignorant human race — so that to impose these standards on the Divine is to try to do what is irrational and impossible. Secondly, this Divine Consciousness behind the apparent personality is concerned with only two things in a fundamental way — the truth above and here below the Lila and the purpose of the incarnation or manifestation, and it does what is necessary for that in the way its greater than human consciousness sees to be the necessary and intended way. But I do not understand how all that can prevent me from answering mental questions. On my own showing, if it is necessary for the divine purpose, it has to be done. Sri Ramakrishna himself answered thousands of questions, I believe. But the answers must be such as he gave and such as I try to give, answers from a higher spiritual experience, from a deeper source of knowledge and not lucubrations of the logical intellect trying to coordinate its ignorance. Still less can there be a placing of a divine truth before the judgments of the intellect to be condemned or acquitted by that authority — for the authority here has no sufficient jurisdiction or competence.

What do you mean by lust? Avatars can be married and have children and that is not possible without sex; they can have friendships, enmities, family feelings, etc., etc., — these are vital things. I think you are under the impression that an Avatar must be a saint or a yogi.

In the yoga we do not strive after greatness. It is not a question of Sri Krishna's disciples but of the earth-consciousness. Rama was a mental man, there is no touch of the overmind consciousness (direct) in anything he said or did, but what he did was done with the greatness of the Avatar. But there have since been men who did live in touch with the planes above mind — higher mind, illumined mind, intuition. There is no question of asking whether they were "greater" than Rama; they might have been less "great", but they were able to live from a new plane of consciousness. And Krishna's opening the overmind certainly made it possible for the attempt at bringing supermind to the earth to be made.

About greater and less, one point. Is Captain John Higgins of S. S. Mauretania a greater man that Christopher Columbus because he can reach America without trouble in a few days? Is a University graduate in philosophy greater than Plato because he can reason about problems and systems which had never even occurred to Plato? No, only humanity has acquired greater scientific power which any good navigator can use or a wider intellectual knowledge which anyone with a philosophic training can use. You will say greater scientific power and wider knowledge is not a change of consciousness. Very well, but there are Rama and Ramakrishna. Rama spoke always from the thinking intelligence, the common property of developed men; Ramakrishna constantly from a swift and luminous spiritual intuition. Can you tell me which is the greater? The Avatar recognised by all India? Or the saint and yogi recognised as an Avatar only by his disciples and some others who follow them?

He [Buddha] had a more powerful vital than Ramakrishna's, a stupendous will and an invincible mind of thought. If he had led the ordinary life, he would have been a great organiser, conqueror and creator. If a man rises to a higher plane of consciousness, it does not necessarily follow that he will be a greater man of action or a greater creator. One may rise to spiritual planes of inspiration undreamed of by Shakespeare and yet not be as great a poetic creator as Shakespeare. "Greatness" is not the object of spiritual realisation any more than fame or success in the world — how are these things the standard of spiritual realisation?

The answer to the question depends on what value we attach to spiritual experience and to the data of other planes of consciousness, other than the physical, as also on the nature of the relations between the cosmic consciousness and the individual and collective consciousness of man. From the point of view of spiritual and occult Truth, what takes shape in the consciousness of man is a reflection and particular kind of formation, in a difficult medium, of things much greater in their light, power and beauty or in their force and range which came to it from the cosmic consciousness of which man is a limited and, in his present state of evolution, a still ignorant part. All this explanation about the genius of the race, of a consciousness of a nation creating the Gods and their forms is a very partial, somewhat superficial and in itself a misleading truth. Man's mind is not an original creator, it is an intermediary; to start creating it must receive an initiating "inspiration", a transmission or a suggestion from the cosmic consciousness and with that it does what it can. God is, but man's conceptions of God are reflections in his own mentality, sometimes of the Divine, sometimes of other Beings and Powers and they are what his mentality can make of the suggestions that come to him, generally very partial and imperfect so long as they are still mental, so long as he has not arrived at a higher and truer, a spiritual or mystic knowledge. The Gods already exist, they are not created by man, even though he does seem to conceive them in his own image; — fundamentally, he formulates as best he can what truth about them he receives from the cosmic Reality. An artist or a bhakta may have a vision of the Gods and it may get stabilised and generalised in the consciousness of the race and in that sense it may be true that man gives their forms to the Gods; but he does not invent these forms, he records what he sees; the forms that he gives are given to him. In the "conventional" form of Krishna men have embodied what they could see of his eternal beauty and what they have seen may be true as well as beautiful, it conveys something of the form, but it is fairly certain that if there is an eternal form of that eternal beauty, it is a thousand times more beautiful than what man had as yet been able to see of it. Mother India is not a piece of earth; she is a Power, a Godhead, for all nations have such a Devi supporting their separate existence and keeping it in being. Such beings are as real and more permanently real than the men they influence, but they belong to a higher plane, are part of the cosmic consciousness and being and act here on earth by shaping the human consciousness on which they exercise their influence. It is natural for man who sees only his own consciousness individual, national or racial at work and does not see what works upon it and shapes it, to think that all is created by him and there is nothing cosmic and greater behind it. The Krishna consciousness is a reality, but if there were no Krishna, there could be no Krishna consciousness; except in arbitrary metaphysical abstractions there can be no consciousness without a Being who is conscious. It is the person who gives value and reality to the personality, he expresses himself in it and is not constituted by it. Krishna is a being, a person and it is as the Divine Person that we meet him, hear his voice, speak with him and feel his presence. To speak of the consciousness of Krishna as something separate from Krishna is an error of the mind, which is always separating the inseparable and which also tends to regard the impersonal, because it is abstract, as greater, more real and more enduring than the person. Such divisions may be useful to the mind for its own purposes, but it is not the real truth; in the real truth the being or person and its impersonality or state of being are one reality.

The historicity of Krishna is of less spiritual importance and is not essential, but it has still a considerable value. It does not seem to me that there can be any reasonable doubt that Krishna the man was not a legend or a poetic invention but actually existed upon earth and played a part in the Indian past. Two facts emerge clearly, that he was regarded as an important spiritual figure, one whose spiritual illumination was recorded in one of the Upanishads, and that he was traditionally regarded as a divine man, one worshipped after his death as a deity; this is apart from the story in the Mahabharata and the Puranas. There is no reason to suppose that the connection of his name with the development of the Bhagavata religion, an important current in the stream of Indian spirituality, was founded on a mere legend or poetic invention. The Mahabharata is a poem and not history, but it is clearly a poem founded on a great historical event, traditionally preserved in memory; some of the figures connected with it, Dhritarashtra, Parikshit, for instance, certainly existed and the story of the part played by Krishna as leader, warrior and statesman can be accepted as probable in itself and to all appearance founded on a tradition which can be

given a historical value and has not the air of a myth or a sheer
poetical invention. That is as much as can be positively said from
the point of view of the theoretical reason as to the historic figure
of the man Krishna; but in my view there is much more than that
in it and I have always regarded the incarnation as a fact and
accepted the historicity of Krishna as I accept the historicity of
Christ.

The story of Brindavan is another matter; it does not enter
into the main story of the Mahabharata and has a Puranic origin
and it could be maintained that it was intended all along to have
a symbolic character. At one time I accepted that explanation,
but I had to abandon it afterwards; there is nothing in the
Puranas that betrays any such intention. It seems to me that it
is related as something that actually occurred or occurs somewhere. The Gopis are to them realities and not symbols. It was
for them at the least an occult truth, and occult and symbolic
are not the same thing; the symbol may be only a significant
mental construction or only a fanciful invention, but the occult
is a reality which is actual somewhere, behind the material scene
as it were and can have its truth for the terrestrial life and its
influence upon it may even embody itself there. The Lila of the
Gopis seems to be conceived as something which is always going
on in a divine Gokul and which projected itself in an earthly
Brindavan and can always be realised and its meaning made
actual in the soul. It is to be presumed that the writers of the
Puranas took it as having been actually projected on earth in the
life of the incarnate Krishna and it has been so accepted by the
religious mind of India.

These questions and the speculations to which they have
given rise have no indispensable connection with the spiritual
life. There what matters is the contact with Krishna and the
growth towards the Krishna consciousness, the presence, the spiritual relation, the union in the soul and till that is reached, the
aspiration, the growth in bhakti and whatever illumination one
can get on the way. To one who has had these things, lived in the
presence, heard the voice, known Krishna as Friend or Lover,
Guide, Teacher, Master or, still more, has had his whole consciousness changed by the contact, or felt the presence within

him, all such questions have only an outer and superficial interest. So also, to one who has had contact with the inner Brindavan and the Lila of the Gopis, made the surrender and undergone the spell of the joy and the beauty or even only turned to the sound of the flute, the rest hardly matters. But from another point of view, if one can accept the historical reality of the incarnation, there is this great spiritual gain that one has a *point d'appui* for a more concrete realisation in the conviction that once at least the Divine has visibly touched the earth, made the complete manifestation possible, made it possible for the divine supernature to descend into this evolving but still very imperfect terrestrial nature.

Of course, X's view about the canalisation of Niagara is my standpoint also. But for the human mind it is difficult to get across the border between mind and spirit without making a forceful rush or push along one line only and that must be some line of pure experience in which, especially if it is the bhakti way, one gets easily swallowed up in the rapids (did not Chaitanya at last disappear in the waters?) and goes no farther. The first thing is to break into the spiritual consciousness, any part of it, anyhow and anywhere, afterwards one can explore the country, to which exploration there can hardly be a limit; one is always going higher and higher, getting wider and wider, but there is a certain intense ecstasy about the first complete plunge which is extraordinarily seizing. It is not only the Bhakta's rapture, but the Jnani's plunge into the Brahma-Nirvana or Brahmananda or release into the still eternity of the Self that is of that seizing and absorbing character — it does not look at first as if one could or would care or need to get beyond into anything else. One cannot find fault with the Sannyasi lost in his *laya* or the Bhakta lost in his ecstasy; they remain there probably because they are constituted for that and it is the limit of their leap. But, all the same, it has always appeared to me that it is a stage and not the end; I subscribe fully to the canalisation of the Niagara.

Adhikara is, of course, a matter of the psychology and the

soul and the nature, it has nothing to do with any outer or artificial standards.

Then as to the Avatar and the symbols. There is, it seems to me, a cardinal error in the modern insistence on the biographical and historical, that is to say, the external factuality of the Avatar, the incidents of his outward life. What matters is the spiritual Reality, the Power, the Influence that come with him or that he brought down by his action and his existence. First of all, what matters in a spiritual man's life is not what he did or what he was outside to the view of the men of his time (that is what historicity or biography comes to, does it not?) but what he was and did within; it is only that that gives any value to his outer life at all. It is the inner life that gives to the outer any power it may have and the inner life of a spiritual man is something vast and full and, at least in the great figures, so crowded and teeming with significant things that no biographer or historian could ever hope to seize it all or tell it. Whatever is significant in the out-ward life is so because it is symbolical of what has been realised within himself and one may go on and say that the inner life also is only significant as an expression, a living representation of the movement of the Divinity behind it. That is why we need not enquire whether the stories about Krishna were transcripts, however loose, of his acts on earth or are symbol-representations of what Krishna was and is for men, of the Divinity expressing itself in the figure of Krishna. Buddha's renunciation, his temp-tation by Mara, his enlightenment under the Bo-tree are such symbols, so too the virgin birth, the temptation in the desert, the crucifixion of Christ are such symbols, true by what they signify, even if they are not scrupulously recorded historical events. The outward facts as related of Christ or Buddha are not much more than what has happened in many other lives — what is it that gives Buddha or Christ their enormous place in the spiritual world? It was because something manifested through them that was more than any outward event or any teaching. The veri-fiable historicity gives us very little of that, yet it is that only that matters. So it seems to me that X is fundamentally right in what he says of the symbols. To the physical mind only the words and facts and acts of a man matter; to the inner mind it is the spiritual happenings in him that matter. Even the teachings of Buddha and Christ are spiritually true not as mere mental teachings but as the expression of spiritual states or happenings in them which by their life on earth they made possible (or even dynamically potential) in others. Also, evidently, sectarian walls are a mistake, an accretion, a mental limiting of the Truth which may serve a mental, but not a spiritual purpose. The Avatar, the Guru have no meaning if they do not stand for the Eternal; it is that that makes them what they are for the worshipper or the disciple.

It is also a fact that nobody can give you any spiritual realisation which does not come from something in one's true Self, it is always the Divine who reveals himself and the Divine is within you; so He who reveals must be felt in your own heart. Your query here simply suggests that this is a truth which can be misinterpreted or misused, but so can every spiritual truth if it is taken hold of in the wrong way — and the human mind has a great penchant for taking Truth by the wrong end and arriving at falsehood. All statements about these things are, after all, mental statements and at the mercy of any mind that interprets them. There is a snag in every such statement created not by the Truth that it expresses but by the mind's interpretation. The snag (what you call the slip) lies not in the statement itself which is quite correct, but in the deflected sense in which it may be taken by ignorant or self-sufficient minds enamoured of their ego. Many have put forward the "own self" gospel without taking the trouble to see whether it is the true Self, have pitted the ignorance of their "own self" — in fact, their ego — against the knowledge of the Guru or made their ego or something that flattered and fostered it the Ishta Devata. The snag in the worship of Guru or Avatar is a sectarian bias which insists on the Representative or the Manifestation but loses sight of the Manifested; the snag in the emphasis on the other side is the ignoring of the need or belittling of the value of the Representative or Manifestation and the substitution, not of the true Self one in all, but of one's "own self" as the guide and light. How many have done that and lost the way through the pull of the magnified ego which is one of the great perils on the way! However that does not lessen the truth of the things said by X, — only in looking at the many sides of Truth one must put each thing in its place in the harmony of the All which is for us the expression of the Supreme.

What X says — the central thing — is very correct, as always, the position of all who have any notion of spirituality, though the religionists seem to find it difficult to get to it. But though Christ and Krishna are the same, they are the same in difference, — that is indeed the utility of so many manifestations instead of there being only one as these missionaries would have it. But is it really because the historical Christ has been made too much the foundation-stone of the Faith that Christianity is failing? It may be something inadequate in the religion itself — perhaps in Religion itself; for all religions are a little off-colour now. The need of a larger opening of the soul into the Light is being felt, an opening through which the expanding human mind and heart can follow.

SECTION EIGHT

REBIRTH

Rebirth

THE soul takes birth each time, and each time a mind, life and body are formed out of the materials of universal nature according to the soul's past evolution and its need for the future.

When the body is dissolved, the vital goes into the vital plane and remains there for a time, but after a time the vital sheath disappears. The last to dissolve is the mental sheath. Finally the soul or psychic being retires into the psychic world to rest there till a new birth is close.

This is the general course for ordinarily developed human beings. There are variations according to the nature of the individual and his development. For example, if the mental is strongly developed, then the mental being can remain; so also can the vital, provided they are organized by and centred around the true psychic being; they share the immortality of the psychic.

The soul gathers the essential elements of its experiences in life and makes that its basis of growth in the evolution; when it returns to birth it takes up with its mental, vital, physical sheaths so much of its Karma as is useful to it in the new life for further experience.

It is really for the vital part of the being that *śrāddha* and rites are done — to help the being to get rid of the vital vibrations which still attach it to the earth or to the vital worlds, so that it may pass quickly to its rest in the psychic peace.

I only said what was originally meant by the ceremonies — the rites. I was not referring to the feeding of the caste or the Brahmins which is not a rite or ceremony. Whether *śrāddha* as performed is actually effective is another matter — for those who perform it have not either the knowledge or the occult power.

After leaving the body, the soul, after certain experiences in other worlds, throws off its mental and vital personalities and goes into rest to assimilate the essence of its past and prepare for a new life. It is this preparation that determines the circumstances of the new birth and guides it in its reconstitution of a new personality and the choice of its materials.

The departed soul retains the memory of its past experiences only in their essence, not in their form of detail. It is only if the soul brings back some past personality or personalities as part of its present manifestation that it is likely to remember the details of the past life. Otherwise, it is only by Yogadrishti that the memory comes.

The Karana-purusha is what is called the central being by us, the Jiva. It stands above the play, supporting it always.

There may be what seems to be retrograde movements but these are only like zigzag movements, not a real falling back, but a return on something not worked out so as to go on better afterwards. The soul does not go back to the animal condition; but a part of the vital personality may disjoin itself and join an animal birth to work out its animal propensities there.

There is no truth in the popular belief about the avaricious man becoming a serpent. These are popular romantic superstitions.

*
**

The soul after it leaves the body travels through several states or planes until the psychic being has shed its temporary sheaths, then it reaches the psychic world where it rests in a kind of sleep till it is ready for reincarnation. What it keeps with it of the human experience in the end is only the essence of all that it has gone through, what it can use for its development. This is the general rule, but it does not apply to exceptional cases or to very developed beings who have achieved a greater consciousness than the ordinary human level.

It is not the soul (the psychic being) that takes a lesser form, it is some part of the manifested being, usually some part of the vital that does it, owing to some desire, affinity, need of particular experience. This happens fairly often to the ordinary man.

At the time of death the being goes out of the body through the head; it goes out in the subtle body and goes to different planes of existence for a short time until it has gone through certain experiences which are the result of its earthly existence. Afterwards it reaches the psychic world where it rests in a kind of sleep, until it is time for it to start a new life on earth. That is what happens usually — but there are some beings who are more developed and do not follow this course.

The soul goes out, after death, in a subtle body.

Recollections last only for a time, not till rebirth — otherwise the stamp would be so strong that remembrance of past births, even after taking a new body, would be the rule rather than the exception.

You say "relationships of one birth persist in successive births, the chances depending on the strength of the attachment". This is possible, but not a law — as a rule the same relationship would not be constantly repeated — the same people often meet again and again on earth in different lives, but the relations are different. The purpose of rebirth would not be served if the same personality with the same relations and experiences are incessantly repeated.

It is not the case that there is complete annihilation of the ego in respect of forms of life lower than man after death.

What was spoken of as being in a static condition of complete rest is not the ego, but the psychic being after it has shed its vital and other sheaths and is resting in the psychic world. Before that it passes through vital and other worlds on its way to the psychic plane.

It is possible to come into direct touch with the departed so long as they are near enough to the earth (it is usually supposed by those who have occult experience that it is for three years only) or if they are earthbound or if they are of those who do not proceed to the psychic plane but linger near the earth and are soon reborn.

Universal statements cannot be easily made about these things — there is a general line, but individual cases vary to an almost indefinite extent.

There is after death a period in which one passes through the vital world and lives there for a time. It is only the first part of this transit that can be dangerous or painful; in the rest one works out, under certain surroundings, the remnant of the vital desires and instincts which one had in the body. As soon as one is tired of these and able to go beyond, the vital sheath is dropped and the soul after a time needed to get rid of some mental survivals passes into a state of rest in the psychic world and remains there till the next life on earth.

One can help the departed souls by one's good will or by occult means, if one has the knowledge. The one thing that one should not do is to hold them back by sorrow for them or longings or by anything else that would pull them nearer to earth or delay their journey to their place of rest.

It may happen to some not to realise for a little time that they are dead, especially if the death has been unforeseen and sudden, but it cannot be said that it happens to all or to most. Some may enter into a state of semi-unconsciousness or obsession by a dark inner condition created by their state of mind at death, in which they realise nothing of where they are, etc., others are quite conscious of the passage. It is true that the departing being in the vital body lingers for some time near the body or the scene of life very often for as many as eight days and, in the ancient religions, mantras and other means were used for the severance. Even after the severance from the body a very earthbound nature or one full of strong physical desires may linger long in the earth-atmosphere up to a maximum period extended to three years.

Afterwards, it passes to the vital worlds, proceeding on its journey which must sooner or later bring it to the psychic rest till the next life. It is true also that sorrow and mourning for the dead impede their progress by keeping them tied to the earth-atmosphere and pulling them back from their passage.

*
**

The movement of the psychic being dropping the outer sheaths on its way to the psychic plane is the normal movement. But there can be any number of variations; one can return from the vital plane and there are many cases of an almost immediate birth, sometimes even attended with a complete memory of the events of the past life.

Hell and heaven are often imaginary states of the soul or rather of the vital which it constructs about it after its passing. What is meant by hell is a painful passage through the vital or lingering there, as for instance, in many cases of suicide where one remains surrounded by the forces of suffering and turmoil created by this unnatural and violent exit. There are, of course, also worlds of mind and vital worlds which are penetrated with joyful or dark experiences. One may pass through these as the result of things formed in the nature which create the necessary affinities, but the idea of reward or retribution is a crude and vulgar conception which is a mere popular error.

There is no rule of complete forgetfulness in the return of the soul to rebirth. There are, especially in childhood, many impressions of the past life which can be strong and vivid enough, but the materialising education and influence of the environments prevent their true nature from being recognised. There are even a great number of people who have definite recollections of a past life. But these things are discouraged by education and the atmosphere and cannot remain or develop; in most cases they are stifled out of existence. At the same time it must be noted that what the psychic being carries away with it and brings back is ordinarily the essence of the experiences it had in former lives, and not the details so that you cannot expect the same memory as one has of the present existence.

A soul can go straight to the psychic world but it depends on the state of consciousness at the time of departure. If the psychic is in front at the time, the immediate transition is quite possible. It does not depend on the acquisition of a mental and vital as well as a psychic immortality — those who have acquired that would rather have the power to move about in the different worlds and even act on the physical world without being bound to it. On the whole, it may be said that there is no one rigid rule for these things, manifold variations are possible depending upon the consciousness, its energies, tendencies and formations, although there is a general framework and design into which all fit and take their place.

It is necessary to understand clearly the difference between the evolving soul (psychic being) and the pure Atman, self or spirit. The pure self is unborn, does not pass through death or birth, is independent of birth or body, mind or life or this manifested Nature. It is not bound by these things, not limited, not affected, even though it assumes and supports them. The soul, on the contrary, is something that comes down into birth and passes through death — although it does not itself die, for it is immortal — from one state to another, from the earth plane to other planes and back again to the earth-existence. It goes on with this progression from life to life through an evolution which leads it up to the human state and evolves through it all a being of itself which we call the psychic being that supports the evolution and develops a physical, a vital, a mental human consciousness as its instruments of world-experience and of a disguised, imperfect, but growing self-expression. All this it does from behind a veil showing something of its divine self only in so far as the imperfection of the instrumental being will allow it. But a time comes when it is able to prepare to come out from behind the veil, to take command and turn all the instrumental nature towards a divine fulfilment. This is the beginning of the true spiritual life. The soul is able now to make itself ready for a higher evolution of manifested consciousness than the mental human — it can pass from the mental to the spiritual and through degrees of the spiritual to the supramental state. Till then there is no reason why it should cease from birth, it cannot in fact do so. If having reached the spiritual state, it wills to pass out of the terrestrial manifestation, it may indeed do so — but there is also possible a higher manifestation, in the Knowledge and not in the Ignorance.

Your question therefore does not arise. It is not the naked spirit, but the psychic being that goes to the psychic plane to rest till it is called again to another life. There is, therefore, no need of a Force to compel it to take birth anew. It is in its nature something that is put forth from the Divine to support the evolution and it must do so till the Divine's purpose in its evolution is accomplished. Karma is only a machinery, it is not the fundamental cause of terrestrial existence — it cannot be, for when the soul first entered this existence, it had no Karma.

What again do you mean by "the all-veiling Maya" or by "losing all consciousness"? The soul cannot lose all consciousness, for its very nature is consciousness though not of the mental kind to which we give the name. The consciousness is merely covered, not lost or abolished by the so-called Inconscience of material Nature and then by the half-conscious ignorance of mind, life and body. It manifests, as the individual mind and life and body grow, as much as may be of the consciousness which it holds in potentiality, manifests it in the outward instrumental nature as far as and in the way that is possible through these instruments and through the outer personality that has been prepared for it and by it — for both are true — for the present life.

I know nothing about any terrible suffering endured by the soul in the process of rebirth; popular beliefs even when they have some foundation are seldom enlightened and accurate.

1. The psychic being stands behind mind, life and body, supporting them; so also the psychic world is not one world in the scale like the mental, vital or physical worlds, but stands behind all these and it is there that the souls evolving here retire for the time between life and life. If the psychic were only one principle

in the rising order of body, life and mind on a par with the others and placed somewhere in the scale on the same footing as the others, it could not be the soul of all the rest, the divine element making the evolution of the others possible and using them as instruments for a growth through cosmic experience towards the Divine. So also the psychic world cannot be one among the other worlds to which the evolutionary being goes for supraphysical experience; it is a plane where it retires into itself for rest, for a spiritual assimilation of what it has experienced and for a replunging into its own fundamental consciousness and psychic nature.

2. For the few who go out of the Ignorance and enter into Nirvana, there is no question of their going straight up into higher worlds of manifestation. Nirvana or Moksha is a liberated condition of the being, not a world — it is a withdrawal from the worlds and the manifestation. The analogy of *pitṛyāna* and *devayāna* can hardly be mentioned in this connection.

3. The condition of the souls that retire into the psychic world is entirely static; each withdraws into himself and is not interacting with the others. When they come out of their trance, they are ready to go down into a new life, but meanwhile they do not act upon the earth life. There are other beings, guardians of the psychic world, but they are concerned only with the psychic world itself and the return of the souls to reincarnation, not with the earth.

4. A being of a psychic world cannot get fused into the soul of a human being on earth. What happens in some cases is that a very advanced psychic being sometimes sends down an emanation which resides in a human being and prepares it until it is ready for the psychic being itself to enter into the life. This happens when some special work has to be done and the human vehicle prepared. Such a descent produces a remarkable change of a sudden character in the personality and the nature.

5. Usually, a soul follows continuously the same line of sex. If there are shiftings of sex, it is, as a rule, a matter of parts of the personality which are not central.

6. As regards the stage at which the soul returning for rebirth enters the new body no rule can be laid down, for the

circumstances vary with the individual. Some psychic beings get into relation with the birth-environment and the parents from the time of conception and determine the preparation of the personality and future in the embryo, others join only at the time of delivery, others even later on in the life and in these cases it is some emanation of the psychic being which upholds the life. It should be noted that the conditions of the future birth are determined fundamentally not during the stay in the psychic world but at the time of death — the psychic being then chooses what it should work out in the next terrestrial appearance and the conditions arrange themselves accordingly.

Note that the idea of rebirth and the circumstances of the new life as a reward or punishment of *puṇya* or *pāpa* is a crude human idea of "justice" which is quite unphilosophical and unspiritual and distorts the true intention of life. Life here is an evolution and the soul grows by experience, working out by it this or that in the nature, and if there is suffering, it is for the purpose of that working out, not as a judgment inflicted by God or Cosmic Law on the errors or stumblings which are inevitable in the Ignorance.

*
**

It is difficult to give a positive answer to these questions, because no general rule can be laid down applicable to all. The mind makes rigid rules or one rigid rule, but the Manifestation is in reality very plastic and various and many-sided. My answers therefore must not be taken as exhaustive of the subject or complete.

1. He [the Jivanmukta] can go wherever his aim was fixed, into a state of Nirvana or one of the divine worlds and stay there or remain, wherever he may go, in contact with the earth-movement and return to it if his will is to help that movement.

This [going direct from the world of the soul's present highest achievement to a still higher world] is doubtful. If originally he is not a being of the evolution but of some higher world, he would go back to that world. If he wants to go higher, it is logical that he should return to the field of evolution so long as he has not evolved the consciousness proper to that higher plane.

The orthodox idea that even the gods have to come to earth if they want salvation may be applied to this ascension also. If he is originally an evolutionary being (Ramakrishna's distinction of the Jivakoti and Ishwarakoti may be extended to this also), he must proceed by the evolutionary path to either the negative withdrawal through Nirvana or some positive divine fulfilment in the increasing manifestation of Sachchidananda.

As to the impossibility of return, that is a knotty question. A divine being can always return — as Ramakrishna said, the Ishwarakoti can at will ascend or descend the stair between Birth and Immortality. For the others, it is probable that they may rest for a relative infinity of time, *śāśvatīḥ samāḥ*, if that is the will in them, but a return cannot be barred out unless they have reached their highest possible status.

No, that [return to the psychic world before a new birth] is part of the evolutionary line only, not obligatory for divine returns.

2. An advanced psychic being may mean here one who has arrived at the soul's freedom and is immersed in the Divine — immersed does not mean abolished. Such a being does not sleep in the psychic world, but may remain in his state of blissful immersion or come back for some purpose.

The word "descend" has various meanings according to the context — I used it here in the sense of the psychic being coming down into the human consciousness and body ready for it; that descent might be at the time of birth or before or it may come down later and occupy the personality it has prepared for itself. I do not quite understand what are these personalities from above — it is the psychic being itself that takes up a body.

3. No, the psychic being cannot take up more than one body. There is only one psychic being for each human being, but the beings of the higher planes, e.g., the Gods of the overmind can manifest in more than one human body at a time by sending different emanations into different bodies. These would be called Vibhutis of these Devatas.

4. These [the Guardians of the psychic world] are not human souls nor is this an office to which they are appointed nor are they functionaries — these are beings of the psychic plane pur-

suing their own natural activity in that plane. My word "guardian" was simply a phrase meant to indicate by an image or metaphor the nature of their action.

The escape from birth was a universal ideal at that time except with one or two sects of the Shaivas, I believe. It is not at all consistent with the Divine taking many births, for the Gita speaks of the highest condition not as a *laya*, but as a dwelling in the Divine. If so there seems to be no reason why the *mukta* and *siddha* who has reached that dwelling in the consciousness of the Divine should fear rebirth and its troubles any more than the Divine does.

The Pitriyan is supposed to lead to inferior worlds attained by the Fathers who still belong to the evolution in the Ignorance. By the Devayan one gets beyond the Ignorance into the light. The difficulty about the Pitris is that in the Puranas they are taken as the Ancestors to whom the Tarpan is given — it is an old Ancestor worship such as still exists in Japan, but in the Veda they seem to be the Fathers who have gone before and discovered the supraphysical worlds.

The psychic being at the time of death chooses what it will work out in the next birth and determines the character and conditions of the new personality. Life is for the evolutionary growth by experience in the conditions of the Ignorance till one is ready for the higher Light.

The dying wish of the man is only something on the surface — it may be determined by the psychic and so help to shape the future but it does not determine the psychic's choice. That is something behind the veil. It is not the outer consciousness's action that determines the inner process, but the other way round. Sometimes, however, there are signs or fragments of the inner action that come up on the surface, e.g. some people have a vision or remembrance of the circumstances of their past in a panoramic flash at the time of death, that is the psychic's review of the life before departing.

The psychic being's choice at the time of death does not *work out* the next formation of personality, it *fixes* it. When it enters the psychic world, it begins to assimilate the essence of its experience and by that assimilation is formed the future psychic personality in accordance with the fixation already made. When this assimilation is over, it is ready for a new birth; but the less developed beings do not work out the whole thing for themselves, there are beings and forces of the higher world who have that work. Also, when it comes to birth, it is not sure that the forces of the physical world will not come across the working out of what it wanted — its own new instrumentation may not be strong enough for that purpose; for, there is the interaction of its own energies and the cosmic forces here. There may be frustration, diversion, a partial working out — many things may happen. All that is not a rigid machinery, it is a working out of complex forces. It may be added, however, that a developed psychic being is much more conscious in this transition and works out much of it itself. The time depends also on the development and on a certain rhythm of the being — for some there is practically immediate rebirth, for others it takes longer, for some it may take centuries; but here, again, once the psychic being is sufficiently developed, it is free to choose its own rhythm and its own intervals. The ordinary theories are too mechanical — and that is the case also with the idea of *puṇya* and *pāpa* and their results in the next life. There are certainly results of the energies put forth in a past life, but not on that rather infantile principle. A good man's suffering in this life would be a proof according to the orthodox theory that he had been a very great villain in his past life, a bad man's prospering would be a proof that he had been quite angelic in his last visit to earth and sown a large crop of virtues and meritorious actions to reap this bumper crop of good fortune. Too symmetrical to be true. The object of birth being growth by experience, whatever reactions come to past deeds must be for the being to learn and grow, not as lollipops for good boys of the class (in the past) and canings for the bad ones. The real sanction for good and ill is not good fortune for the one and bad fortune for the other, but this that good leads us towards a higher nature which is eventually lifted above suffering, and ill pulls us towards the lower nature which remains always in the circle of suffering and evil.

***

There is no such thing as an insuperable difficulty from past lives. There are formations that help and formations that hamper; the latter have to be dismissed and dissolved, not to be allowed to repeat themselves. The Mother told you that to explain the origin of this tendency and the necessity of getting rid of it — there was no hint of any insuperable difficulty, quite the contrary.

***

These words [*mūḍhayoniṣu* or *adho gacchanti*] do not necessarily refer to the animal birth, but it is true that there has been a general belief of that kind not only in India but wherever "transmigration" or "metempsychosis" was believed in. Shakespeare is referring to Pythagoras's belief in transmigration when he speaks of the passage of somebody's grandmother into an animal. But the soul, the psychic being, once having reached the human consciousness cannot go back to the inferior animal consciousness any more than it can go back into a tree or an ephemeral insect. What is true is that some part of the vital energy or the formed instrumental consciousness or nature can and very frequently does so, if it is strongly attached to anything in the earth life. This may account for some cases of immediate rebirth with full memory in human forms also. Ordinarily. it is only by yogic development or by clairvoyance that the exact memory of past lives can be brought back.

It is when the vital gets broken up, some strong movements of it, desires, greeds, may precipitate themselves into animal forms, e.g., sexual desire with the part of the vital consciousness under its control into a dog or some habitual movement of excessive greed may carry part of the vital consciousness into a pig. The animals represent the vital consciousness with mind involved in the vital, so that it is naturally there that such things would gravitate for satisfaction.

The fragments [of a dead person] are not of the inner being (who goes on his way to the psychic world) but of his vital sheath which falls away after death. These can join for birth the vital of some other Jiva who is being born or they can be used by a vital being to enter a body in process of birth and partly possess it for the satisfaction of its propensities. The junction can also take place after birth.

All human incarnations or births have naturally a psychic being. It is only other types like the vital beings that have not, and that is precisely the reason why they want to possess men and enjoy physical life without being themselves born here, for so they escape the psychic law of evolution and spiritual progress and change. But these formations [vital fragments of a dead person] are different, they are things that do not leave the earth and do not possess but simply attach themselves to some human rebirth (of course with a psychic in it) which has some affinity and therefore does not object to or resist their inclusion.

Āsuriṣu[1] cannot possibly mean "animal". The Gita uses precise terms and if it had meant animal it would have said animal and not Asuric. As for the punishment, it is that they go down in their nature to more depths of Asurism till they touch bottom as it were. But that is a natural result of their uncontrolled tendencies which they freely indulge without any effort to rise out of them while in the cultivation of the higher side of personality one naturally rises and develops towards godhead or the Divine. In the Gita the Divine is regarded as the controller of the whole cosmic action through Nature, so the "I cast" is in harmony with its ideas! The world is a mechanism of Nature, but a mechanism regulated by the presence of the Divine.

As far as I know, the births follow usually one line or the other and do not alternate — that, I think, is the Indian tradition also, though there are purposeful exceptions like Shikhandi's. If there is a change of sex, it is only part of the being that associates itself with the change, not the central being.

What do you mean by the popular idea? All the instances I have heard of in the popular accounts of rebirth are of man becoming man and woman becoming woman in the next life — except when they become animal, but even then I think the male becomes a male animal and the female a female animal. There are only stray cases quoted like Shikhandi's in the Mahabharata for variations of sex. The Theosophist conception is full of raw imagination, one Theosophist even going so far as to say that if you are a man in this birth you are obliged to be a woman in the next and so on.

Not sex exactly, but what might be called the masculine and

---

[1] *Kṣipāmyajasram aśubhàn asurīṣveva yoniṣu.* "I cast down continually into more and more Asuric births." *Gita,* Ch. XVI. 19.

feminine principle [is there in the psychic being]. It is a difficult question [whether sex is altered in rebirth]. There are certain lines the reincarnation follows and so far as my experience goes and general experience goes, one follows usually a single line. But the alteration of sex cannot be declared impossible. There may be some who do alternate. The presence of feminine traits in a male does not necessarily indicate a past feminine birth — they may come in the general play of forces and their formations. There are besides qualities common to both sexes. Also a fragment of the psychological personality may have been associated with a birth not one's own. One can say of a certain person of the past, "that was not myself, but a fragment of my psychological personality was present in him." Rebirth is a complex affair and not so simple in its mechanism as in the popular idea.

The question as put in your letter seems to me to be too rigidly phrased and not to take into sufficient account the plasticity of the facts and forces of existence. It sounds like the problem which one might raise on the strength of the most recent scientific theories — if all is made up of protons and electrons, all exactly similar to each other (except for the group numbers, and why should a difference of quantity make such an extraordinary difference or any difference of quality?) how does their action result in such stupendous differences of degree, kind, power, everything? But why should we assume that the psychic seeds or sparks all started in a race at the same time, equal in conditions, equal in power and nature? Granted that the One Divine is the source of all and the Self is the same in all; but in manifestation why should not the Infinite throw itself out in infinite variety, why must it be in an innumerable sameness? How many of these psychic seeds started long before others and have a great past of development behind them and how many are young and raw and half-grown only? And even among those who started together, why should not there be some who ran at a great speed and others who loitered and grew with difficulty or went about in circles? And then there is an evolution, and it is only at a certain stage in the evolution that the animal belt is past and there is a human beginning; what constitutes the human beginning, which represents a very considerable revolution or turnover? Up to the animal line it is the vital and physical that have been developing — for the human to begin is it not necessary that there should be the descent of a mental being to take up the vital and physical evolution? And may it not well be that the mental beings who descend are not all of the same power and stature and, besides, do not take up equally developed vital and physical consciousness-material? There is also the occult tradition of a hierarchy of beings who stand above the present manifestation and put themselves into it with results which will obviously be just such a stupendous difference of degrees, and even intervene by descending into the play through the gates of birth in human Nature. There are many complexities and the problem cannot be put with the rigidity of a mathematical formula.

A great part of the difficulty of these problems, I mean especially the appearance of inexplicable contradiction, arises from the problem itself being badly put. Take the popular account of reincarnation and Karma — it is based on the mere mental assumption that the workings of Nature ought to be moral and proceed according to an exact morality of equal justice — a scrupulous, even mathematical law of reward and punishment or, at any rate, of results according to a human idea of right correspondences. But Nature is non-moral — she uses forces and processes moral, immoral and amoral pell-mell for working out her business. Nature in her outward aspect seems to care for nothing except to get things done — or else to make conditions for an ingenious variety of the play of life. Nature in her deeper aspect as a conscious spiritual Power is concerned with the growth, by experience, the spiritual development of the souls she has in her charge — and these souls themselves have a say in the matter. All these good people lament and wonder that unaccountably they and other good people are visited with such meaningless sufferings and misfortunes. But are they really visited with them by an outside Power or by a mechanical Law of Karma? Is it not possible that the soul itself — not the outward mind, but the spirit within — has accepted and chosen these things as part of its development in order to get through the necessary experience at a rapid rate, to hew through, *durchhauen*, even at the risk or the cost of much damage to the outward life and the body? To the growing soul, to the spirit within us, may not difficulties, obstacles, attacks be a means of growth, added strength, enlarged experience, training for spiritual victory? The arrangement of things may be that and not a mere question of the pounds, shillings and pence of a distribution of rewards and retributory misfortunes!

It is the same with the problem of the taking of animal life under the circumstances put forward by your friend in the letter. It is put on the basis of an invariable ethical right and wrong to be applied to all cases — is it right to take animal life at all, under any circumstances, is it right to allow an animal to suffer under your eyes when you can relieve it by an euthanasia? There can be no indubitable answer to a question put like that, because the answer depends on data which the mind has not before it. In fact there are many other factors which make people incline to this short and merciful way out of the difficulty — the nervous inability to bear the sight and hearing of so much suffering, the unavailing trouble, the disgust and inconvenience — all tend to give force to the idea that the animal itself would want to be out of it. But what does the animal really feel about it — may it not be clinging to life in spite of the pain? Or may not the soul have accepted these things for a quicker evolution into a higher state of life? If so, the mercy dealt out may conceivably interfere with the animal's Karma. In fact the right decision might vary in each case and depend on a knowledge which the human mind has not — and it might very well be said that until it has it, it has not the right to take life. It was some dim perception of this truth that made religion and ethics develop the law of Ahimsa — and yet that too becomes a mental rule which it is found impossible to apply in practice. And perhaps the moral of it all is that we must act for the best according to our lights in each case, as things are, but that the solution of these problems can only come by pressing forward towards a greater light, a greater consciousness in which the problems themselves, as now stated by the human mind, will not arise because we shall have a vision which will see the world in a different way and a guidance which at present is not ours. The mental or moral rule is a stop-gap which men are obliged to use, very uncertainly and stumblingly, until they can see things whole in the light of the spirit.

You must avoid a common popular blunder about reincarnation. The popular idea is that Titus Balbus is reborn again as John Smith, a man with the same personality, character, attainments as he had in his former life with the sole difference that he wears coat and trousers instead of a toga and speaks in cockney English instead of popular Latin. That is not the case. What would be the earthly use of repeating the same personality or character a million times from the beginning of time till its end? The soul comes into birth for experience, for growth, for evolution till it can bring the Divine into Matter. It is the central being that in-carnates, not the outer personality — the personality is simply a mould that it creates for its figures of experience in that one life. In another birth it will create for itself a different personality, different capacities, a different life and career. Supposing Virgil is born again, he may take up poetry in one or two other lives, but he will certainly not write an epic but rather perhaps slight but elegant and beautiful lyrics such as he wanted to write, but did not succeed, in Rome. In another birth he is likely to be no poet at all, but a philosopher and a yogin seeking to attain and to express the highest truth — for that too was an unrealised trend of his consciousness in that life. Perhaps before he had been a warrior or ruler doing deeds like Aeneas or Augustus before he sang them. And so on — on this side or that the central being develops a new character, a new personality, grows, deve-lops, passes through all kinds of terrestrial experience.

As the evolving being develops still more and becomes more rich and complex, it accumulates its personalities, as it were. Sometimes they stand behind the active elements, throwing in some colour, some trait, some capacity here and there, — or they stand in front and there is a multiple personality, a many-sided character or a many-sided, sometimes what looks like a universal capacity. But if a former personality, a former capacity is brought fully forward, it will not be to repeat what was already done, but to cast the same capacity into new forms and new shapes and fuse it into a new harmony of the being which will not be a reproduction of what was before. Thus you must not expect to be what the warrior and the poet were. Something of the outer characteristics may reappear but very much changed and new-cast in a new combination. It is in a new direction that the energies will be guided to do what was not done before.

Another thing. It is not the personality, the character that is of the first importance in rebirth — it is the psychic being who stands behind the evolution of the nature and evolves with it. The psychic when it departs from the body, shedding even the mental and vital on its way to its resting place, carries with it the heart of its experiences, — not the physical events, not the vital movements, not the mental buildings, not the capacities or cha-racters, but something essential that it gathered from them, what might be called the divine element for the sake of which the rest existed. That is the permanent addition, it is that that helps in the growth towards the Divine. That is why there is usually no memory of the outward events and circumstances of past lives— for this memory there must be a strong development towards un-broken continuance of the mind, the vital, even the subtle physi-cal; for though it all remains in a kind of seed memory, it does not ordinarily emerge. What was the divine element in the mag-nanimity of the warrior, that which expressed itself in his loyalty, nobility, high courage, what was the divine element behind the harmonious mentality and generous vitality of the poet and expressed itself in them, that remains and in a new harmony of character may find a new expression or, if the life is turned towards the Divine, be taken up as powers for the realisation or for the work that has to be done for the Divine.

The non-materialistic European idea makes a distinction between soul and body — the body is perishable, the mental-vital con-sciousness is the immortal soul and remains always the same (horrible idea!) in heaven as on earth or if there is rebirth it is also the same damned personality that comes back and makes a similar fool of itself.

The being as it passes through the series of its lives takes on various kinds of personalities and passes through various types of experiences, but it does not carry these on to the next life, as a rule. It takes on a new mind, vital and body. The mental capacities, occupations, interests, idiosyncrasies of the past mind and vital are not taken over by the new mind and vital, except to the extent that is useful for the new life. One may have the power of poetic expression in one life, but in the next not have any such power or any interest in poetry. On the other hand, tendencies suppressed or missed or imperfectly developed in one life may come out in the next. There would be therefore nothing surprising in the contrast which you noted. The essence of past experiences is kept by the psychic being but the forms of experience or of personality are not, except such as are needed for the new stage in the soul's progress.

The being in its long course of experience may permit for a time the search after sensual pleasure and afterwards discard it and turn to higher things. This can happen even in the course of a life-time, *a fortiori* in a second life where the old personalities would not be carried over.

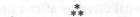

I do not remember the context in which the phrase ["other forces"] was used. But what you suggest is true — that is to say when it is some past personality which or part of which is strongly carried over into the present life. It is, I believe, true that you were a revolutionary in a past life or if not a revolutionary, engaged in a violent political action. I can't put a name or a precise form on it. But it was not only the sudden angers and violences, but probably also the desire to help, to reform, to purify and other intensities and vehemences that came from there. When a personality is carried over like that it is not only the un-

desirable sides that are carried over but things that purified and
chastened can be useful.

Certainly, the subconscient is formed for this life only and is not
carried with it by the soul from one life to another. The memory
of past lives is not something that is active anywhere in the
being — if by memory is meant the memory of details. That
memory of details is quiescent and untraceable except in so far
as certain constituent personalities taken over from the past
retain the memories of the particular life in which they were
manifest. E.g. if some personality that was put forth by one in
Venice or Rome remembers from time to time a detail or details
of what happened then. But usually it is only the essence of past
lives that is activised in the being, not any particular memories.
So it is impossible to say that the memory is located in a particular part of the consciousness or in a particular plane.

No, the subconscient is the instrument for the physical life and
disappears [after death]. It is too incoherent to be an organized
enduring existence.

For most people the vital dissolves after a time as it is not sufficiently formed to be immortal. The soul descending makes a
new vital formation suitable for the new life.

If one has had a strong spiritual development that makes it easier
to retain the developed mental or vital after death. But it is not
absolutely necessary that the person should have been a Bhakta
or a Jnani. One like Shelley or like Plato for instance could be
said to have a developed mental being centred round the psychic
— of the vital the same can hardly be said. Napoleon had a

strong vital, but not one organised round the psychic being.

[Survival of the "centres" after death:] Not *as* they are. What remains and to what degree depends on the development in each case. Of course the centres themselves remain — for they are in the subtle body and it is from there that they act on the corresponding physical centres.

As there are many personalities in a man in his conscious ordinary planes of consciousness, so also several beings can associate themselves with his consciousness as it develops afterwards — descending into his higher mind or other higher planes of being and connecting themselves with his personality. That is for the principle. But as for the particular information, it is inaccurate. It has probably reference to the period when Mother was bringing down beings to aid in the work.

It is always possible for a being of the higher planes to take birth on earth — in that case they create a mind or vital for themselves or else they join a mind, vital and body which has already been prepared under their influence — there are indeed many ways and not one only in which they can manifest here.

But too much importance must not be given to past lives. For the purpose of this yoga one is what one is and, still more, what one will be. What one was has a minor importance.

Seriously, these historical identifications are a perilous game and open a hundred doors to the play of imagination. Some may, in the nature of things must, be true; but once people begin, they don't know where to stop. What is important is the lines, rather than the lives, the incarnation of Forces that explain what one now is — and, as for the particular lives or rather personalities, those alone matter which are very definite in one and have powerfully contributed to what one is developing now. But it is not always possible to put a name upon these; for not one hundred-thousandth part of what has been has still a name preserved by human Time.

It is a little difficult to explain. When one gets a new body, the nature which inhabits it, nature of mind, nature of vital, nature of physical, is made up of many personalities, not one simple personality as is supposed — although there is one central being. This complex personality is formed partly by bringing together personalities of past lives, but also by gathering experiences, tendencies, influences from the earth atmosphere — which are taken up by one of the constituent personalities as suitable to his own nature. Such an influence left behind by X or one of his disciples may have been taken up by you without your being an incarnation of either.

These things [seeing Buddha, Ramakrishna, Vivekananda, Shankara frequently in vision] are the result of past thoughts and influences. They are of various kinds — sometimes merely thought-forms created by one's own thought-force to act as a vehicle for some mental realisation — sometimes Powers of different planes that take these forms as a support for their work through the individual, — but sometimes one is actually in communion with that which had the name and form and personality of Buddha or Ramakrishna or Vivekananda or Shankara.

It is not necessary to have an element akin to these personalities — a thought, an aspiration, a formation of the mind or vital are enough to create the connection — it is sufficient for a vibration of response anywhere to what these Powers represent.

The Mother only speaks to people about their past births when she sees definitely some scene or memory of their past in concentration; but this happens rarely nowadays.

What is remembered mainly from past lives is the nature of the personality and the subtle results of the life-experience. Names, events, physical details are remembered only under exceptional circumstances and are of a very minor importance. When people try to remember these outward things they usually build up a number of romantic imaginations which are not true.

I think you should dismiss this idea about the past lives. If the memory of past personalities comes of itself (without a name or mere outward details) that is sometimes important as giving a clue to something in the present development, but to know the nature of that personality and its share in the present constitution of the character is quite enough. The rest is of little use.

It is not necessary to attach any entire belief to these ideas of past births. X's idea of Y's rebirth is evidently a mere idea — nothing else.

When there is any truth in these things, it is most often a perception that some Force once represented in a certain person has also some part in one's own nature — not that the same personality is here.

Of course, there is rebirth, but to establish that one is such a one reborn, a deeper experience is necessary, not a mere mental intuition which may easily be an error.

Ideas of this kind about X and Y are ideas of the mind to which the vital strongly attaches itself — the truth of the past lives cannot be discovered in that way. These mental ideas are not true. You must wait for direct knowledge in a liberated nature before you can know who in past lives you were.

The psychic does not give up the mental and other sheaths (apart from the physical) immediately at death. It is said that it takes three years on the whole to get clear away from the zone of communicability with the earth — though there may be cases of slower or quicker passage. The psychic world does not communicate with earth — at any rate, not in that way. And the ghost or spirit who turns up at seances is not the psychic being. What comes through the medium is a mixture of the medium's subconscient (using subconscient in the ordinary, not in the yogic sense) and that of the sitters, vital sheaths left by the departed or perhaps occupied or used by some spirit or some vital being, the departed himself in his vital sheath or else something assumed for the occasion (but it is the vital part that communicates), elementals, spirits of the lowest vital physical world near earth, etc., etc. A horrible confusion for the most part — a hotch-potch of all sorts of things coming through a medium of "astral" grey light and shadow. Many communicants seem to be people who have just gone across into a subtle world where they feel surrounded by an improved edition of the earthly life and think that that is the real and definitive other world after earth — but it is a mere optimistic prolongation of the ideas and images and associations of the human plane. Hence the next world as depicted by the spiritualist "guides" and other seance communicants.

Not much confidence can be placed in all that [communications from spirit guides]. If examined closely it will be seen that these spirit guides only suggest to their subjects what is in the mind of the sitter or sitters or in the air and it comes to very little. Influences from the other worlds there are of course and any number of them, but the central guidance is not of this kind except in very rare cases.

**

Automatic writings and spiritualistic seances are a very mixed affair. Part comes from the subconscious mind of the medium and part from that of the sitters. But it is not true that all can be accounted for by a dramatising imagination and memory. Sometimes there are things none present could know or remember; sometimes even, though that is rare, glimpses of the future. But usually these seances etc. put one into *rapport* with a very low world of vital beings and forces, themselves obscure, incoherent or tricky and it is dangerous to associate with them or to undergo any influence. Ouspensky and others must have gone through these experiments with too "mathematical" a mind, which was no doubt their safeguard but prevented them from coming to anything more than a surface intellectual view of their significance.

**

What do you mean by a ghost? The word "ghost" as used in popular parlance covers an enormous number of distinct phenomena which have no necessary connection with each other. To name a few only:

1. An actual contact with the soul of a human being in its subtle body and transcribed to our mind by the appearance of an image or the hearing of a voice.

2. A mental formation stamped by the thoughts and feelings of a departed human being on the atmosphere of a place or locality, wandering about there or repeating itself, till that formation either exhausts itself or is dissolved by one means or another. This is the explanation of such phenomena as the haunted house in which the scenes attending or surrounding or preceding a murder are repeated over and over again and many other similar phenomena.

3. A being of the lower vital planes who has assumed the discarded vital sheath of a departed human being or a fragment of his vital personality and appears and acts in the form and perhaps

with the surface thoughts and memories of that person.

4. A being of the lower vital plane who by the medium of a living human being or by some other means or agency is able to materialise itself sufficiently so as to appear and act in a visible form or speak with an audible voice or, without so appearing, to move about material things, e.g., furniture or to materialise objects or to shift them from place to place. This accounts for what are called *poltergeists,* phenomena of stone-throwing, tree-inhabiting Bhutas, and other well-known phenomena.

5. Apparitions which are the formations of one's own mind and take to the senses an objective appearance.

6. Temporary possession of people by vital beings who sometimes pretend to be departed relatives etc.

7. Thought-images of themselves projected, often by people at the moment of death, which appear at that time or a few hours afterwards to their friends or relatives.

You will see that in only one of these cases, the first, can a soul be posited and there no difficulty arises.

Each person follows in the world his own line of destiny which is determined by his own nature and actions — the meaning and necessity of what happens in a particular life cannot be understood except in the light of the whole course of many lives. But this can be seen by those who can get beyond the ordinary mind and feelings and see things as a whole, that even errors, misfortunes, calamities are steps in the journey, — the soul gathering experience as it passes through and beyond them until it is ripe for the transition which will carry it beyond these things to a higher consciousness and higher life. When one comes to that line of crossing, one has to leave behind one the old mind and feelings. One looks then on those who are still fixed in the pleasures and sorrows of the ordinary world with sympathy and wherever it is possible with spiritual helpfulness, but no longer with attachment. One learns that they are being led through all their stumblings and trusts to the Universal Power that is watching and supporting their existence to do for them whatever for them is the best. But the one thing that is really important for us is to get into the greater Light and the Divine Union — to turn to the Divine alone, to put our trust there alone whether for ourselves or for others.

It is a very intricate and difficult question to tackle and it can hardly be answered in a few words. Moreover, it is impossible to give a general rule as to why there are these close inner contacts followed by a physical separation through death — in each case there is a difference and one would have to know the persons and be familiar with their soul history to tell what was behind their meeting and separation. In a general way, a life is only one brief episode in a long history of spiritual evolution in which the soul follows the curve of the line set for the earth, passing through many lives to complete it. It is an evolution out of material inconscience to consciousness and towards the Divine Consciousness, from ignorance to Divine Knowledge, from darkness through half-light to Light, from death to Immortality, from suffering to the Divine Bliss. Suffering is due first to the Ignorance, secondly to the separation of the individual consciousness from the Divine Consciousness and Being, a separation created by the Ignorance — when that ceases, when one lives in the Divine and no more in one's separated smaller self, then only suffering can altogether cease. Each soul follows its own line and these lines meet, journey together for a space, then part to meet again perhaps hereafter — they meet once more to help each other on the journey in one way or another. As for the after-death period, the soul passes into other planes of existence, staying there for a while till it reaches its place of rest where it remains until it is ready for another terrestrial existence. This is the general law, but for the connections of embodied souls, that is a matter of personal evolution of the two on which nothing general can be said, as it is intimate to the soul stories of the two and needs a personal knowledge. That is all I can say, but I don't know that it will be of much help to her as these things are helpful usually only when one enters into the consciousness in which they become not mere ideas but realities. Then one grieves no longer because one has entered into the Truth and the Truth brings calm and peace.

There is a vital connection generally — the psychic is comparatively rare. It is something in past lives usually that determines these connections in this one, but the connection in this life is seldom the same as that of the past which determined it.

I can understand the shock your wife's catastrophic death must have been to you. But you are now a seeker and sadhak of the Truth and must set your mind to rise above the normal reactions of the human being and see things in a larger greater light. Regard your lost wife as a soul that was progressing through the vicissitudes of the life of Ignorance — like all others here; in that progress things happen that seem unfortunate to the human mind and a sudden accidental or violent death cutting short prematurely this always brief spell of terrestrial experience we call life seems to it especially painful and unfortunate. But one who gets behind the outward view knows that all that happens in the progress of the soul has its meaning, its necessity, its place in the series of experiences which are leading it towards the turning-point where one can pass from the Ignorance to the Light. He knows that whatever happens in the Divine Providence is for the best, even though it may seem to the mind otherwise. Look on your wife as a soul that has passed the barrier between two states of existence. Help her journey towards her place of rest by calm thoughts and the call to the Divine Help to aid her upon it. Grief too long continued does not help but delays the journey of the departed soul. Do not brood on your loss, but think only of her spiritual welfare.

What has happened must now be accepted calmly as the thing decreed and best for his soul's progress from life to life, though not the best in human eyes which look only at the present and at outside appearance. For the spiritual seeker death is only a passage from one form of life to another, and none is dead but only departed. Look at it as that and shaking from you all reactions of vital grief, — that cannot help him in his journey, — pursue steadfastly the path to the Divine.

Of course, that is the real fact — death is only a shedding of the body, not a cessation of the personal existence. A man is not dead because he goes into another country and changes his clothes to suit that climate.

FATE AND FREE-WILL, KARMA
AND HEREDITY, ETC.

Fate and Free-Will, Karma
and Heredity, etc.

YOUR extracts taken by themselves are very impressive, but when one reads the book, the impression made diminishes and fades away. You have quoted Cheiro's successes, but what about his failures? I have looked at the book and was rather staggered by the number of prophecies that have failed to come off. You can't deduce from a small number of predictions, however accurate, that all is predestined down to your putting the questions in the letter and my answer. It may be, but the evidence is not sufficient to prove it. What is evident is that there is an element of the predictable, predictable accurately and in detail as well as in large points, in the course of events. But that was already known; it leaves the question still unsolved whether all is predictable, whether destiny is the sole factor in existence or there are other factors also that can modify destiny, — or, destiny being given, there are not different sources or powers or planes of destiny and we can modify the one with which we started by calling in another destiny source, power or plane and making it active in our life. Metaphysical questions are not so simple that they can be trenchantly solved either in one sense or in another contradictory to it — that is the popular way of settling things, but it is quite summary and inconclusive. All is free-will or else all is destiny — it is not so simple as that. This question of free-will or determination is the most knotty of all metaphysical questions and nobody has been able to solve it — for a good reason that both destiny and will exist and even a free-will exists somewhere; the difficulty is only how to get at it and make it effective.

Astrology? Many astrological predictions come true, quite a mass of them, if one takes all together. But it does not follow that the stars rule our destiny; the stars merely record a destiny that has been already formed, they are a hieroglyph, not a Force, — or if their action constitutes a force, it is a transmitting energy, not an originating Power. Someone is there who has determined or something is there which is Fate, let us say; the stars are only indicators. The astrologers themselves say that there are two forces, *daiva* and *puruṣakāra*, fate and individual energy, and the individual energy can modify and even frustrate fate. Moreover, the stars often indicate several fate-possibilities; for example that one may die in mid-age, but that if that determination can be overcome, one can live to a predictable old age. Finally, cases are seen in which the predictions of the horoscope fulfil themselves with great accuracy up to a certain age, then apply no more. This often happens when the subject turns away from the ordinary to the spiritual life. If the turn is very radical, the cessation of predictability may be immediate; otherwise certain results may still last on for a time, but there is no longer the same inevitability. This would seem to show that there is or can be a higher power or higher plane or higher source of spiritual destiny which can, if its hour has come, override the lower power, lower plane or lower source of vital and material fate of which the stars are indicators. I say vital because character can also be indicated from the horoscope much more completely and satisfactorily than the events of the life.

The Indian explanation of fate is Karma. We ourselves are our own fate through our actions, but the fate created by us binds us; for what we have sown, we must reap in this life or another. Still we are creating our fate for the future even while undergoing old fate from the past in the present. That gives a meaning to our will and action and does not, as European critics wrongly believe, constitute a rigid and sterilising fatalism. But again, our will and action can often annul or modify even the past Karma, it is only certain strong effects, called *utkaṭa karma*, that are non-modifiable. Here too the achievement of the spiritual consciousness and life is supposed to annul or give the power to annul Karma. For we enter into union with the Will Divine, cosmic or transcendent, which can annul what it had sanctioned for certain conditions, new-create what it had created, the narrow fixed lines disappear, there is a more plastic freedom and wideness. Neither Karma nor Astrology therefore points to a rigid and for ever immutable fate.

As for prophecy, I have never met or known of a prophet, however reputed, who was infallible. Some of their predictions come true to the letter, others do not, — they half-fulfil or misfire entirely. It does not follow that the power of prophecy is unreal or the accurate predictions can be all explained by probability, chance, coincidence. The nature and number of those that cannot is too great. The variability of fulfilment may be explained either by an imperfect power in the prophet sometimes active, sometimes failing or by the fact that things are predictable in part only, they are determined in part only or else by different factors or lines of power, different series of potentials and actuals. So long as one is in touch with one line, one predicts accurately, otherwise not — or if the lines of power change, one's prophecy also goes off the rails. All the same, one may say, there must be, if things are predictable at all, some power or plane through which or on which all is foreseeable; if there is a divine Omniscience and Omnipotence, it must be so. Even then what is foreseen has to be worked out, actually is worked out by a play of forces, — spiritual, mental, vital and physical forces — and in that plane of forces there is no absolute rigidity discoverable. Personal will or endeavour is one of those forces. Napoleon when asked why he believed in Fate, yet was always planning and acting, answered, "Because it is fated that I should work and plan"; in other words, his planning and acting were part of Fate, contributed to the results Fate had in view. Even if I foresee an adverse result, I must work for the one that I consider should be; for it keeps alive the force, the principle of Truth which I serve and gives it a possibility to triumph hereafter so that it becomes part of the working of the future favourable Fate, even if the fate of the hour is adverse. Men do not abandon a cause because they have seen it fail or foresee its failure; and they are spiritually right in their stubborn perseverance. Moreover, we do not live for outward result alone; far more the object of life is the growth of the soul, — not outward success of the hour or even of the near future. The soul can grow against or even by a material destiny that is adverse.

Finally, even if all is determined, why say that life is, in Shakespeare's phrase or rather Macbeth's, "a tale told by an idiot full of sound and fury, signifying nothing"? Life would rather be that if it were all chance and random incertitude. But if it is something foreseen, planned in every detail, does it not rather mean that life does signify something, that there must be a secret Purpose that is being worked up to, powerfully, persistently, through the ages, and ourselves are a part of it and fellow-workers in the fulfilment of that invincible Purpose?

P.S. Well, one of the greatest ecstasies possible is to feel oneself carried by the Divine, not by the stars or Karma, for the latter is a bad business, dry and uncomfortable — like being turned on a machine, "*yantrārūḍhāni māyayā*".

I am afraid I have no great confidence in Cheiro's ideas and prophecies — some prophecies are fulfilled but most have gone wrong. The idea about the Jews is an old Jewish and Christian belief; not much faith can be put in it. As for the numbers, it is true that according to occult science numbers have a mystic meaning. It is also true that there are periods and cycles in life as well as in world-life. But too exact a meaning cannot always be put in these things.

I have not said that everything is rigidly predetermined. Play of forces does not mean that. What I said was that behind visible events in the world there is always a mass of invisible forces at work unknown to the outward minds of men, and by yoga, (by going inward and establishing a conscious connection with the Cosmic Self and Force and forces,) one can become conscious of these forces, intervene consciously in the play, and to some extent at least determine things in the result of the play. All that has nothing to do with predetermination. On the contrary, one watches how things develop and gives a push here and a push there when possible or when needed. There is nothing in all that to contradict the dictum of the great scientist Sir C. V.

Raman. Raman said once that all these scientific discoveries are only games of chance. Only, when he says that scientific discoveries are games of chance, he is merely saying that human beings don't know how it works out. It is not rigid predetermination, but it is not a blind inconscient Chance either. It is a play in which there is a working out of the possibilities in Time.

It is difficult indeed to make out what Planck means in these pages — what is his conclusion and how he arrives at it; he has probably so condensed his arguments that the necessary explanatory links are missing. The free-will affair, I see by glancing through the previous pages, arises only incidentally from his position that the new discoveries grouped round the quantum theory do not make a radical difference in physics. If there is a tendency to regard laws as statistical, — in which case there is no "strict causality" and no determinism — still there is nothing to prove that they cannot be treated and may not be advantageously treated as dynamical also — in which case determinism can stand; the uncertainty of individual behaviour (electrons, quanta) does not really undermine determinism, but only brings a new feature into it. That seems from a hasty glance to be his position. Certain scientific thinkers consider this uncertainty of individual behaviour to be a physical factor correspondent to the element of free-will in individual human beings. It is here that Planck brings in the question of free-will to refute the conclusion that it affects strict causality and the law of determinism. His argument, as far as I can make it out, is this:

1. The law of strict causality stands because any given action or inner happening of the individual human being is an effect determined completely by two causes, (a) the previous state of his mind taken as a whole, (b) external influences.

2. The will is a mental process completely determined by these two factors; therefore it is not free, it is part of the chain of strict causality — as are also the results of the free-will.

3. What is important is not the actual freedom of the will, but the man's consciousness of freedom. This creates an inner

experience of conscious motive which again creates fresh motives
and so on indefinitely. For this reason it is impossible for a man
to predict his future action — for at any moment a fresh motive
may arise. But when we look back at the past, then the concate-
nation of cause and effect becomes apparent.

4. The fact of strict causality (or at least the theory of it)
stands therefore unshaken by the consciousness of free-will of
the individual. It is only obscured by the fact that a man cannot
predict his own actions or grasp the causes of his present state;
but that is because here the subject and object are the same and
this subject-object is in a state of constant alternative motion
unlike an object outside, which is supposed not to change as a
result of the inner movements of the knower.

There is a reference to causal law and ethical law which
baffles me. Is the "ethical law" something outside the strict chain
of effects and causes? Is there such a thing at all? If "strict
causality" rules all, what is such an ethical law doing there?

That is the argument so far as I can follow it, but it does not
seem to me very conclusive. If a man's conduct cannot be predicted by himself, neither can it be predicted by anyone else,
though here the subject and object are not the same; if not predictable, then it must be for the same reason, the element of free-
will and the mobility created by the possible indefinite intrusion
of fresh motives. If that is so, strict causality cannot be affirmed,
— though a plastic causality in which the power of choice called
by us free-will is an element (either as one among many contri-
butory causes or as an instrument of a cause beyond itself) can
still be asserted as possible.

The statement that the action of the individual is strictly
determined by his total mental state plus external influences is
doubtful and does not lead very far. It is possible to undermine
the whole idea of inevitable causality by holding that the total
existing state before a happening is only the condition under
which it happens — there are a mass of antecedents and there is
a sequent, if it may be so called, or a mass of sequences, but
nothing proves that the latter are inevitable consequences of the
mass of antecedents. Possibly, this total existing state is a matrix
into which some seed of happening is thrown or becomes active,

so that there may be many possible results, and in the case of human action it is conceivable that free-will is the or at least a determining factor.

I do not think therefore that these arguments of Planck carry us very far. There is also, of course, the question raised in the book itself whether, granting determinism, a local state of things is an independent field of causality or all is so bound together that it is the whole that determines the local result. A man's action then would be determined by universal forces and his state of mind and apparent choice would be part of the instrumentation of the Universal Force.

In the case of Socrates and that of the habitual drunkard raised by you, the difference you make is correct. The weak-willed man is governed by his vital and physical impulsions, his mental being is not dynamic enough to make its will prevail over them. His will is not "free" because it is not strong enough to be free, it is the slave of the forces that act on or in his vital and physical nature. In the case of Socrates the will is so far free that it stands above the play of these forces and he determines by his mental idea and resolve what he shall or shall not do. The question remains whether the will of Socrates is only free in this sense, itself being actually determined by something larger than the mentality of Socrates, something of which it is the instrument — whether the Universal Force or a Being in him of which his daemon was the voice and which not only gave his mind that decisive awareness of the mental ideal but imposed on it the drive to act in obedience to the awareness. Or it may be subject to a nexus between the inner Purusha and the Universal Force. In the latter case there would be an unstable balance between the determinism of Nature and a self-determination from within. If we start from the Sankhya view of things, that being (viz., the one of which his daemon was the voice) would be the soul or Purusha and both in the strong-willed Socrates and in the weak-willed slave of vital impulse, the action and its results would be determined by the assent or refusal of the Purusha. In the latter the Purusha gives its assent to and undergoes the play of the forces of Nature, the habit of the vital impulse, through a vital submission while the mind looks on helpless. In Socrates the Purusha has begun to emancipate itself and decide what it shall accept or shall not accept — the conscious being has begun to impose itself on the forces that act on it. This mastery has become so complete that he can largely determine his own actions and can even within certain limits not only forecast but fix the results — so that what he wants shall happen sooner or later.

As for the Superman, that is the conscious being whose emancipation is complete by his rising to a station beyond the limits of mind. He can determine his action in complete accord with an awareness which perceives all the forces acting in and on and around him and is able, instead of undergoing, to use them and even to determine.

After reading X's cogent exposition, I saw what might be said from the intellectual point of view on this question so as to link the reality of the supreme Freedom with the phenomenon of the Determinism of Nature — in a different way from his, but to the same purpose. In reality, the freedom and the determination are only two sides of the same thing — for the fundamental truth is self-determination of the cosmos and in it a secret self-determination of the individual. The difficulty arises from the fact that we live in the surface mind of ignorance, do not know what is going on behind and see only the phenomenal process of Nature. There the apparent fact is an overwhelming determinism of Nature and as our surface consciousness is part of that process, we are unable to see the other term of the biune reality. For practical purposes, on the surface there is an entire determinism in Matter — though this is now disputed by the latest school of Science. As Life emerges a certain plasticity sets in, so that it is difficult to predict anything exactly as one predicts material things that obey a rigid law. The plasticity increases with the growth of Mind, so that man can have at least a sense of free-will, of a choice of his action, of a self-movement which at least helps to determine circumstances. But this freedom is dubious because it can be declared to be an illusion, a device of Nature, part of its machinery of determination, only a seeming freedom or at most a restricted, relative and subject independence. It is only when one goes behind away from Prakriti to Purusha and upward away from Mind to spiritual Self that the side of freedom comes to be first evident and then, by unison with the Will which is above Nature, complete.

In life all sorts of things offer themselves. One cannot take anything that comes with the idea that it is sent by the Divine. There is a choice and a wrong choice produces its consequences.

Destiny in the rigid sense applies only to the outer being so long as it lives in the Ignorance. What we call destiny is only in fact the result of the present condition of the being and the nature and energies it has accumulated in the past acting on each other and determining the present attempts and their future results. But as soon as one enters the path of spiritual life, this old predetermined destiny begins to recede. There comes in a new factor, the Divine Grace, the help of a higher Divine Force other than the force of Karma, which can lift the sadhak beyond the present possibilities of his nature. One's spiritual destiny is then the divine election which ensures the future. The only doubt is about the vicissitudes of the path and the time to be taken by the passage. It is here that the hostile forces playing on the weaknesses of the past nature strive to prevent the rapidity of the progress and to postpone the fulfilment. Those who fall, fall not because of the attacks of the vital forces, but because they put themselves on the side of the hostile Force and prefer a vital ambition or desire (ambition, vanity, lust, etc.) to the spiritual siddhi.

Neither Nature nor Destiny nor the Divine work in the mental way or by the law of the mind or according to its standards — that is why even to the scientist and the philosopher Nature, Destiny, the way of the Divine all remain a mystery. The Mother does not act by the mind, so to judge her action with the mind is futile.

Nature is very largely what you make of her or can make of her.

Each has his own destiny and his entering into a particular family in one life is only an incident.

Consciousness is not a mechanical dead thing to cut in that way. Hereditary influence creates an affinity and affinity is a long thing. It is only when the hereditary part is changed that the affinity ceases.

[Stamp of heredity, race, caste and family:] A very big stamp in most cases — it is in the physical vital and physical material that the stamp chiefly exists — and it is increased by education and upbringing.

Many things in the body and some in the mind and vital are inherited from the father and mother or other ancestors — that everybody is supposed to know. There are other things that are not inherited, but peculiar to one's own nature or developed by the happenings of this life.

Karma and heredity are the two main causes [which determine

the temperament at birth]. According to some heredity is also subject to Karma, but that may be only in a general way, not in all the details.

All energies put into activity — thought, speech, feeling, act — go to constitute Karma. These things help to develop the nature in one direction or another, and the nature and its actions and reactions produce their consequences inward and outward: they also act on others and create movements in the general sum of forces which can return upon oneself sooner or later. Thoughts unexpressed can also go out as forces and produce their effects. It is a mistake to think that a thought or will can have effect only when it is expressed in speech or act: the unspoken thought, the unexpressed will are also active energies and can produce their own vibrations, effects or reactions.

Exact? How can one measure exactly where vital, mental and spiritual factors come in? In dealing with a star and atom you may (though it appears you can't with an electron) but not with a man and his living mind, soul and body.

II

What X said is true, the play of the forces is very complex and one has to be conscious of them and, as it were, see and watch how they work before one can really understand why things happen as they do. All action is surrounded by a complexity of forces and if one puts a force for one of them to succeed, one must be careful to do it thoroughly and maintain it and not leave doors open for the other contrary ones to find their way in. Each man is himself a field of many forces — some were working for his sadhana, some were working for his ego and desires. There are besides powers which seek to make a man an instrument for purposes not his own without his knowing it. All of these may combine to bring about a particular result. These forces work each for the fulfilment of its own drive — they need not be at all what we call hostile forces, — they are simply forces of Nature.

The feeling of jealousy and *abhimāna* was of course a survival from the past movements of the nature. It is so that these things go out if they are rejected; they lose their force, can stay less and less, can affect less and less the consciousness, — finally, they are able to touch no longer and so come no longer.

Anyone with some intelligence and power of observation who lives more in an inward consciousness can see the play of invisible forces at every step which act on men and bring about events without their knowing about the instrumentation. The difference created by yoga or by an inner consciousness — for there are people like Socrates who develop or have some inner consciousness without yoga — is that one becomes conscious of these invisible forces and can also consciously profit by them or use and direct them. That is all.

[Vital interchange:] Difficult to specify. There is always a drawing of vital forces from one to another in all human social mixture that takes place automatically. Love-making is one of the most powerful ways of each drawing upon the other's vital force, or of one drawing the other's, which also often happens in a one-sided way to the great detriment of the "other". In the passage come many things good and bad, elation, feeling of strength and support, infiltration of good or bad qualities, interchange of psychological moods, states and movements, depressions, exhaustion — the whole gamut. People don't know it — which is a mercy of God upon them — but when one gets into a certain yogic consciousness, one becomes very much aware and sensitive to all this interchange and action and reaction, but also one can build a wall against, reject etc. etc.

It is a wall of consciousness that one has to build. Consciousness is not something abstract, it is like existence itself or Ananda or mind or *prāṇa*, something very concrete. If one becomes aware of the inner consciousness, one can do all sorts of things with it, send it out as a stream of force, erect a circle or wall of consciousness around oneself, direct an idea so that it shall enter somebody's head in America etc. etc.

His new consciousness makes him feel more strongly the opposite forces that one contacts when one moves in the world and has to do affairs and meet with others and he is afraid of a response in the vital which will upset his sadhana or create difficulties. Evidently he is a man who is psychically sensitive or has become so to that thing which you blindly refuse to recognise even when you are in the midst of it — the play of forces. You can feel your friend's atmosphere through the letter "so beautiful, so strengthening, so refreshing" and it has an immediate effect on you. But your mind stares like an owl and wonders "What the hell can this be ?", I suppose, because your medical books never told you about it and how can things be true which are not known either to the ordinary mind or science? It is by an incursion of an opposite kind of forces that you fall into the Old Man's clutches, but you can only groan and cry, "What's this ?" and when they are swept aside in a moment by other forces blink and mutter, "Well, that's funny!" Your friend can feel and know at once when he is being threatened by the opposite forces and so he can be on his guard and resist old Nick, because he can detect at once one of his principal means of attack.

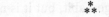

The consciousness of these things [influences of people] is intended for knowledge — a psycho-occult knowledge, necessary for the fullness of consciousness and experience. It is not intended that what is felt should be allowed to become an influence, whether a good one or a bad one.

As for the other matter, there are two different things. Some
people have a faculty for receiving impressions about others
which is not by any means infallible, but often turns out
to be right. That is one thing and the yogic intuition by which
one directly knows or feels what is in a man, his capacities,
character, temperament is another. The first may help for developing the other, but it is not the same thing. The yogic faculty
has to be and it can be complete only with a great development
of the inner consciousness.

Leave aside the question of Divine or undivine, no spiritual man
who acts dynamically is limited to physical contact — the idea
that physical contact through writing, speech, meeting is indispensable to the action of the spiritual force is self-contradictory,
for then it would not be a spiritual force. The spirit is not limited
by physical things or by the body. If you have the spiritual force,
it can act on people thousands of miles away who do not know
and never will know that you are acting on them or that they are
being acted upon — they only know that there is a force enabling
them to do things and may very well suppose it is their own great
energy and genius.

The Divine Forces are meant to be used — the mistake of man
individualised in the Ignorance is to use it for the ego and not
for the Divine. It is that that has to be set right by the union with
the Divine Consciousness and also by the widening of the individual being so that it can live consciously in the universal. Difficult it is owing to the fixed ego-habit, but it is not impossible.

All force comes from the Divine but it is more usually misused
than used spiritually or rightly.

It is certainly possible to have consciousness of things at a distance and to intervene.

The idea that yogins do not or ought not to use these powers I regard as an ascetic superstition. I believe that all yogins who have these powers do use them whenever they find that they are called on from within to do so. They may refrain if they think the use in a particular case is contrary to the Divine Will or see that preventing one evil may be opening the door to a worse or for any other valid reason, but not from any general prohibitory rule. What is forbidden to anyone with a strong spiritual sense is to be a miracle-monger, performing extraordinary things for show, for gain, for fame, out of vanity or pride. It is forbidden to use powers from mere vital motives, to make an Asuric ostentation of them or to turn them into a support for arrogance, conceit, ambition or any other of the amiable weaknesses to which human nature is prone. It is because half-baked yogins so often fall into these traps of the hostile forces that the use of yogic powers is sometimes discouraged as harmful to the user.

But it is mostly people who live much in the vital that so fall; with a strong and free and calm mind and a psychic awake and alive, such pettinesses are not likely to occur. As for those who can live in the true Divine Consciousness, certain powers are not powers at all in that sense, not, that is to say, supernatural or abnormal, but rather their normal way of seeing and acting, part of the consciousness — and how can they be forbidden or refuse to act according to their consciousness and its nature?

I suppose I have had myself an even more completely European education than you, and I have had too my period of agnostic denial, but from the moment I looked at these things I could never take the attitude of doubt and disbelief which was for so long fashionable in Europe. Abnormal, otherwise supraphysical experiences and powers, occult or yogic, have always seemed to me something perfectly natural and credible. Consciousness in its very nature could not be limited by the ordinary physical human-animal consciousness, it must have other ranges. Yogic or occult powers are no more supernatural or incredible than is supernatural or incredible the power to write a great poem or compose great music; few people can do it, as things are, — not even one in a million; for poetry and music come from the inner being and to write or to compose true and great things one has to have the passage clear between the outer mind and something in the inner being. That is why you got the poetic power as soon as you began yoga, — yogic force made the passage clear. It is the same with yogic consciousness and its powers; the thing is to get the passage clear, — for they are already within you. Of course, the first thing is to believe, aspire and, with the true urge within, make the endeavour.

Jādu (magic) is a special practice which is done by professional magicians or those who learn the art of the magician, but it is no part of yoga. What happens in yoga is that sometimes or even very commonly certain powers develop in the sadhak by which he can influence others or make them do things or make things happen that he wants. This and other yogic powers should never be used by the sadhak for egoistic purposes or to satisfy his vital desires. They can only be used when they become part of the realised divine consciousness by the Mother herself or at her command for good and unselfish purposes. There is no harm in yogic powers that come naturally as a part of the new conscious-ness and are not used for a wrong personal purpose. For instance you see something in vision or dream and that happens afterwards in the waking state. Well, that is a yogic power of prevision, knowing future things which often occurs as the con-sciousness grows; there is nothing wrong in its happening; it is part of the growth in sadhana. So with other powers. Only one must not get proud or boast or misuse the powers for the sake of desire, pride, power or the satisfaction of the ego.

The vision you saw of the man and the fire at his feet was probably a vision of the God Agni from whom flows the fire of tapasya and purification in the sadhana.

When the sadhana progresses, one almost always gets the power of vision; what one sees is true if one remains in the right consciousness. There are also wrong voices and experiences. The people who have gone mad, went mad because they were egoistic, began to think themselves great sadhaks and attach an exaggerated importance to themselves and their experiences; this made them get a wrong consciousness and wrong voices and visions and inspirations. They attached so much importance to them that they refused to listen to the Mother and finally became hostile to her because she told them they were in error and checked their delusions. Your visions and experiences are very true and good and I have explained to you what they signify — the wrong ones tried to come but you threw them away, because you were not attached to them and are fixed on the true aim of sadhana. One must not get attached to these things, but observe them simply and go on; then they become a help and cannot be a danger.

By black magic is meant the occultism of the adverse powers — the occultism of the divine Powers is quite different. One is based on unity, the other on division.

It is difficult to say [why Christ healed people] — it looks from the Bible account as if he did it as a sign that he was one sent by the Divine with power.

You are quite right. She [Madame Blavatsky] was an occultist, not a spiritual personality. What spiritual teaching she gave, seemed to be based on intellectual knowledge, not on realisation. Her attitude was Tibetan Buddhistic. She did not believe in God, but in Nirvana, miraculous powers and the Mahatmas.

It is not possible to put any credence in the stories about this Swami.... It is possible that he has practised some kind of Tantric Yoga and obtained a few occult powers, but in all that you have said about him and in the printed papers there is no trace of any spiritual realisation or experience. All that he seems to think about is occult powers and feats of thaumaturgy. Those who take their stand on occult powers divorced from spiritual experiences are not yogis of a high plane of achievement. There are yogis who behave as if they had no control over themselves — the theory is that they separate the spirit from the nature and live in their inner realisation leaving the nature to a disordered action "like a child, mad man, *piśāca* or inert object". There are others who deliberately use rough or violent speech to keep people at a distance or to test them. But the outbreak of rage of this Swami which you recount seems to have been simply an outburst of fury due to offended egoism. His judgment about Ramana Maharshi is absurd in the extreme.[1] As to his asking for the nail, hair etc. and his presenting of clothes or jumper, it was probably to establish a physical means of establishing an occult influence on you and your wife possibly by some Tantric or magic *kriyā* — in Tibet such magic processes are well-known and in common use.

I don't know whether I can throw any positive light on X's mystic experiences. The description, at any rate the latter part is not very easy to follow as it is very allusive in its expressions and not always precise enough to be clear. The first part of the experience indicates a native power of healing of whose action she herself does not know the process. It seems from her account to come from something in herself which should be from the terms she uses a larger and higher and brighter and more powerful consciousness with which she is in occasional communion but in which she does not constantly live. On the other hand another sentence seems to point to a Godhead or Divine Presence giving commands to her to guide others so that they might grow in consciousness. But she distinctly speaks of it as a greater "me" standing behind a blue diamond force. We must fall back then on the idea of a greater consciousness very high up with a feeling of divinity, a sense of considerable light and spiritual

---

[1] Absurd because the greatness of a yogi does not depend at all on how long he lives or his state of health, but on the height or the depth of his spiritual realisation and experience.

authority — perhaps in one of those higher spiritual mental planes of which I speak in *The Life Divine* and the *Letters*. The diamond light could well be native to these planes; it is usually white, but there it might well be blue; it is a light that dispels or drives away all impure things, especially a demoniac possession or the influence of some evil force. Evidently, the use of a power like this should be carefully guarded from the intrusion of any wrong element such as personal love of power, but that need not cause any apprehension as a keen inlook into oneself would be sufficient to reject it or keep it aloof. I think that is all I can say upon the data given in her letter.

About spiritism, I think, I can say this much for the present. It is quite possible for the dead or rather the departed — for they are not dead — who are still in regions near the earth to have communication with the living; sometimes it happens automatically, sometimes by an effort at communication on one side of the curtain or the other. There is no impossibility of such communication by the means used by the spiritists; usually, however, genuine communications or a contact can only be with those who are yet in a world which is a sort of idealised replica of the earth-consciousness and in which the same personality, ideas, memories persist that the person had here. But all that pretends to be communications with departed souls is not genuine, especially when it is done through a paid professional medium. There is there an enormous amount of mixture of a very undesirable kind — for apart from the great mass of unconscious suggestions from the sitters or the contributions of the medium's subliminal consciousness, one gets into contact with a world of beings which is of a very deceptive or self-deceptive illusory nature. Many of these come and claim to be the departed souls of relatives, acquaintances, well-known men, famous personalities, etc. There are also beings who pick up the discarded feelings and memories of the dead and masquerade with them. There are a great number of beings who come to such seances only to play with the consciousness of men or exercise their

powers through this contact with the earth and who dope the
mediums and sitters with their falsehoods, tricks and illusions.
(I am supposing, of course, the case of mediums who are not
themselves tricksters.) A contact with such a plane of spirits
can be harmful (most mediums become nervously or morally
unbalanced) and spiritually dangerous. Of course, all pretended
communications with the famous dead of long-past times are
in their very nature deceptive and most of those with the recent
ones also — that is evident from the character of these communications. Through conscientious mediums one may get sound
results (in the matter of the dead), but even these are very
ignorant of the nature of the forces they are handling and have
no discrimination which can guard them against trickery from the
other side of the veil. Very little genuine knowledge of the
nature of the after-life can be gathered from these seances;
a true knowledge is more often gained by the experience of
individuals who make serious contact or are able in one way
or another to cross the border.

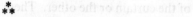

They [mediums, clairvoyants, etc.] are most of them in contact
with the vital-physical or subtle physical worlds and do not
receive anything higher at all.

III

The view taken by the Mahatma in these matters is
Christian rather than Hindu — for the Christian, self-abasement,
humility, the acceptance of a low status to serve humanity
or the Divine are things which are highly spiritual and
the noblest privilege of the soul. This view does not admit any
hierarchy of castes; the Mahatma accepts castes but on the
basis that all are equal before the Divine; a Bhangi doing his
dharma is as good as the Brahmin doing his, there is division
of function but no hierarchy of functions. That is one view of
things and the hierarchic view is another, both having a stand-

point and logic of their own which the mind takes as wholly valid but which only corresponds to a part of the reality. All kinds of work are equal before the Divine and all men have the same Brahman within them is one truth, but that development is not equal in all is another. The idea that it needs a special *puṇya* to be born as a Bhangi is, of course, one of those forceful exaggerations of an idea which are common with the Mahatma and impress greatly the mind of his hearers. The idea behind is that his function is an indispensable service to the society, quite as much as the Brahmin's, but, that being disagreeable, it would need a special moral heroism to choose it voluntarily and he thinks as if the soul freely chose it as such a heroic service and as reward of righteous acts — but that is hardly likely. The service of the scavenger is indispensable under certain conditions of society, it is one of those primary necessities without which society can hardly exist and the cultural development of which the Brahmin life is part could not have taken place. But obviously the cultural development is more valuable than the service of the physical needs for the progress of humanity as opposed to its first static condition, and that development can even lead to the minimising and perhaps the entire disappearance by scientific inventions of the need for the functions of the scavenger. But that, I suppose, the Mahatma would not approve of, as it would come by machinery and would be a departure from the simple life. In any case, it is not true that the Bhangi life is superior to the Brahmin life and the reward of a special righteousness. On the other hand, the traditional conception that a man is superior to others because he is born a Brahmin is not rational or justifiable. A spiritual or cultured man of pariah birth is superior in the divine values to an unspiritual and worldly-minded or a crude and uncultured Brahmin. Birth counts, but the basic value is in the man himself, in the soul behind, and the degree to which it manifests itself in his nature.

Sacrifice has a moral and psychological value always. This

value is the same no matter what may be the cause for which the sacrifice is made, provided the one who makes it believes in the truth or justice or other worthiness of his cause. If one makes the sacrifice for a cause one knows to be wrong or unworthy, all depends on the motive and spirit of the sacrifice. Bhishma accepting death in a cause he knew to be unjust, obeyed the call of loyalty to what he felt to be his personal duty. Many have done that in the past, and the moral and psychic value of their act lies, irrespective of the nature of the cause, in the nobility of the motive.

As to the other question, in this sense of the word 'sacrifice', there is none for the man who gives up something which he does not value, except in so far as he undergoes loss, defies social ban or obloquy or otherwise pays a price for his liberation. I may say, however, that without being cold and unloving a man may be so seized by a spiritual call or the call of a great human cause that the family or other ties count for nothing beside it, and he leaves all joyfully, without a pang, to follow the summoning Voice.

In the spiritual sense, however, sacrifice has a different meaning — it does not so much indicate giving up what is held dear as an offering of oneself, one's being, one's mind, heart, will, body, life, actions to the Divine. It has the original sense of "making sacred" and is used as an equivalent of the word *yajña*. When the Gita speaks of the "sacrifice of knowledge", it does not mean a giving up of anything, but a turning of the mind towards the Divine in the search for knowledge and an offering of oneself through it. It is in this sense, too, that one speaks of the offering or sacrifice of works. The Mother has written somewhere that the spiritual sacrifice is joyful and not painful in its nature. On the spiritual path, very commonly, if a seeker still feels the old ties and responsibilities strongly he is not asked to sever or leave them, but to let the call in him grow till all within is ready. Many, indeed, come away earlier because they feel that to cut loose is their only chance, and these have to go sometimes through a struggle. But the pain, the struggle, is not the essential character of this spiritual self-offering.

*
**

It simply means that your sacrifice is still mental and has not yet become spiritual in its character. When your vital being consents to give up its desires and enjoyments, when it offers itself to the Divine, then the Yajna will have begun. What I meant was that the European sense of the word is not the sense of the word "Yajna" or the sense of "sacrifice" in such phrases as "the sacrifice of works". It doesn't mean that you give up all works for the sake of the Divine — for there would be no sacrifice of works at all. Similarly the sacrifice of knowledge doesn't mean that you painfully and resolutely make yourself a fool for the sake of the Lord. Sacrifice means an inner offering to the Divine and the real spiritual sacrifice is a very joyful thing. Otherwise one is only trying to make oneself fit and has not yet begun the real Yajna. It is because your mind is struggling with your vital, the unwilling animal and asking it to allow itself to be immolated that there is the pain and struggle. If the spiritual will (or psychic) were more in the front then you would not be lamenting over the loss of the ghee and butter and curds thrown into the Fire or trying to have a last lick at it before casting it. The only difficulty would be about bringing down the gods fully enough (a progressive labour), not about lamentations over the ghee. By the way, do you think that the Mother or myself or others who have taken up the spiritual life had not enjoyed life and that it is therefore that the Mother was able to speak of a joyous sacrifice to the Divine as a true spirit of spiritual sacrifice? Or do you think we spent the preliminary stages in longings for the lost fleshpots of Egypt and that it was only later on we felt the joy of the spiritual sacrifice? Of course we did not; we and many others had no difficulty on the score of giving up anything we thought necessary to give up and no hankering afterwards. Your rule is as usual a stiff rule that does not at all apply generally.

Sacrifice depends on the inner attitude. If one has nothing outward to sacrifice one has always oneself to give.

There is nothing noble besides in fanaticism — there is no nobility of motive, though there may be a fierce enthusiasm of motive. Religious fanaticism is something psychologically low-born and ignorant — and usually in its action fierce, cruel and base. Religious ardour like that of the martyr who sacrifices himself only is a different thing.

IV

There has been almost continuous war in the world — it is as in the history of the Roman Republic when the gates of the temple of Janus were closed only once or twice in its many centuries — a sign that the Republic was at peace with all the world. There have been in modern times long intervals between long wars, but small ones have been generally going on somewhere or another. Man is a quarrelling and fighting animal and so long as he is so how can there be peace?

War and conquest are part of the economy of vital Nature, it is no use blaming this or that people for doing it — everybody does it who has the power and the chance. China who now complains was herself an imperialist and colonising country through all the centuries in which Japan kept religiously within her own borders.... If it were not profitable, I suppose nobody would do it. England has grown rich on the plundered wealth of India. France depends for many things on her African colonies. Japan needs an outlet for her over-abundant population and safe economic markets nearby. Each is pushed by forces that use the minds of rulers and peoples to fulfil themselves — unless human nature changes no amount of moralizing will prevent it.

I would prefer to avoid all public controversy especially if it touches in the least on politics. Gandhi's theories are like other mental theories built on a basis of one-sided reasoning and claiming for a limited truth (that of non-violence and passive resistance) a universality which it cannot have. Such theories will always exist so long as the mind is the main instrument of human truth-seeking. To spend energy trying to destroy such theories is of little use; if destroyed they are replaced by others equally limited and partial.

As for imperialism, that is no new thing — it is as old as the human vital; there was never a time in known human history when it was not in existence. To get out of it means to change human nature or at least to curb it by a superior power. Our work is not to fight these things but to bring down a higher nature and a Truth-creation which will make spiritual Light and Power the chief force in terrestrial existence.

There is a truth in Ahimsa, there is a truth in destruction also. I do not teach that you should go on killing everybody every day as a spiritual dharma. I say that destruction can be done when it is part of the divine work commanded by the Divine. Non-violence is better than violence as a rule, and still sometimes violence may be the right thing. I consider dharma as relative; unity with the Divine and action from the Divine Will, the highest way. Buddha did not aim at action in the world but at cessation from the world-existence. For that he found the Eightfold Path a necessary preparatory discipline and so proclaimed it.

It [Ahimsa] had nothing to do with the yoga, but with the path towards liberation found by Buddha. There are many paths and all need not be one and the same in their teaching.

[Re Vivisection:] I feel inclined to back out of the arena or take refuge in the usual saving formula, "there is much to be said on both sides". Your view is no doubt correct from the common-sense or what might be called the "human" point of view.

Krishnaprem takes the standpoint that we must not only consider the temporary good to humanity, but certain inner laws.
He thinks the harm, violence or cruelty to other beings is not
compensated and cannot be justified by some physical good to
a section of humanity or even to humanity as a whole; such
methods awake, in his opinion, a sort of Karmic reaction
apart from the moral harm to the men who do these things.
He is also of the opinion that the cause of disease is psychic,
that is to say, subjective and the direction should be towards
curing the inner causes much more than patching up by physical
means. These are ideas that have their truth also. I fully recog-
nize the psychic law and methods and their preferability, but the
ordinary run of humanity is not ready for that rule and, while
it is so, doctors and their physical methods will be there. I
have also supported justifiable violence on justifiable occasions,
e.g., Kurukshetra and the war against Hitler and all he means.
The question then, from this middle point of view, about the
immediate question is whether this violence is justifiable and
the occasion justifiable. I back out.

Destruction in itself is neither good nor evil. It is a fact of
Nature, a necessity in the play of forces, as things are in this
world. The Light destroys the Darkness and the Powers of
Darkness, and that is not a movement of Ignorance!

It all depends on the character of the destruction and the
forces that enter into it. All dread of fire or other violent forces
should be overcome. For dread shows a weakness — the free
spirit can stand fearless before even the biggest forces of Nature.

Why should earthquakes occur by some wrong movement of
man? When man was not there, did not earthquakes occur?
If he were blotted out by poison gas or otherwise, would they
cease? Earthquakes are a perturbation in Nature due to some
pressure of forces; frequency of earthquakes may coincide

with a violence of upheavals in human life but the upheavals of
earth and human life are both results of a general clash or
pressure of forces, one is not the cause of the other.

It seems to be very foolish, these fasts — as if they could
alter anything at all. A fast can at most affect one's own condition, but how can it "atone" for the doings of others or change
their nature?

It is a world which has emerged from the Inconscient and
these things [poverty and misery] are results of the imperfect
working of the human mind which, being born into the ignorant
life and matter has to learn by effort and experience. Ignorance
and ego have to be outgrown before there can be a true uti-
lisation of the resources of Nature.

V

The idea of time may be a mental construction, but the sense
of it may not be. Savages have the idea of time but it is
in connection with the sun and stars and the lapse of day
and night and the seasons, not perhaps a separate construction
— but one is not sure for they have metaphysical conceptions
of their own. Animals are not, I think, so limited in their
consciousness — they have not only sensations, but an acute
memory of certain things, observation, clear associations, an
intelligence that plans, a very accurate sense of place and memory
of place, an initial power of reasoning (not reflectively as the
human mind does, but practically as any vital mind can do).
I have seen a young kitten observing, coming at a correct
conclusion, proceeding to do what was necessary for her purpose, a necessity imposed by that conclusion, just as a human
child might do. We cannot therefore say that animals have no

ideas. No clear measure of yesterday and tomorrow, perhaps, but the perception of past and future needs is there and of right times and seasons also — all vital, practical, not reflectively mental in the human way.

But it is true that when one gets beyond the mind, this sense of time changes into timelessness, into the eternal present.

[Time sense in the animals:] A very strong time sense — at least some of them — but usually it works only in connection with strong desires or habits, e.g. food.

No doubt the physical regulated time consciousness belongs mainly to the waking state but it can be subliminal as well as of the mental waking consciousness. E.g., sometimes one wills at night to get up at a fixed time in the morning and wakes exactly at that hour and minute — it is something in the subliminal being that recorded the time and vigilantly executed it.

It is the change in the consciousness. When one begins to feel the inner being and live in it (the result of the experience of peace and silence) the ordinary time sense disappears or becomes purely external.

Time is to the Intuition an extension of consciousness in which happenings are arranged and has not the same rigidity that it has to the intellect.

You are right. The present is a convention or only a constant movement out of the past into the future.

VI

By greatness is meant an exceptional capacity of one kind or another which makes a man eminent among his fellows.

That kind of greatness has nothing to do with the psychic. It consists in a special mental capacity (Raman, Tagore) or in a great vital force which enables them to lead men and dominate them. These faculties are often but not always accompanied by something in the personality Daivic or Asuric which supports their action and gives to men an impression of greatness apart even from the special capacity — the sense of a great personality.

People have begun to try to prove that great men were not great, which is a very big mistake. If greatness is not appreciated by men, the world will become mean, small, dull, narrow and tamasic.

Obviously, outer greatness is not the aim of yoga. But that is no reason why one should not recognise the part played by greatness in the order of the universe or the place of great men of action, great poets and artists, etc.

It is the power in them [the great men] that is great and that power comes from the Divine — by their actions and greatness they help the world and aid the cosmic purpose. It does not matter whether they have ego or not — they are not doing yoga.

I don't think it can be said that Napoleon had little of ego — he was exceedingly ego-centric. He made himself a dictator from Brumaire, and as a dictator he should always have acted — but he felt the need of support and made the error of seeking it in the democratic way – a way for which he was utterly unfit. He had the capacities of a ruler but not of a politician — as a politician he would have been an entire failure. His hesitations were due to this defect — if it can be called one. He could not have dealt successfully with parties or a parliamentary assembly.

Why should the Divine not care for the outer greatness? He cares for everything in the universe. All greatness is the Vibhuti of the Divine, says the Gita.

It is not only the very very big people who are of importance to the Divine. All energy, strong capacity, power of effectuation are of importance.

As for Napoleon, Caesar and Shakespeare, not one of them was a virtuous man, but they were great men, and that was your contention that only virtuous men are great men and those who have vices are not great, which is an absurd contention. All of them went after women — two were ambitious, unscrupulous. Napoleon was most arrogant and violent.

Shakespeare stole deer, Napoleon lied freely, Caesar was without scruples.

Are you in a position to make a judgment as to what will or will not help God's work? You seem to have very elementary ideas in these matters. What is your idea of divinisation — to be a virtuous man, a good husband, son, father, a good citizen, etc.? In that case, I myself must be undivine, — for I have never been these things. Men like X or Y would then be the great Transformed Divine Men.

But do you really believe that men like Napoleon, Caesar, Shakespeare were not great men and did nothing for the world or for the cosmic purpose? that God was deterred from using them for His purpose because they had defects of character and vices? What an absurd idea!

Why should the Divine care for the vices of great men? Is he a policeman? So long as one is in the ordinary nature, one has capacities and defects, virtues and vices. When one goes beyond, there are no virtues and vices, — for these things do not belong to the Divine Nature.

Vice and virtue have nothing to do with darkness or light, truth and falsehood. The spiritual man rises above vice and virtue, he does not rise above truth and light, unless you mean by truth and light, human truth and mental light. They have to be transcended, just as virtue and vice have to be transcended.

Vices are simply an overflow of energy in irregulated channels.

Great men have more energy (mental, vital, physical, all kinds of energy) and the energy comes out in what men call vices as well as in what men call virtues.

Men with great capacities or a powerful mind or a powerful vital have very often more glaring defects of character than ordinary men or at least the defects of the latter do not show so much, being like themselves, smaller in scale.

Yes, certainly. Many great men even have often very great vices and many of them. Great men are not usually model characters.

Great or dazzling or small in their field, ambition is ambition and it is necessary for most for an energetic action. What is the use of calling a thing a vice when it is small and glorifying it when it is big?

When vanity is there on a big scale, it usually works like that. The man feels the energy in all he does, and mistakes the energy for high accomplishment. It is a common error. The high accomplishment is in only one or two fields.

It is a vanity, but it is not humbug, unless he does not believe in it. If he does not believe in it, it is humbug, but it is not vanity.

Most great men know perfectly well that they are great.

VII

[The seeking of animals:] The satisfaction of their emotions and desires and their bodily needs — mostly. Animals are predominantly the vital creation on earth — the mind in them also is a vital mind — they act according to the push of the forces and have a vital but not a mental will.

Even the animal is more in touch with a certain harmony in things than man. Man's only superiority is a more complex consciousness and capacity (but terribly perverted and twisted by misuse of Mind) and the ability (not much used as yet) of reaching towards higher things.

Human life and mind are neither in tune with Nature like the animals nor with Spirit — it is disturbed, incoherent, conflicting with itself, without harmony and balance. We can then regard it as diseased, if not itself a disease.

The plants are very psychic, but they can express it only by silence and beauty.

[Beauty of a flower:] Form, colour, scent and something else which is indefinable.

The rose is not the only beautiful flower, there are hundreds of others; most flowers are beautiful.

There are degrees and kinds of beauty, that is all.

The rose is among the first of flowers because of the richness of its colour, the intensity of sweetness of its scent and the grace and magnificence of its form.

It is true that the plant world — even the animals if one takes them the right way — can be much better than human beings. It is the mental distortion that makes men worse.

Yes, it is a more simple and honest consciousness — that of the animal. Of course it expects something, but even if it does not get, the affection remains. Many animals, even if ill-treated, do not lose their love which means remarkable psychic development in the vital.

The emotional being of animals is often much more psychic than that of men who can be very insensitive. There were recently pictures of the tame tigress kept by a family and afterwards given by them to a Zoo. The look of sorrow on the face of the tigress in her cage at once gentle and tragically poignant is so intense as to be heart-breaking.

Most animals do not usually attack unless they are menaced or frightened or somehow made angry — and they can feel the atmosphere of people.

Cats have a very sure vital perception.

There are people who can move the ears without doing yoga at all or calling upon the resources of the Kundalini. I suppose it is simply a movement that man has lost through disuse, not having had like the animals to prick up his ear at every moment to listen to sounds that might indicate danger. I suppose he could revive the faculty if it were of any use.

[Responsibility for suffering:] Why man's? What about the animals? They too suffer. You can say that suffering is a distortion of the lower consciousness, but you cannot make man or human nature alone responsible for it.

Yes — to watch the animals with the right perception of their consciousness helps to get out of the human mental limitations and see the Cosmic Consciousness on earth individualising itself in all forms — plant, animal, man and growing towards what is beyond man.

VIII

I am not aware that highly evolved personalities have no sense of humour or how the person can be said to be integrated when this sense is lacking. "Looseness" applies only to a frivolous levity without any substance behind it. There is no law that wisdom should be something rigidly solemn and without a smile.

Sense of humour? It is the salt of existence. Without it the world would have got utterly out of balance — it is unbalanced enough already — and rushed to blazes long ago.

People are exceedingly silly — but I suppose they can't help themselves. The more I see of humanity, the more that forces itself on me. The abysses of silliness of which its mind is capable....

*
**

My opinion is that Allah is great and great is the mystery of the universe and things are not what they seem, etc.

END OF PART ONE